Gestational Diabetes: Nutrition, Complications and Treatment

Gestational Diabetes: Nutrition, Complications and Treatment

Editor: Solomon Fleming

AMERICAN
MEDICAL PUBLISHERS
www.americanmedicalpublishers.com

AMERICAN
MEDICAL PUBLISHERS
www.americanmedicalpublishers.com

Cataloging-in-Publication Data

Gestational diabetes : nutrition, complications and treatment / edited by Solomon Fleming.
p. cm.
Includes bibliographical references and index.
ISBN 978-1-63927-676-9
1. Diabetes in pregnancy. 2. Diabetes in pregnancy--Treatment. 3. Pregnancy--Complications.
4. Diabetes--Complications. 5. Pregnancy--Nutritional aspects. 6. Diabetes--Nutritional aspects.
I. Fleming, Solomon.
RG580.D5 G47 2023
618.3--dc23

American Medical Publishers,
41 Flatbush Avenue,
1st Floor, New York,
NY 11217, USA

ISBN 978-1-63927-676-9 (Hardback)

Contents

Preface VII

Chapter 1 **Vitamin D and Gestational Diabetes Mellitus: Is there a Link?** 1
Gianluca Rizzo, Simone Garzon, Michele Fichera, Marco Marzio Panella, Ursula Catena, Antonio Schiattarella, Pasquale de Franciscis, George Vilos, Jan Tesarik, Péter Török and Giuseppe Grosso

Chapter 2 **Exploring the Feasibility of Use of an Online Dietary Assessment Tool (myfood24) in Women with Gestational Diabetes** 14
Carla Gianfrancesco, Zoe Darwin, Linda McGowan, Debbie M. Smith, Roz Haddrill, Michelle Carter, Eleanor M. Scott, Nisreen A. Alwan, Michelle A. Morris, Salwa A. Albar and Janet E. Cade

Chapter 3 **Dietary Intake and Beliefs of Pregnant Women with Gestational Diabetes in Cape Town, South Africa** 30
Stephanie M. Krige, Sharmilah Booley, Naomi S. Levitt, Tawanda Chivese, Katherine Murphy and Janetta Harbron

Chapter 4 **Gestational Diabetes Mellitus: The Impact of Carbohydrate Quality in Diet** 51
Tiziana Filardi, Francesca Panimolle, Clara Crescioli, Andrea Lenzi and Susanna Morano

Chapter 5 **The Role of Dietary Carbohydrates in Gestational Diabetes** 60
Vikkie A. Mustad, Dieu T.T. Huynh, José M. López-Pedrosa, Cristina Campoy and Ricardo Rueda

Chapter 6 **Self-Reported Eating Speed and Incidence of Gestational Diabetes Mellitus: The Japan Environment and Children's Study** 77
Jia-Yi Dong, Satoyo Ikehara, Takashi Kimura, Meishan Cui, Yoko Kawanishi, Tadashi Kimura, Kimiko Ueda and Hiroyasu Iso

Chapter 7 **How can Maternal Lifestyle Interventions Modify the Effects of Gestational Diabetes in the Neonate and the Offspring?** 85
Delphine Mitanchez, Cécile Ciangura and Sophie Jacqueminet

Chapter 8 **Temporal Trends in Maternal Food Intake Frequencies and Associations with Gestational Diabetes: The Cambridge Baby Growth Study** 102
Clive J. Petry, Ken K. Ong, Ieuan A. Hughes, Carlo L. Acerini and David B. Dunger

Chapter 9 **Effect of High Versus Low Carbohydrate Intake in the Morning on Glycemic Variability and Glycemic Control Measured by Continuous Blood Glucose Monitoring in Women with Gestational Diabetes Mellitus** 117
Louise Rasmussen, Maria Lund Christensen, Charlotte Wolff Poulsen, Charlotte Rud, Alexander Sidelmann Christensen, Jens Rikardt Andersen, Ulla Kampmann and Per Glud Ovesen

Chapter 10 **Bisphenol A and Phthalates in Diet: An Emerging Link with Pregnancy Complications** 129
Tiziana Filardi, Francesca Panimolle, Andrea Lenzi and Susanna Morano

Chapter 11 **Influence of GDM Diagnosis and Treatment on Weight Gain, Dietary Intake and Physical Activity in Pregnant Women with Obesity: Secondary Analysis of the UPBEAT Study** 144
La'Shay Atakora, Lucilla Poston, Louise Hayes, Angela C. Flynn and Sara L. White

Chapter 12 **Methylglyoxal, Glycated Albumin, PAF and TNF-α: Possible Inflammatory and Metabolic Biomarkers for Management of Gestational Diabetes** 155
Gabriele Piuri, Katia Basello, Gabriele Rossi, Chiara Maria Soldavini, Silvia Duiella, Giulia Privitera, Angela Spadafranca, Andrea Costanzi, Emiliana Tognon, Mattia Cappelletti, Paola Antonia Corsetto, Angela Maria Rizzo, Attilio Francesco Speciani and Enrico Ferrazzi

Chapter 13 **Leptin and Nutrition in Gestational Diabetes** 167
Antonio Pérez-Pérez, Teresa Vilariño-García, Pilar Guadix, José L. Dueñas and Víctor Sánchez-Margalet

Chapter 14 **Influence of Diabetes during Pregnancy on Human Milk Composition** 185
Chiara Peila, Diego Gazzolo, Enrico Bertino, Francesco Cresi and Alessandra Coscia

Chapter 15 **Ketonuria is Associated with Changes to the Abundance of *Roseburia* in the Gut Microbiota of Overweight and Obese Women at 16 Weeks Gestation** 200
Helen Robinson, Helen Barrett, Luisa Gomez-Arango, H. David McIntyre, Leonie Callaway and Marloes Dekker Nitert

Chapter 16 **Dietary Patterns and Dietary Adaptations in Women with and without Gestational Diabetes: Evidence from the Growing Up in New Zealand Study** 210
Robyn L. Lawrence, Clare R. Wall and Frank H. Bloomfield

Permissions

List of Contributors

Index

Preface

Gestational diabetes is one of the types of diabetes diagnosed during pregnancy for the first time. It affects the cell's capability to use sugar, resulting in high blood sugar levels, which can affect the pregnancy and health of the baby. The most common cause of gestational diabetes is a change in hormone levels that make it difficult for the body to efficiently process blood sugar. There are several complications associated with gestational diabetes, such as increased risk of breathing difficulties in infants, hypoglycemia, excessive birth weight, preterm birth and obesity. In certain cases it may also result in still birth. Diagnosis involves a screening test between 24 and 28 weeks of pregnancy. Initial glucose challenge test and follow-up glucose tolerance testing are routine screening procedures for gestational diabetes. Treatment and management for gestational diabetes includes medication, blood sugar monitoring and certain lifestyle changes. Repeated ultrasounds for examining the growth and development of an infant become paramount in the course of treatment. This book provides comprehensive insights into gestational diabetes. It presents researches and studies on the nutritional aspects of this disease as well as its complications and treatment. This book will serve as a valuable source of reference for graduate and post graduate students.

This book has been the outcome of endless efforts put in by authors and researchers on various issues and topics within the field. The book is a comprehensive collection of significant researches that are addressed in a variety of chapters. It will surely enhance the knowledge of the field among readers across the globe.

It gives us an immense pleasure to thank our researchers and authors for their efforts to submit their piece of writing before the deadlines. Finally in the end, I would like to thank my family and colleagues who have been a great source of inspiration and support.

Editor

1

Vitamin D and Gestational Diabetes Mellitus: Is there a Link?

Gianluca Rizzo [1], Simone Garzon [2], Michele Fichera [3], Marco Marzio Panella [3], Ursula Catena [4], Antonio Schiattarella [5], Pasquale de Franciscis [5], George Vilos [6], Jan Tesarik [7], Péter Török [8] and Giuseppe Grosso [9,*]

1 Independent Researcher; gianlucarizzo@email.it
2 Department of Obstetrics and Gynecology, "Filippo del Ponte" Hospital, University of Insubria, 21100 Varese, Italy; simone.garzon@yahoo.it
3 Department of General Surgery and Medical Surgical Specialties, University of Catania, 95124 Catania, Italy; fichera.michele@policlinico.unict.it (M.F.); mpanella@unict.it (M.M.P.)
4 Division of Gynecologic Oncology, Fondazione Policlinico Universitario Agostino Gemelli, IRCCS, 00168 Rome, Italy; ursula.catena@gmail.com
5 Department of Woman, Child and General and Specialized Surgery, University of Campania "Luigi Vanvitelli", 81100 Naples, Italy; aschiattarella@gmail.com (A.S.); pasquale.defranciscis@unicampania.it (P.d.F.)
6 Department of Obstetrics and Gynecology, Division of Reproductive Endocrinology and Infertility, Western University, London, ON N6H5W9, Canada; George.Vilos@lhsc.on.ca
7 MARGen Clinic, 18006 Granada, Spain; jtesarik@clinicamargen.com
8 Faculty of Medicine, Institute of Obstetrics and Gynaecology, University of Debrecen, H-4032 Debrecen, Hungary; drtorokp@freemail.hu
9 Department of Biomedical and Biotechnological Sciences, University of Catania, 95123 Catania, Italy
* Correspondence: giuseppe.grosso@unict.it

Abstract: Gestational diabetes mellitus (GDM) is a very common condition among pregnant women worldwide with important metabolic implications on the mother and the offspring. Vitamin D status has been suggested to potentially play a role in GDM risk with no documented consequences for the offspring. The purpose of this article was to review currently available evidence on the relationship between vitamin D and GDM. Current evidence shows an association between vitamin D blood levels and risk of GDM, despite heterogeneity of results across studies limit the conclusions. Moreover, data from randomized controlled trials is scarce and resulting in null findings. Among the limitations to be noted, improving the standardization of dosages, the characteristics of individuals in the sample, and the appropriate outcome measurement could provide a more effective approach in understanding the relationship between vitamin D and GDM. In conclusions, despite observational studies may suggest that adequate vitamin D levels may decrease the risk of GDM compared to deficiency status, evidence from clinical trials is inadequate to draft any definitive conclusion regarding its supplementation. Future better designed randomized clinical trials taking into account a more integrated approach could provide clearer and definitive data on the outcomes of such a multifactorial condition.

Keywords: vitamin D; gestational diabetes mellitus; pregnancy; nutrition; supplements; antenatal care; food fortification

1. Introduction

Interest in vitamin D has increased in the last decades with the improvement of the knowledge regarding its wide implication in several physiological processes. In fact, although its involvement in bone metabolism and calcium management in bone health processes is widely confirmed, literature repeatedly suggested non-musculoskeletal targets such as the immune system, regulation of cell proliferation and differentiation, and glucose metabolism [1–4]. Interestingly, recent evidence demonstrated that vitamin D may also influence metabolic parameters in both menopausal and postmenopausal women [5,6], and, consequently, being potentially associated with human reproduction [7–9] and birth outcomes [10].

In pregnancy, external *stimuli* can affect mother-foetus dyad with possible consequences for both the mother and the offspring [11,12]. Thus, nutritional recommendations in this condition may be specific and significantly different from those referring to adult women in general, taking into account that adaptation for relevant nutrients would affect both mother and foetal health [13–16]. The need of vitamin D could be higher in pregnancy [17]; in fact, many populations, both among developing and industrialized countries, still suffer from vitamin D deficiency in pregnancy with a variable incidence ranging from 40% to 100% [18–22]. Interestingly, vitamin D has been suggested as a potential candidate for prevention of gestational diabetes mellitus (GDM), despite conflicting current opinions [23–25]. The purpose of this review is to summarize current evidence on the possible link between vitamin D and GDM, briefly discussing the potential mechanisms underlying this relation and providing data from meta-analysis and systematic reviews.

2. Potential Role of Vitamin D on GDM Pathogenesis

Increased blood glucose levels stimulate pancreatic β-cells secretion of insulin. Peripheral tissues respond to this hormone by activating glucose transport inside the cells. The balance between insulin secretion and its peripheral sensitivity represents the modulation system for carbohydrates tolerance [26]. The chronic stimulation of this modulation system by high glycaemic levels and consequent insulin resistance leads to an exhaustion of pancreatic secretion competence that provokes alteration of insulinemia, leading to glucose intolerance and even type-2 diabetes mellitus (T2DM).

GDM is defined as an alteration of glucose tolerance with variable severity, with the first onset during pregnancy, in the absence of a diagnosis of T2DM [27]. The GDM prevalence ranges from 1% to 25% depending on population reference and diagnostic cut-offs [28,29]. It represents the leading cause of complications for mother and offspring [30]. Moreover, GDM is a determinant for serious long-term complications such as obesity, T2DM, metabolic syndrome for both mother and the offspring, with a risk for the establishment of a trans-generational predisposition [31].

Pregnancy is a condition that promotes physiological insulin resistance. Higher maternal glucose levels allow the adequate delivery to the foetus through the placental syncytium. This well-known phenomenon is mediated by steroid hormones and by the anti-insulin action of placental tissues [32], which in turn can modulate insulin signalling, glucose transport and peroxisome proliferator-activated receptor (PPAR) function [33,34], which placenta expression has been directly associated with GDM in female population [35]. However, if there is latent and pre-existing glucose intolerance, the pregnancy can uncover a pancreas inadequacy for compensating the secretion in response to the peripheral insulin resistance, resulting in a β-cells dysfunction through a physio-pathological continuum [36].

Vitamin D can influence glucose homeostasis with multiple mechanisms:

- Functional pancreatic alteration can be associated with immune cell infiltration among glandular cells with consequent inflammation [37]. Vitamin D exerts anti-inflammatory properties that can drive the recovery of physiological insulin secretion [38].
- Insulin receptor of peripheral cells drives receptor-mediated endocytosis routing calmodulin-dependent intracellular signalling [39]. Vitamin D enhances duodenal absorption and renal resorption of calcium that is therefore available to the intracellular signalling activated by insulin [40].
- Interaction between insulin-like growth factor (IGF) and molecular partners of vitamin D pathways could play a role in glucose homeostasis.

- Vitamin D receptors (VDRs) were described in different extra-bones peripheral tissues which explains the wide non-musculoskeletal functions of vitamin D, including the action on insulin receptor that promotes insulin sensitivity [41]. Pancreatic β-cells show VDRs with a possible modulating action of vitamin D on insulin secretion [42,43].
- Vitamin D can act indirectly through the reduction of risk factors common to GDM such as obesity. Vitamin D is a fat-soluble vitamin and its migration from the bloodstream to fat deposits can reduce its availability [44]. Moreover, obese patients have higher levels of vitamin D binding protein (VDBP) that can reduce vitamin D bioactive fractions [45].

3. Cut-offs and Methods of Detection

Diagnosis of GDM includes fasting blood glucose concentration and/or oral glucose tolerance test (OGTT), depending on the organization releasing the diagnostic procedure and cut-offs [46–49]. Specifically, the American College of Obstetricians and Gynaecologists (ACOG) recommendations require two or more threshold values for the diagnosis, while the Canadian Diabetes Association (CDA), the International Association of Diabetes and Pregnancy Study Groups Consensus Panel (IADPSG), and the World Health Organization (WHO) require only one. About cut-offs, fasting plasma glucose ≥ 5.3 mmol/L (95 mg/dL) is adopted by CDA and ACOG, while 5.1 mmol/L (92 mg/dL) is adopted by WHO and IADPSG. Except for ACOG that use 100 g of glucose, all organizations use 75 g of glucose for the OGTT. The 1h plasma glucose cut-off of ≥ 10.0 mmol/L (180 mg/dL) is adopted by all but CDA that uses 10.6 mmol/L (191 mg/dL) value. There is great variability in 2 h plasma glucose cut-offs: ≥ 8.5 (153 mg/dL) for IADPSG and WHO; ≥ 9 (162 mg/dL) for CDA; and ≥ 8.6 (155 mg/dL) for ACOG. A 3 h plasma glucose is adopted only by ACOG with a cut-off of 7.8 mmol/L (140 mg/dL). The American Diabetes Association (ADA) adopted two different strategy for the screening of GDM: A one-step method requiring only one glucose plasma value exceeding fasting, 75 g OGTT at 1 or 2 h with cut-offs equivalent to IADPSG; or a two-step method requiring a first non-fasting 50 g OGTT evaluation, followed by a 100 g OGTT with criteria, and cut-offs equivalent to ACOG. A 2 h 75 g OGTT adoption for GDM diagnosis were confirmed in the international and multicentre HAPO Study, based on 25,505 pregnant women outcomes [50].

Even the vitamin D cut-offs are widely debated with no shared consensus, especially for pregnancy. Indeed, it is not clear whether blood levels of vitamin D during pregnancy are stable through all phases of gestation and also if they can be the same for adults in a general population.

There are some difficulties in choosing the adequate gold standard to set the cut-off for the vitamin D. In the attempt to validate vitamin D blood levels of adequacy, the value above which the parathyroid hormone (PTH) reaches its plateau in response to the vitamin D was chosen [51]. This plateau seems to be reached in adults with 25-hydroxyvitamin D (25(OH)D) blood concentrations ranges from 30 to 40 ng/ml (75–100 nmol/L). However, the reverse correlation between vitamin D and PTH blood levels is not accepted by all researchers [52–55]. PTH concentration depends on the duration of vitamin D deficiency and on calcium that can mask vitamin D insufficiency [56]. In pregnancy, PTH levels do not seem to correlate with vitamin D [57,58]. However, Kramer at al. highlighted a link between PTH and GDM with the finding that the prevalence of GDM increased while increasing the PTH [59].

Cut-offs of vitamin D were also evaluated on calcium absorption that shown an increased intestinal efficiency when postmenopausal women increased their 25(OH)D blood levels from 20 ng/ml (50 nmol/L) to 32 ng/ml (80 nmol/L) [60]. In a review on clinical practice by Holick and co-workers, routine population screening for vitamin D was not recommended with the higher straight of evidence and the maximum quality for the statement [61]. However, pregnancy was considered an "at risk" condition for vitamin D insufficiency. The American Institute of Medicine and the European Food Safety Authority (EFSA) defined the same cut-off of vitamin D for adults and pregnant women fixing the value of sufficiency blood levels of 25(OH)D above 20 ng/mL (50 nmol/L) [55,62]. Nevertheless, some researchers debated the possibility that pregnancy would need higher concentrations of vitamin D [24].

Insufficiency and deficiency for vitamin D are common among pregnant women worldwide, due to foetal growth, low exposure to sunlight, and low dietary intake [63]. A comprehensive analysis of existing studies conducted on pregnant and lactating women worldwide showed low serum vitamin D levels especially in Asia, with the highest prevalence of deficiency in Kuwait (38–41%), Pakistan (45%), Turkey (50%), and India (60%) [64]. In Europe, also the Netherlands and Belgium had a relevant percentage of deficiency (23% and 12%, respectively); low vitamin D status was also found in some high-income countries such as Spain (20%), Canada (24%), America (33%), UK (35%), Netherlands (44%), Belgium (45%), and Germany (77%), suggesting that there is a potential global insufficient vitamin D consumption resulting in a common deficiency especially during pregnancy [64].

Deficiency criteria may depend also on methods used because of the wide availability of different analytical techniques for the detection of markers for vitamin D. Even the preparations (i.e., solvent extraction or the sample pre-treatment) adopted in different laboratories for the same protocol may affect results [65,66]. Currently, there is a massive use of immunoassays methods thanks to automation, however, there is the need of a consensus that harmonizes the cut-offs of various techniques used such as high-performance liquid chromatography (HPLC), liquid chromatography-tandem mass spectrometry (LC-MS/MS), chemiluminescence immunoassays (CLIA), enzyme-linked immunosorbent assays (ELISA), competitive protein binding assays (CPBA), and radioimmunoassays (RIA) [67–70]. It seems that other methods with respect to HPLC or LC-MS/MS underestimate serum levels of vitamin D [71]. However, all methods could suffer from the lack of a common standard and differences of methods applied among different laboratories.

4. Evidences of Relation between Vitamin D and GDM

4.1. Observational Studies

Table 1 summarize the main data from meta-analyses of observational studies: Poel, et al. in a systematic review and meta-analysis of seven studies including 2146 participants found an association between 25(OH)D blood concentration and GDM (Odds Ratio (OR) 1.61, 95% Confidence Interval (CI): 1.19–2.17) [72]. Aghajafari, et al. have conducted a meta-analysis of 31 observational studies and have found a correlation between low levels of 25(OH)D and risk for GDM (OR 1.49, 95% CI: 1.18–1.89) [24]. Similar, Wei, et al. have conducted a meta-analysis of 12 studies with 5,615 patients and have found a moderate correlation between 25(OH)D concentrations below 50 nmol/L of pregnant women and an increased risk of GDM (OR 1.38, 95% CI: 1.12–1.70) [73]. More recently, Zhang and colleagues found similar conclusions after a meta-analysis of 20 studies conducted in Europe, Australia, North America, and Asia with different study design including cross-sectional, case-control, nested case-control, and cohort studies including 9209 participants [74]. Quality assessment indicated a homogeneous high-quality score among studies and, even if seven different criteria for GDM diagnosis and five different assay techniques for serum vitamin D detection were used, an overall association between vitamin D deficiency and risk of GDM was found (OR 1.53, 95% CI: 1.33–1.75) with 4.93 nmol/L decreased levels of 25(OH)D in case of GDM. There was a high diversity of participant characteristics with a prevalence of vitamin D deficiency from 3.1% to 94.7% with a 25(OH)D concentration ranged from 16.5 to 97.0 nmol/L with a median of 49.30 nmol/L. Unfortunately, not all studies provided analysis adjusted for confounding factors such as skin tone and BMI, thus heterogeneity was high ($I^2 = 61\%$). Lu, et al. in 2016 published a wider and more updated meta-analysis of 20 observational studies with 16,515 individuals and found an association between vitamin D insufficiency and GDM risk (RR 1.45, 95% CI: 1.15–1.83) [75]. Even in this meta-analysis the geographical origin was heterogeneous, accounting for studies from Australia, UK, Iran, Spain, Turkey, China, Korea, India, America, and Canada that may contribute to the differences in the subgroup analysis associations together with differences in adjusted models, study design, and assessment of vitamin D (laboratory techniques used and cut-offs). Again, heterogeneity was high ($I^2 = 66\%$). Characteristics of the studies were crucial to notice the association: In fact, vitamin D insufficiency was associated with GDM in studies using HPLC-MS assay but not when radioimmunoassay was used. Similarly, in a systematic review and meta-analysis of 26 observational studies by Amraei and coworkers, a relation between vitamin D deficiency and risk of GDM (OR 1.18, 95% CI: 1.01–1.35) was shown [76]. Serum 25(OH)D in GDM patients were lower than controls with no significant association with population nationality of the studies. However, study design (cross-sectional, prospective, nested case-control, retrospective, or prospective cohort), in the subgroup analysis showed a variable association. Interestingly, there was limited evidence of heterogeneity among the reviewed studies ($I^2 = 8.1\%$, $p = 0.346$). Standardized mean difference (SMD) between vitamin D levels in women with GDM and those with normal glucose tolerance was −0.26 (95% CI: From −0.39 to −0.14) with high heterogeneity ($I^2 = 68.8\%$). Limitations of this study were the heterogeneity of GDM criteria, vitamin D cut-offs, and the lack of important information in some studies such as skin color, socio-economic status, weight gain in pregnancy, exposure to sunlight, and vitamin D intakes. The association between increased risk of GDM and vitamin D insufficiency was also confirmed by Hu at al. in a meta-analysis of 29 observational studies that included 28,982 participants (OR 1.39, 95% CI: 1.20–1.60) with significant high heterogeneity ($I^2 = 50.2\%$) [77]. Moreover, differences of 25(OH)D levels between patients with GDM and patients without any issue of glucose tolerance was significant but with high heterogeneity (−4.79 nmol/L, 95% CI: From −6.43 to −3.15, $I^2 = 65.0\%$). 72% of studies were conducted in developed countries but there was no homogeneity for GDM and 25(OH)D cut-offs, as can be expected. As for other meta-analyses, also in this work the adjustments for confounding factors such as BMI, ethnicity, season, gestational age, physical activity, pregnancy weight gain, parity, vitamin D intake, alcohol, and socioeconomic status. were in different combinations. Interestingly, stratification of the studies in the meta-analysis showed that the correlation between vitamin D insufficiency and risk of GDM was significant (i) for developed countries rather than for the developing ones; (ii) for GDM cut-offs of ADA, ADPS, and WHO but not for those from other organizations; and (iii) in case of significant difference of 25(OH)D levels between GDM and control but not when difference was not significant.

Table 1. Association between insufficient vitamin D and risk of Gestational Diabetes Mellitus in selected meta-analyses of observational studies.

References	No. Studies	No. Participants	Risk (95% CI)	I^2
Poel, et al. 2012 [72]	7	2146	OR 1.61 (1.19–2.17)	5.8%
Aghajafari, et al. 2013 [25]	31	4112	OR 1.49 (1.18–1.89)	0.0%
Wei, et al. 2013 [73]	12	5615	OR 1.38 (1.12–1.70)	0.0%
Zhang, et al. 2015 [74]	20	9209	OR 1.53 (1.33–1.75)	16.2%
Lu, et al. 2016 [75]	20	16,515	RR 1.45 (1.15–1.83)	66.6%
Amraei, et al. 2018 [76]	26	20,503	OR 1.18 (1.01–1.35)	8.1%
Hu, et al. 2018 [77]	29	28,982	OR 1.39 (1.20–1.60)	50.2%

OR: Odds Ratio, RR: Risk Ratio, I^2: Heterogeneity.

4.2. Clinical Trials

Vitamin D supplementation for GDM seems to ameliorate different metabolic markers including blood glucose levels, insulin resistance and inflammatory biomarkers [78–80]. Supplementation with 50,000 International Units (IU) twice monthly has been shown to improve insulin resistance significantly [79], while 5000 IU daily has failed to improve glucose levels in another trial [81]. Table 2 summarises the results of selected meta-analyses of Randomized Controlled Trials (RCTs). A meta-analysis in 2012 showed the protective efficacy of vitamin D supplementation (800–1000 IU daily) for mother and child's health outcomes [82]. Yap at al. found no change in glucose concentration among Australian first-trimester pregnant patients with a high dosage intervention of vitamin D supplementation [81]. However, the study was not adequately designed to explore the incidence of GDM and it was based on a low-risk population for vitamin D deficiency. In fact, in a randomized controlled trial, Sablok and co-workers showed about half of the GDM prevalence among vitamin D treated group with respect to non-intervention in 200 Indian pregnant women [83]. Unfortunately, in two recent meta-analyses about oral supplementation of vitamin D, there was no association with GDM, even if vitamin D assumption led to higher levels of 25(OH)D compared to control [84,85]. Pérez-Lòpez, et al. published a systematic review and meta-analysis of 13 RCTs (2299 participants) on the effect of vitamin D in pregnancy [85]: Vitamin D supplementation was associated with increased circulating 25(OH)D levels (mean difference 66.5 nmol/L, 95% CI: 66.2–66.7), but it did not influence GDM and other maternal outcomes including pre-eclampsia, short for gestational age, caesarean section, and low birth weight. Besides the moderate heterogeneity (possibly due to different geographical areas investigated, dosage, duration, type of supplementation, or method of measurement), some methodological issues should be taken into account, including intervention in the second semester of pregnancy and lack of correction for some confounding factors, such as nutritional aspects that may be crucial when considering developing countries. Palacios and co-workers conducted an updated meta-analysis about the supplementation of vitamin D during pregnancy that included 15 RCT involving 2,833 women regarding multiple outcomes in pregnancy [84]: Supplementation with vitamin D raised serum 25(OH)D levels compared to placebo (mean difference 54.7 nmol/L, 95% CI: 36.6–72.9): Coherently with the work of Pérez-Lòpez, the biomarker for vitamin D was affected by the intervention but no difference in the risk of GDM was found. However, studies that explored the risk of GDM were only two with low quality, thus the lack of association was not definitive. In a Cochrane review of 15 randomized and quasi-randomized trials including a total of 2833 women on vitamin D efficacy on pregnant outcomes, only three studies investigated GDM with no association, but these trials were the same described above by Palacios [86]. The rise of circulating 25(OH)D after supplementation, particularly on a daily basis, is confirmed, but with a high heterogeneous response. Data on the safety of supplementation was lacking in all studies. In 2017, Akbari and co-workers conducted a systematic review and meta-analysis of 11 RCT on the effects of vitamin D supplementation on glucose metabolism and lipid profiles in GDM patients (187 subjects and 184 controls) and found a significant effect of vitamin D on metabolic homeostasis models [87]: Researchers observed an improvement of homeostatic model assessment of insulin resistance (HOMA-IR) (SMD −0.66, 95% CI: From −1.14 to −0.18) and quantitative insulin sensitivity check index (QUICKI) (SMD 0.73, 95% CI: From 0.26 to 1.20), despite supplementation resulted in a worsening of the homeostatic model assessment β-cells function (HOMA-B) (SMD −0.52, 95% CI: From −0.79 to −0.25). Fasting plasma glucose, insulin, and HbA1c were not significantly affected. High heterogeneity was reported, possibly depending on study duration and participants' characteristics and, more importantly, on vitamin D dosage.

Table 2. Association between intervention with vitamin D and GDM outcomes in meta-analyses of RCTs.

References	No. Studies	No. Participant	Outcomes	I^2
Pérez-Lòpez, et al. 2015 [85]	13	2299	Circulating 25-OHD: (MD 66.46, CI 95% 66.22 to 66.71)	100.0%
			Preeclampsia: (RR 0.88, CI 95% 0.51 to 1.52)	24.0%
			Gestational diabetes: (RR 1.05, CI 95% 0.60 to 1.84)	0.0%
			Small for gestational age: (RR 0.78, CI 95% 0.50 to 1.21)	15%
			Low birth weight: (RR 0.72, CI 95% 0.44 to 1.16)	0.0%
			Preterm birth: (RR 1.26, CI 95% 0.60 to 2.63)	0.0%
			Birth weight: (MD 107.60, CI 95% 59.86 to 155.33)	0.0%
			Birth length: (MD 0.30, CI 95% 0.19 to 0.41)	84.0%
			Cesarean section: (RR 0.94, CI 95% 0.78 to 1.13)	0.0%
Palacios, et al. 2016 [84]	7	868	Serum 25-OHD: (MD 54.73, CI 95% 23.76 to 70.39)	99.0%
			Preeclampsia: (RR 0.52, CI 95% 0.25 to 1.05)	15.5%
			Gestational diabetes: (RR 0.43, CI 95% 0.05 to 3.45)	NR
de-Regil, et al. 2016 [86]	3	273	Circulating 25-OHD: (MD 47.08, CI 95% 36.60 to 72.86)	98.0%
			Low birth weight: (RR 0.48, CI 95% 0.23 to 1.01)	53.0%
			Birth length: (MD 0.97, CI 95% −0.41 to 2.34)	84.0%
			Head circumference: (MD 0.43, CI 95% 0.06 to 0.79)	50.0%
			Birth weight: (MD 39.55, CI 95% −240.68 to 319.78)	96.0%
Akbari, et al. 2017 [87]	11	371	HOMA-IR: (SMD −0.66, CI 95% −1.14 to -0.18)	57.4%
			QUICKI: (SMD 0.73, CI 95% 0.26 to 1.20)	64.9%
			HOMA-B: (SMD −0.52, CI 95% −0.79 to −0.25)	0.0%

OR: Odds Ratio, RR: Risk Ratio, MD: Mean Difference, SMD: Standardized Mean Difference, I^2: Heterogeneity, NS: Not Significant.

5. Limitations of Current Evidence and Future Perspectives

Despite the summary results of observational studies seem convincing, their relevance in the evidence hierarchy and the frequent presence of heterogeneity (probably due to ethnicity, geographical characteristics, skin tone, gestational age, cut-offs, and laboratory methods used) makes difficult the transfer this knowledge into clinical practice. Without considering the evaluation of the quality of the meta-analyses included in this review (which is out of the scope of the present article), there is a gap between observational and intervention studies investigating the role of vitamin D in preventing GDM or ameliorating its clinical presentation. This is often observed in nutritional epidemiology, and it is currently the topic of a recent diatribe, which will not be discussed in this article neither. However, it is noteworthy to discuss the meaning of the findings here reviewed: A disagreement in findings between observational studies measuring vitamin D levels in association with occurrence of GDM and studies evaluating the efficacy of vitamin D supplementation (with no univocal methodology across studies included in the meta-analysis) in decreasing the risk of GDM is not necessarily equivalent to ambivalent results. Specifically, the observational studies assessed a clinical condition occurring following physiological processes (i.e., dietary consumption of vitamin D-rich foods, and sun exposure) while the RCTs showed the effect of dietary supplementation, which actually differ from the previous condition.

The highest level of evidence for efficacy of supplementation could be provided by the results of randomized, double-blind, placebo-controlled clinical trials. However, meta-analyses of clinical trials may still be influenced by potential confounding factors that ultimately affect the conclusions derived from these studies [88,89]. For instance, the gestational age of intervention can be crucial for restoring a situation of repletion. In fact, while 25(OH)D blood levels seem to promptly respond to supplementation, peripheral cellular deficiency may require more time, and intervention studies designed during the late gestational age may not consider sufficient time to restore physiological conditions useful for the prevention of dysfunctions [90]. The selection of factors to be controlled in the experimental setting is of great importance since it is well known that some aspects such as reduced physical activity, BMI, and high mother age are risk factors for both GDM and vitamin D deficiency [91,92]. Other factors strictly related to vitamin D, such as endogenous biosynthesis, type and dosage of vitamin D (including matrix used in the supplement and other substances), diet, etc, should ideally be taken into account when planning a trial. Dose-response studies can be crucial to design efficient intervention [93]. Dosage and duration of supplementation could be critical to establishing a relationship between intervention and outcomes. In fact, even large *boli* are rapidly absorbed and undetectable, while during the supplementation vitamin D levels reach a plateau after three to four months of continuous provision [94,95]. In a relatively short window like pregnancy, this aspect could be crucial. The specific vitamin D isoform used could play a role in the conflicting results. Though vitamin D_2 and vitamin D_3 follow the same metabolic fate after absorption, the latter isoform seems to provoke a more marked increase of 25(OH)D blood levels after supplementation [23,96]. The same dosage of vitamin D_3 rises two-fold the serum levels of 25(OH)D in respect to vitamin D_2 supplement [23,96]. This phenomenon occurs both in the short-term and in the long-term administration [97–99]. The greater efficiency of the vitamin D_3 form seems to depend on the more marked affinity towards the vitamin D binding protein [100–102]. The current state of the art suggests that, although the D_3 form could be a preferential substrate for the hepatic hydroxylation, and therefore in raising the circulating levels more efficiently in the case of high bolus doses, at physiological daily concentrations there do not seem to be any differences between the two isoforms [103].

6. Conclusions

There is a need for larger well-designed RCTs that evaluate interventions together with the evaluation of numerous confounding factors. However, first of all, it would be useful to define the cut-offs, detection methods, and dosages for a more homogeneous analysis of such complex phenomenon as the GDM. The choice of the population is decisive, therefore, to obtain a clear and convincing result. Populations replete for vitamin D and with an effective program of preventive supplementation may not respond to vitamin supplementation while other factors such as smoking, weight, and gestational age, may mask the outcomes of the intervention. Supplementation should be calibrated on the variation of circulating 25(OH)D and not on the intervention dosage.

Because GDM establishes in a very early stage of pregnancy, even the first trimester could be too late for interventional supplementation and periconceptional period could be the most suitable for interventions. The role of PTH in GDM must be elucidated and therefore intervention studies should be able to discriminate from the possible phenomenon of PTH suppression by vitamin D during pregnancy supplementation. Understanding the adaptive mechanisms in pregnancy and also the bioavailability of vitamin D in its isoforms and in relation to the expression of vitamin D binding protein and receptor could increase the interpretative power in clinical trials. Taking into account the diffused vitamin D insufficiency among pregnant women, vitamin D can be a good candidate for the prevention and management of GDM with no relevant risks in case of intervention protocols at physiological dosages. However, it must be integrated into broader approaches that take into consideration other determinants that can effectively influence the multifactorial nature of the disease.

Author Contributions: G.R. conceived the paper and drafted the manuscript; G.G. drafted the paper and provided insights on the nutritional part; S.G., M.F., M.M.P., and U.C. provided insights on the clinical part; A.S., P.d.F., G.V., J.T., and P.T. provided insights on the epidemiological data and clinical limitations; all authors revised the overall content.

References

1. Bikle, D. Nonclassic actions of Vitamin D. *J. Clin. Endocrinol. Metab.* **2009**, *94*, 26–34. [CrossRef] [PubMed]
2. Holick, M.F.; Chen, T.C. Vitamin d deficiency: A worldwide problem with health consequences. *Am. J. Clin. Nutr.* **2008**, *87*, 1080S–1086S. [CrossRef] [PubMed]
3. Lacroix, M.; Battista, M.C.; Doyon, M.; Houde, G.; Menard, J.; Ardilouze, J.L.; Hivert, M.F.; Perron, P. Lower vitamin d levels at first trimester are associated with higher risk of developing gestational diabetes mellitus. *Acta Diabetol.* **2014**, *51*, 609–616. [CrossRef] [PubMed]
4. Weyland, P.G.; Grant, W.B.; Howie-Esquivel, J. Does sufficient evidence exist to support a causal association between vitamin d status and cardiovascular disease risk? An assessment using hill's criteria for causality. *Nutrients* **2014**, *6*, 3403–3430. [CrossRef] [PubMed]
5. Vitale, S.G.; Caruso, S.; Rapisarda, A.M.C.; Cianci, S.; Cianci, A. Isoflavones, calcium, vitamin d and inulin improve quality of life, sexual function, body composition and metabolic parameters in menopausal women: Result from a prospective, randomized, placebo-controlled, parallel-group study. *Prz Menopauzalny* **2018**, *17*, 32–38. [CrossRef]
6. Cianci, A.; Colacurci, N.; Paoletti, A.M.; Perino, A.; Cicinelli, E.; Maffei, S.; Di Martino, M.; Daguati, R.; Stomati, M.; Pilloni, M.; et al. Soy isoflavones, inulin, calcium, and vitamin d3 in post-menopausal hot flushes: An observational study. *Clin. Exp. Obs. Gynecol.* **2015**, *42*, 743–745.
7. Lagana, A.S.; Vitale, S.G.; Ban Frangez, H.; Vrtacnik-Bokal, E.; D'Anna, R. Vitamin d in human reproduction: The more, the better? An evidence-based critical appraisal. *Eur. Rev. Med. Pharm. Sci.* **2017**, *21*, 4243–4251.
8. Colonese, F.; La Rosa, V.L.; Lagana, A.S.; Vitale, S.G.; Cortinovis, D.; Bidoli, P. Comment on: "Is there a role for vitamin d in human reproduction?". *Horm. Mol. Biol. Clin. Investig.* **2017**, *29*, 37–38.
9. Fichera, M.; Török, P.; Tesarik, J.; Della Corte, L.; Rizzo, G.; Garzon, S.; Carlea, A.; Di Angelo Antonio, S.; Zito, G.; Panella, M.M. Vitamin d, reproductive disorders and assisted reproduction: Evidences and perspectives. *Int. J. Food Sci. Nutr.* **2019**, in press. [CrossRef]
10. Amegah, A.K.; Klevor, M.K.; Wagner, C.L. Maternal vitamin d insufficiency and risk of adverse pregnancy and birth outcomes: A systematic review and meta-analysis of longitudinal studies. *PLoS ONE* **2017**, *12*, e0173605. [CrossRef]
11. Drever, N.; Saade, G.R.; Bytautiene, E. Fetal programming: Early-life modulations that affect adult outcomes. *Curr. Allergy Asthma Rep.* **2010**, *10*, 453–459. [CrossRef] [PubMed]

12. Poston, L. Influences of maternal nutritional status on vascular function in the offspring. *Curr. Drug Targets* **2007**, *8*, 914–922. [CrossRef] [PubMed]
13. Berti, C.; Cetin, I.; Agostoni, C.; Desoye, G.; Devlieger, R.; Emmett, P.M.; Ensenauer, R.; Hauner, H.; Herrera, E.; Hoesli, I.; et al. Pregnancy and infants' outcome: Nutritional and metabolic implications. *Crit. Rev. Food Sci. Nutr.* **2016**, *56*, 82–91. [CrossRef] [PubMed]
14. Kulkarni, B.; Hills, A.P.; Byrne, N.M. Nutritional influences over the life course on lean body mass of individuals in developing countries. *Nutr. Rev.* **2014**, *72*, 190–204. [CrossRef]
15. Società Italiana di Nutrizione Umana (SINU). *LARN: Livelli di Assunzione di Riferimento di Nutrienti ed Energia per la Popolazione Italiana*; IV Revisione; SICS Editore; Società Italiana di Nutrizione Umana: Firenze, Italy, 2014; ISBN 978-88-906852-2-4.
16. US Department of Agriculture (USDA). United States Department Of Agriculture. Agricultural research service (USDA). Food composition databases. Available online: https://ndb.nal.usda.gov/ndb/search/list (accessed on 7 September 2017).
17. Shahgheibi, S.; Farhadifar, F.; Pouya, B. The effect of vitamin d supplementation on gestational diabetes in high-risk women: Results from a randomized placebo-controlled trial. *J. Res. Med. Sci.* **2016**, *21*, 2.
18. Marwaha, R.K.; Tandon, N.; Chopra, S.; Agarwal, N.; Garg, M.K.; Sharma, B.; Kanwar, R.S.; Bhadra, K.; Singh, S.; Mani, K.; et al. Vitamin d status in pregnant indian women across trimesters and different seasons and its correlation with neonatal serum 25-hydroxyvitamin d levels. *Br. J. Nutr.* **2011**, *106*, 1383–1389. [CrossRef]
19. Perampalam, S.; Ganda, K.; Chow, K.A.; Opie, N.; Hickman, P.E.; Shadbolt, B.; Hennessy, A.; Grunstein, H.; Nolan, C.J. Vitamin d status and its predictive factors in pregnancy in 2 australian populations. *Aust. N. Z. J. Obs. Gynaecol.* **2011**, *51*, 353–359. [CrossRef]
20. Saaf, M.; Fernell, E.; Kristiansson, F.; Barnevik Olsson, M.; Gustafsson, S.A.; Bagenholm, G. Severe vitamin d deficiency in pregnant women of somali origin living in sweden. *Acta Paediatr.* **2011**, *100*, 612–614. [CrossRef]
21. Shibata, M.; Suzuki, A.; Sekiya, T.; Sekiguchi, S.; Asano, S.; Udagawa, Y.; Itoh, M. High prevalence of hypovitaminosis d in pregnant japanese women with threatened premature delivery. *J. Bone Min. Metab.* **2011**, *29*, 615–620. [CrossRef]
22. Tao, M.; Shao, H.; Gu, J.; Zhen, Z. Vitamin d status of pregnant women in Shanghai, China. *J. Matern. Fetal. Neonatal. Med.* **2012**, *25*, 237–239. [CrossRef]
23. Triunfo, S.; Lanzone, A. Potential impact of maternal vitamin d status on obstetric well-being. *J. Endocrinol. Investig.* **2016**, *39*, 37–44. [CrossRef] [PubMed]
24. Aghajafari, F.; Nagulesapillai, T.; Ronksley, P.E.; Tough, S.C.; O'Beirne, M.; Rabi, D.M. Association between maternal serum 25-hydroxyvitamin d level and pregnancy and neonatal outcomes: Systematic review and meta-analysis of observational studies. *BMJ* **2013**, *346*, f1169. [CrossRef]
25. Senti, J.; Thiele, D.K.; Anderson, C.M. Maternal vitamin d status as a critical determinant in gestational diabetes. *J. Obs. Gynecol. Neonatal. Nurs.* **2012**, *41*, 328–338. [CrossRef] [PubMed]
26. Kahn, S.E.; Prigeon, R.L.; McCulloch, D.K.; Boyko, E.J.; Bergman, R.N.; Schwartz, M.W.; Neifing, J.L.; Ward, W.K.; Beard, J.C.; Palmer, J.P.; et al. Quantification of the relationship between insulin sensitivity and beta-cell function in human subjects. Evidence for a hyperbolic function. *Diabetes* **1993**, *42*, 1663–1672. [CrossRef] [PubMed]
27. American Diabetes. Diagnosis and classification of diabetes mellitus. *Diabetes Care* **2013**, *36* (Suppl. 1), S67–S74. [CrossRef]
28. Hao, M.; Lin, L. Fasting plasma glucose and body mass index during the first trimester of pregnancy as predictors of gestational diabetes mellitus in a chinese population. *Endocr. J.* **2017**, *64*, 561–569. [CrossRef]
29. Moyer, V.A.; Force, U.S.P.S.T. Screening for gestational diabetes mellitus: U.S. Preventive services task force recommendation statement. *Ann. Intern. Med.* **2014**, *160*, 414–420. [CrossRef]
30. Hunt, K.J.; Schuller, K.L. The increasing prevalence of diabetes in pregnancy. *Obs. Gynecol. Clin. North Am.* **2007**, *34*, 173–199. [CrossRef]
31. Reece, E.A.; Leguizamon, G.; Wiznitzer, A. Gestational diabetes: The need for a common ground. *Lancet* **2009**, *373*, 1789–1797. [CrossRef]
32. Triunfo, S.; Lanzone, A.; Lindqvist, P.G. Low maternal circulating levels of vitamin d as potential determinant in the development of gestational diabetes mellitus. *J. Endocrinol. Investig.* **2017**, *40*, 1049–1059. [CrossRef]

33. Vitale, S.G.; Lagana, A.S.; Nigro, A.; La Rosa, V.L.; Rossetti, P.; Rapisarda, A.M.; La Vignera, S.; Condorelli, R.A.; Corrado, F.; Buscema, M.; et al. Peroxisome proliferator-activated receptor modulation during metabolic diseases and cancers: Master and minions. *PPAR Res.* **2016**, *2016*, 6517313. [CrossRef] [PubMed]
34. Lagana, A.S.; Vitale, S.G.; Nigro, A.; Sofo, V.; Salmeri, F.M.; Rossetti, P.; Rapisarda, A.M.; La Vignera, S.; Condorelli, R.A.; Rizzo, G.; et al. Pleiotropic actions of peroxisome proliferator-activated receptors (ppars) in dysregulated metabolic homeostasis, inflammation and cancer: Current evidence and future perspectives. *Int. J. Mol. Sci.* **2016**, *17*, 999. [CrossRef] [PubMed]
35. Gao, Y.; She, R.; Sha, W. Gestational diabetes mellitus is associated with decreased adipose and placenta peroxisome proliferator-activator receptor gamma expression in a chinese population. *Oncotarget* **2017**, *8*, 113928–113937. [CrossRef] [PubMed]
36. Kautzky-Willer, A.; Prager, R.; Waldhausl, W.; Pacini, G.; Thomaseth, K.; Wagner, O.F.; Ulm, M.; Streli, C.; Ludvik, B. Pronounced insulin resistance and inadequate beta-cell secretion characterize lean gestational diabetes during and after pregnancy. *Diabetes Care* **1997**, *20*, 1717–1723. [CrossRef] [PubMed]
37. Marchetti, P. Islet inflammation in type 2 diabetes. *Diabetologia* **2016**, *59*, 668–672. [CrossRef] [PubMed]
38. Alvarez, J.A.; Ashraf, A. Role of vitamin d in insulin secretion and insulin sensitivity for glucose homeostasis. *Int. J. Endocrinol.* **2010**, *2010*, 351385. [CrossRef]
39. Carpentier, J.L.; Gorden, P.; Lew, D.P. Calcium ions are required for the intracellular routing of insulin and its receptor. *Exp. Cell Res.* **1992**, *198*, 144–149. [CrossRef]
40. Xuan, Y.; Zhao, H.Y.; Liu, J.M. Vitamin d and type 2 diabetes mellitus (d2). *J. Diabetes* **2013**, *5*, 261–267. [CrossRef]
41. Vaidya, A.; Williams, J.S. Vitamin d and insulin sensitivity: Can gene association and pharmacogenetic studies of the vitamin d receptor provide clarity? *Metabolism* **2012**, *61*, 759–761. [CrossRef]
42. Chiu, K.C.; Chu, A.; Go, V.L.; Saad, M.F. Hypovitaminosis d is associated with insulin resistance and beta cell dysfunction. *Am. J. Clin. Nutr.* **2004**, *79*, 820–825. [CrossRef]
43. Norman, A.W.; Frankel, J.B.; Heldt, A.M.; Grodsky, G.M. Vitamin d deficiency inhibits pancreatic secretion of insulin. *Science* **1980**, *209*, 823–825. [CrossRef] [PubMed]
44. Wamberg, L.; Christiansen, T.; Paulsen, S.K.; Fisker, S.; Rask, P.; Rejnmark, L.; Richelsen, B.; Pedersen, S.B. Expression of vitamin d-metabolizing enzymes in human adipose tissue—The effect of obesity and diet-induced weight loss. *Int. J. Obes.* **2013**, *37*, 651–657. [CrossRef] [PubMed]
45. Karlsson, T.; Osmancevic, A.; Jansson, N.; Hulthen, L.; Holmang, A.; Larsson, I. Increased vitamin d-binding protein and decreased free 25(oh)d in obese women of reproductive age. *Eur. J. Nutr.* **2014**, *53*, 259–267. [CrossRef] [PubMed]
46. American Diabetes Association. 2. Classification and diagnosis of diabetes: Standards of medical care in diabetes-2019. *Diabetes Care* **2019**, *42*, S13–S28. [CrossRef]
47. Diabetes Canada Clinical Practice Guidelines Expert; Feig, D.S.; Berger, H.; Donovan, L.; Godbout, A.; Kader, T.; Keely, E.; Sanghera, R. Diabetes and pregnancy. *Can. J. Diabetes* **2018**, *42* (Suppl. 1), S255–S282. [CrossRef]
48. International Association of Diabetes; Pregnancy Study Groups Consensus Panel; Metzger, B.E.; Gabbe, S.G.; Persson, B.; Buchanan, T.A.; Catalano, P.A.; Damm, P.; Dyer, A.R.; Leiva, A.; et al. International association of diabetes and pregnancy study groups recommendations on the diagnosis and classification of hyperglycemia in pregnancy. *Diabetes Care* **2010**, *33*, 676–682. [CrossRef]
49. WHO. *Who/Nmh/Mnd Diagnostic Criteria and Classification of Hyperglycaemia First Detected in Pregnancy*; WHO: Geneva, Switzerland, 2013.
50. Coustan, D.R.; Lowe, L.P.; Metzger, B.E.; Dyer, A.R. International Association of Pregnancy Study. The hyperglycemia and adverse pregnancy outcome (hapo) study: Paving the way for new diagnostic criteria for gestational diabetes mellitus. *Am. J. Obs. Gynecol.* **2010**, *202*, 654. [CrossRef]
51. Chapuy, M.C.; Preziosi, P.; Maamer, M.; Arnaud, S.; Galan, P.; Hercberg, S.; Meunier, P.J. Prevalence of vitamin d insufficiency in an adult normal population. *Osteoporos. Int.* **1997**, *7*, 439–443. [CrossRef]
52. Chapuy, M.C.; Schott, A.M.; Garnero, P.; Hans, D.; Delmas, P.D.; Meunier, P.J. Healthy elderly french women living at home have secondary hyperparathyroidism and high bone turnover in winter. Epidos study group. *J. Clin. Endocrinol. Metab.* **1996**, *81*, 1129–1133.

53. Holick, M.F.; Siris, E.S.; Binkley, N.; Beard, M.K.; Khan, A.; Katzer, J.T.; Petruschke, R.A.; Chen, E.; de Papp, A.E. Prevalence of vitamin d inadequacy among postmenopausal north american women receiving osteoporosis therapy. *J. Clin. Endocrinol. Metab.* **2005**, *90*, 3215–3224. [CrossRef]
54. Thomas, M.K.; Lloyd-Jones, D.M.; Thadhani, R.I.; Shaw, A.C.; Deraska, D.J.; Kitch, B.T.; Vamvakas, E.C.; Dick, I.M.; Prince, R.L.; Finkelstein, J.S. Hypovitaminosis d in medical inpatients. *N. Engl. J. Med.* **1998**, *338*, 777–783. [CrossRef] [PubMed]
55. Ross, A.C.; Taylor, C.L.; Yaktine, A.L.; Del Valle, H.B. *Dietary Reference Intakes for Calcium and Vitamin D*; National Academies Press: Washington, DC, USA, 2011.
56. Adami, S.; Viapiana, O.; Gatti, D.; Idolazzi, L.; Rossini, M. Relationship between serum parathyroid hormone, vitamin d sufficiency, age, and calcium intake. *Bone* **2008**, *42*, 267–270. [CrossRef] [PubMed]
57. Holick, M.F. Sunlight and vitamin d for bone health and prevention of autoimmune diseases, cancers, and cardiovascular disease. *Am. J. Clin. Nutr.* **2004**, *80*, 1678S–1688S. [CrossRef] [PubMed]
58. Holick, M.F. Vitamin d: Importance in the prevention of cancers, type 1 diabetes, heart disease, and osteoporosis. *Am. J. Clin. Nutr.* **2004**, *79*, 362–371. [CrossRef]
59. Kramer, C.K.; Swaminathan, B.; Hanley, A.J.; Connelly, P.W.; Sermer, M.; Zinman, B.; Retnakaran, R. Vitamin d and parathyroid hormone status in pregnancy: Effect on insulin sensitivity, beta-cell function, and gestational diabetes mellitus. *J. Clin. Endocrinol. Metab.* **2014**, *99*, 4506–4513. [CrossRef]
60. Heaney, R.P.; Dowell, M.S.; Hale, C.A.; Bendich, A. Calcium absorption varies within the reference range for serum 25-hydroxyvitamin d. *J. Am. Coll. Nutr.* **2003**, *22*, 142–146. [CrossRef]
61. Holick, M.F. Vitamin d deficiency. *N. Engl. J. Med.* **2007**, *357*, 266–281. [CrossRef]
62. EFSA panel on dietetic products, nutrition and allergies (nda) dietary reference values for vitamin d. *EFSA J.* **2016**, *14*, e04547. [CrossRef]
63. Cashman, K.D.; Dowling, K.G.; Skrabakova, Z.; Gonzalez-Gross, M.; Valtuena, J.; De Henauw, S.; Moreno, L.; Damsgaard, C.T.; Michaelsen, K.F.; Molgaard, C.; et al. Vitamin d deficiency in europe: Pandemic? *Am. J. Clin. Nutr.* **2016**, *103*, 1033–1044. [CrossRef]
64. Palacios, C.; Gonzalez, L. Is vitamin d deficiency a major global public health problem? *J. Steroid Biochem. Mol. Biol.* **2014**, *144 Pt A*, 138–145. [CrossRef]
65. Hollis, B.W.; Wagner, C.L. Vitamin d requirements during lactation: High-dose maternal supplementation as therapy to prevent hypovitaminosis d for both the mother and the nursing infant. *Am. J. Clin. Nutr.* **2004**, *80*, 1752S–1758S. [CrossRef] [PubMed]
66. Lankes, U.; Elder, P.A.; Lewis, J.G.; George, P. Differential extraction of endogenous and exogenous 25-oh-vitamin d from serum makes the accurate quantification in liquid chromatography-tandem mass spectrometry assays challenging. *Ann. Clin. Biochem.* **2015**, *52*, 151–160. [CrossRef] [PubMed]
67. Naughton, D.; Petroczi, A. Vitamin d status and ill health. *Lancet Diabetes Endocrinol.* **2014**, *2*, 274–275. [CrossRef]
68. Shah, I.; James, R.; Barker, J.; Petroczi, A.; Naughton, D.P. Misleading measures in vitamin d analysis: A novel lc-ms/ms assay to account for epimers and isobars. *Nutr. J.* **2011**, *10*, 46. [CrossRef] [PubMed]
69. Shah, I.; Petroczi, A.; Naughton, D.P. Method for simultaneous analysis of eight analogues of vitamin d using liquid chromatography tandem mass spectrometry. *Chem. Cent. J.* **2012**, *6*, 112. [CrossRef]
70. Shah, I.; Petroczi, A.; Naughton, D.P. Exploring the role of vitamin d in type 1 diabetes, rheumatoid arthritis, and alzheimer disease: New insights from accurate analysis of 10 forms. *J. Clin. Endocrinol. Metab.* **2014**, *99*, 808–816. [CrossRef]
71. Wootton, A.M. Improving the measurement of 25-hydroxyvitamin d. *Clin. Biochem. Rev.* **2005**, *26*, 33–36.
72. Poel, Y.H.; Hummel, P.; Lips, P.; Stam, F.; van der Ploeg, T.; Simsek, S. Vitamin d and gestational diabetes: A systematic review and meta-analysis. *Eur. J. Intern. Med.* **2012**, *23*, 465–469. [CrossRef]
73. Wei, S.Q.; Qi, H.P.; Luo, Z.C.; Fraser, W.D. Maternal vitamin d status and adverse pregnancy outcomes: A systematic review and meta-analysis. *J. Matern. Fetal Neonatal. Med.* **2013**, *26*, 889–899. [CrossRef]
74. Zhang, M.X.; Pan, G.T.; Guo, J.F.; Li, B.Y.; Qin, L.Q.; Zhang, Z.L. Vitamin d deficiency increases the risk of gestational diabetes mellitus: A meta-analysis of observational studies. *Nutrients* **2015**, *7*, 8366–8375. [CrossRef]
75. Lu, M.; Xu, Y.; Lv, L.; Zhang, M. Association between vitamin d status and the risk of gestational diabetes mellitus: A meta-analysis. *Arch. Gynecol. Obs.* **2016**, *293*, 959–966. [CrossRef] [PubMed]

76. Amraei, M.; Mohamadpour, S.; Sayehmiri, K.; Mousavi, S.F.; Shirzadpour, E.; Moayeri, A. Effects of vitamin d deficiency on incidence risk of gestational diabetes mellitus: A systematic review and meta-analysis. *Front Endocrinol.* **2018**, *9*, 7. [CrossRef] [PubMed]
77. Hu, L.; Zhang, Y.; Wang, X.; You, L.; Xu, P.; Cui, X.; Zhu, L.; Ji, C.; Guo, X.; Wen, J. Maternal vitamin d status and risk of gestational diabetes: A meta-analysis. *Cell Physiol. Biochem.* **2018**, *45*, 291–300. [CrossRef]
78. Asemi, Z.; Hashemi, T.; Karamali, M.; Samimi, M.; Esmaillzadeh, A. Effects of vitamin d supplementation on glucose metabolism, lipid concentrations, inflammation, and oxidative stress in gestational diabetes: A double-blind randomized controlled clinical trial. *Am. J. Clin. Nutr.* **2013**, *98*, 1425–1432. [CrossRef] [PubMed]
79. Soheilykhah, S.; Mojibian, M.; Moghadam, M.J.; Shojaoddiny-Ardekani, A. The effect of different doses of vitamin d supplementation on insulin resistance during pregnancy. *Gynecol. Endocrinol.* **2013**, *29*, 396–399. [CrossRef] [PubMed]
80. Asemi, Z.; Samimi, M.; Tabassi, Z.; Shakeri, H.; Esmaillzadeh, A. Vitamin d supplementation affects serum high-sensitivity c-reactive protein, insulin resistance, and biomarkers of oxidative stress in pregnant women. *J. Nutr.* **2013**, *143*, 1432–1438. [CrossRef] [PubMed]
81. Yap, C.; Cheung, N.W.; Gunton, J.E.; Athayde, N.; Munns, C.F.; Duke, A.; McLean, M. Vitamin d supplementation and the effects on glucose metabolism during pregnancy: A randomized controlled trial. *Diabetes Care* **2014**, *37*, 1837–1844. [CrossRef]
82. Thorne-Lyman, A.; Fawzi, W.W. Vitamin d during pregnancy and maternal, neonatal and infant health outcomes: A systematic review and meta-analysis. *Paediatr. Perinat. Epidemiol.* **2012**, *26* (Suppl. 1), 75–90. [CrossRef] [PubMed]
83. Sablok, A.; Batra, A.; Thariani, K.; Batra, A.; Bharti, R.; Aggarwal, A.R.; Kabi, B.C.; Chellani, H. Supplementation of vitamin d in pregnancy and its correlation with feto-maternal outcome. *Clin. Endocrinol.* **2015**, *83*, 536–541. [CrossRef]
84. Palacios, C.; De-Regil, L.M.; Lombardo, L.K.; Pena-Rosas, J.P. Vitamin d supplementation during pregnancy: Updated meta-analysis on maternal outcomes. *J. Steroid Biochem. Mol. Biol.* **2016**, *164*, 148–155. [CrossRef]
85. Perez-Lopez, F.R.; Pasupuleti, V.; Mezones-Holguin, E.; Benites-Zapata, V.A.; Thota, P.; Deshpande, A.; Hernandez, A.V. Effect of vitamin d supplementation during pregnancy on maternal and neonatal outcomes: A systematic review and meta-analysis of randomized controlled trials. *Fertil Steril.* **2015**, *103*, 1278–1288. [CrossRef] [PubMed]
86. De-Regil, L.M.; Palacios, C.; Lombardo, L.K.; Pena-Rosas, J.P. Vitamin d supplementation for women during pregnancy. *Sao Paulo Med. J.* **2016**, *134*, 274–275. [CrossRef] [PubMed]
87. Akbari, M.; Moosazaheh, M.; Lankarani, K.B.; Tabrizi, R.; Samimi, M.; Karamali, M.; Jamilian, M.; Kolahdooz, F.; Asemi, Z. The effects of vitamin d supplementation on glucose metabolism and lipid profiles in patients with gestational diabetes: A systematic review and meta-analysis of randomized controlled trials. *Horm. Metab. Res.* **2017**, *49*, 647–653. [PubMed]
88. Karras, S.N.; Anagnostis, P.; Annweiler, C.; Naughton, D.P.; Petroczi, A.; Bili, E.; Harizopoulou, V.; Tarlatzis, B.C.; Persinaki, A.; Papadopoulou, F.; et al. Maternal vitamin d status during pregnancy: The mediterranean reality. *Eur. J. Clin. Nutr.* **2014**, *68*, 864–869. [CrossRef] [PubMed]
89. Xiang, F.; Jiang, J.; Li, H.; Yuan, J.; Yang, R.; Wang, Q.; Zhang, Y. High prevalence of vitamin d insufficiency in pregnant women working indoors and residing in guiyang, china. *J. Endocrinol. Investig.* **2013**, *36*, 503–507.
90. Karras, S.N.; Anagnostis, P.; Naughton, D.; Annweiler, C.; Petroczi, A.; Goulis, D.G. Vitamin d during pregnancy: Why observational studies suggest deficiency and interventional studies show no improvement in clinical outcomes? A narrative review. *J. Endocrinol. Investig.* **2015**, *38*, 1265–1275. [CrossRef]
91. Prentice, A.; Goldberg, G.R.; Schoenmakers, I. Vitamin d across the lifecycle: Physiology and biomarkers. *Am. J. Clin. Nutr.* **2008**, *88*, 500S–506S. [CrossRef]
92. Tobias, D.K.; Zhang, C.; van Dam, R.M.; Bowers, K.; Hu, F.B. Physical activity before and during pregnancy and risk of gestational diabetes mellitus: A meta-analysis. *Diabetes Care* **2011**, *34*, 223–229. [CrossRef]
93. Smith, J.E.; Goodman, D.S. The turnover and transport of vitamin d and of a polar metabolite with the properties of 25-hydroxycholecalciferol in human plasma. *J. Clin. Investig.* **1971**, *50*, 2159–2167. [CrossRef]
94. Heaney, R.P. Guidelines for optimizing design and analysis of clinical studies of nutrient effects. *Nutr. Rev.* **2014**, *72*, 48–54. [CrossRef]

95. Vieth, R.; Chan, P.C.; MacFarlane, G.D. Efficacy and safety of vitamin d3 intake exceeding the lowest observed adverse effect level. *Am. J. Clin. Nutr.* **2001**, *73*, 288–294. [CrossRef] [PubMed]
96. Haddad, J.G.; Stamp, T.C. Circulating 25-hydroxyvitamin d in man. *Am. J. Med.* **1974**, *57*, 57–62. [CrossRef]
97. Binkley, N.; Gemar, D.; Engelke, J.; Gangnon, R.; Ramamurthy, R.; Krueger, D.; Drezner, M.K. Evaluation of ergocalciferol or cholecalciferol dosing, 1600 iu daily or 50,000 iu monthly in older adults. *J. Clin. Endocrinol. Metab.* **2011**, *96*, 981–988. [CrossRef] [PubMed]
98. Heaney, R.P.; Recker, R.R.; Grote, J.; Horst, R.L.; Armas, L.A. Vitamin d(3) is more potent than vitamin d(2) in humans. *J. Clin. Endocrinol. Metab.* **2011**, *96*, E447–E452. [CrossRef]
99. Tjellesen, L.; Hummer, L.; Christiansen, C.; Rodbro, P. Serum concentration of vitamin d metabolites during treatment with vitamin d2 and d3 in normal premenopausal women. *Bone Min.* **1986**, *1*, 407–413.
100. Armas, L.A.; Hollis, B.W.; Heaney, R.P. Vitamin d2 is much less effective than vitamin d3 in humans. *J. Clin. Endocrinol. Metab.* **2004**, *89*, 5387–5391. [CrossRef]
101. Logan, V.F.; Gray, A.R.; Peddie, M.C.; Harper, M.J.; Houghton, L.A. Long-term vitamin d3 supplementation is more effective than vitamin d2 in maintaining serum 25-hydroxyvitamin d status over the winter months. *Br. J. Nutr.* **2013**, *109*, 1082–1088. [CrossRef]
102. McCullough, M.L. Vitamin d deficiency in pregnancy: Bringing the issues to light. *J. Nutr.* **2007**, *137*, 305–306. [CrossRef]
103. Tripkovic, L.; Lambert, H.; Hart, K.; Smith, C.P.; Bucca, G.; Penson, S.; Chope, G.; Hypponen, E.; Berry, J.; Vieth, R.; et al. Comparison of vitamin d2 and vitamin d3 supplementation in raising serum 25-hydroxyvitamin d status: A systematic review and meta-analysis. *Am. J. Clin. Nutr.* **2012**, *95*, 1357–1364. [CrossRef]

2

Exploring the Feasibility of Use of an Online Dietary Assessment Tool (myfood24) in Women with Gestational Diabetes

Carla Gianfrancesco [1,2], Zoe Darwin [3], Linda McGowan [3], Debbie M. Smith [4], Roz Haddrill [5], Michelle Carter [1], Eleanor M. Scott [6], Nisreen A. Alwan [7,8], Michelle A. Morris [9], Salwa A. Albar [10] and Janet E. Cade [1,*]

1 Nutritional Epidemiology Group, School of Food Science and Nutrition, University of Leeds, Leeds LS2 9JT, UK; carla.gianfrancesco@sth.nhs.uk (C.G.); michellecarter.uk@hotmail.co.uk (M.C.)

2 Sheffield Diabetes and Endocrine Centre, Sheffield Teaching Hospitals NHSF Trust, Sheffield S5 7AU, UK

3 School of Healthcare, University of Leeds, Leeds LS2 9JT, UK; Z.J.Darwin@leeds.ac.uk (Z.D.); L.McGowan@leeds.ac.uk (L.M.)

4 School of Social and Health Sciences, Leeds Trinity University, Leeds LS18 5HD, UK; D.Smith@leedstrinity.ac.uk

5 Department of Nursing, Midwifery & Health, Northumbria University, Newcastle upon Tyne NE7 7XA, UK; Roz.Haddrill@northumbria.ac.uk

6 Leeds Institute of Cardiovascular and Metabolic Medicine, University of Leeds, Leeds LS2 9JT, UK; e.m.scott@leeds.ac.uk

7 Academic Unit of Primary Care and Population Sciences, Faculty of Medicine, University of Southampton, Southampton General Hospital, Southampton SO16 6YD, UK; n.a.alwan@soton.ac.uk

8 NIHR Southampton Biomedical Research Centre, University of Southampton and University Hospital Southampton NHS Foundation Trust, Southampton SO16 6YD, UK

9 Leeds Institute for Data Analytics, School of Medicine, University of Leeds, Leeds LS2 9JT, UK; m.morris@leeds.ac.uk

10 Department of Food Science and Nutrition, King Abdul-Aziz University, P.O. Box 42807, Jeddah 21551, Saudi Arabia; salbar1@kau.edu.sa

* Correspondence: j.e.cade@leeds.ac.uk

Abstract: myfood24 is an online 24 hr dietary recall tool developed for nutritional epidemiological research. Its clinical application has been unexplored. This mixed methods study explores the feasibility and usability of myfood24 as a food record in a clinical population, women with gestational diabetes (GDM). Women were asked to complete five myfood24 food records, followed by a user questionnaire (including the System Usability Scale (SUS), a measure of usability), and were invited to participate in a semi-structured interview. Of the 199 participants, the mean age was 33 years, mean booking body mass index (BMI) 29.7 kg/m^2, 36% primiparous, 57% White, 33% Asian. Of these, 121 (61%) completed myfood24 at least once and 73 (37%) completed the user questionnaire; 15 were interviewed. The SUS was found to be good (mean 70.9, 95% CI 67.1, 74.6). Interviews identified areas for improvement, including optimisation for mobile devices, and as a clinical management tool. This study demonstrates that myfood24 can be used as an online food record in a clinical population, and has the potential to support self-management in women with GDM. However, results should be interpreted cautiously given the responders' demographic characteristics. Further research to explore the barriers and facilitators of uptake in people from ethnic minority and lower socioeconomic backgrounds is recommended.

Keywords: 24-h recall; nutrition assessment; technology assisted dietary assessment; gestational diabetes

---

1. Introduction

Gestational diabetes mellitus (GDM) has onset or detection in pregnancy, most commonly in the third trimester. Universal screening for GDM is conducted in some countries such as Australia. However, in the UK, screening targets those with one or more established risk factors. i.e., women with body mass index (weight kg/height m^2) above 30, previous large baby >4.5 kg, previous GDM, ethnic family origin with a higher prevalence of diabetes, or a family history of diabetes [1]. It is performed at around 24–28 weeks gestation and uses an oral glucose tolerance test following fasting, to detect raised blood glucose levels.

The main treatment aim is to maintain healthy blood glucose levels throughout pregnancy to reduce the risks of complications for the mother and child; for example: macrosomia, stillbirth, and birth-related trauma [2]. After giving birth, blood glucose levels usually revert to normal; however, 50% of women with GDM will develop Type 2 diabetes within five years [1]. As with Type 2 diabetes, the treatment of GDM initially focuses on dietary and lifestyle changes with a healthy diet being recommended [1]. To achieve blood glucose targets, emphasis is placed on optimising the type of carbohydrate by encouraging low glycaemic index choices; and on reducing the portion size. If within one to two weeks of dietary modification, blood glucose levels are above the target range for pregnancy (fasting blood glucose below 5.3 mmol/L and one hour after meals below 7.8 mmol/L), women will then require medication for diabetes for the remainder of pregnancy; for example, metformin tablets or insulin injections. The self-management behaviours that are required to achieve these levels, including dietary modification, and frequent self-blood glucose monitoring, are demanding and are associated with increased levels of distress [3].

Standard care at diagnosis for women with GDM includes a dietary assessment, usually by a dietitian, from which education and negotiations for dietary changes will be based; progress may be reviewed at subsequent appointments with further dietary assessments [1]. As with other clinical populations requiring dietary management, typical dietary assessment methods include 24 h dietary recalls that are undertaken with a dietitian or with self-completion of paper food records. The level of detail acquired is variable, and it may include the frequency, amount, and type of food. Gathering and interpreting this information requires time and skills for both health professionals and patients. Such dietary assessment methods are known to have limitations. For example, interviewer-led 24 h dietary recalls can introduce reporting bias as subjects under-report certain foods due to social desirability [4].

The development and implementation of technology-assisted dietary assessment, including, for example the use of websites, mobile phone cameras, and mobile apps to log food intake, is proving to be an alternative to these traditional methods [5–9]. Such technologies in healthy populations are being shown to reduce costs [10], improve completion rates, and increase the accuracy of the dietary assessment [5,7,10–12]. Automated self-administered dietary assessment tool provides participants with more privacy than interviewer-led assessments; hence reducing judgment bias, which is associated with omissions in reporting and underestimation of portion sizes of unhealthy foods [13]. Therefore, minimising contact with the interviewer may encourage more participants to report all food items [14].

Given these favourable findings when using technology-assisted dietary assessment in healthy populations, their application in the management of medical conditions has begun to be explored [15,16]. This data can be instantly analysed and provide feedback to the user and health professional. These features can provide additional support and education outside of the clinic setting [15,17,18], and a study in primary care reported that technology-assisted dietary assessment may promote self-efficacy and increase empowerment in users [17]. Such tools also enable remote monitoring and follow up, potentially reducing the number of face-to-face appointments; therefore, there could be substantial clinical benefits and cost reductions associated with their use.

myfood24 is a self-completed online 24 h dietary recall tool, incorporating elements of an automated multiple pass methodology [19]. Foods consumed are entered on the system, by selecting from a list of options; portion size is then selected, and the food is added to a meal event or time. Prior to submitting the completed recall, it prompts the user to check for omissions, e.g., snacks. The recall is completed at one time, inputting all information from the previous 24 h period. The myfood24 food database contains 45,000 foods including both generic and branded items, 5600 with associated portion size images, and provides the user with an immediate nutritional analysis of their dietary intake. The tool was developed for large scale epidemiological studies in the UK population. Usability and acceptability testing of myfood24 has shown it is suitable to be used in healthy UK teenager (System Usability Score (SUS) Median score 80) and adult populations (SUS Median score 73) and relative validity testing in teenagers showed good agreement with interviewer-administered 24 h multiple-pass recall (MPR)s [19–21]. A validation study in healthy adults that includes the use of biomarkers has been undertaken [22]. Whilst myfood24 is currently used as a 24 h recall tool for nutritional assessment in epidemiological research, its application in healthcare as a food record has not been explored.

This study examined the introduction of myfood24 in a clinical population for the first time. Women with GDM, who are routinely required to complete food records, were requested to use myfood24 as an alternative tool for self-recording dietary intake. The aim of this observational study was to explore the feasibility of using the tool as an electronic food record and the usability of the tool software. Therefore, providing direction for the ongoing development and evaluation of this tool, both for use in clinical research, and ultimately, as an electronic food diary in routine clinical practice. The study also addressed wider aims, including the association between dietary components and blood glucose levels, and the broader experiences of women with GDM, which are the subject of other publications.

2. Materials and Methods

2.1. Ethics

All subjects gave their informed consent for inclusion before they participated in the study. The study was conducted in accordance with the Declaration of Helsinki, and the protocol and subsequent amendments were approved by the South Central Oxford Research Ethics Committee C (reference 14/SC/1267).

2.2. Eligibility

Women attending for their initial appointment following the diagnosis of GDM at Leeds Teaching Hospitals NHS Trust Diabetes in Pregnancy Clinic, were eligible to participate, provided they could read and understand English and were not to be commenced on any diabetes medication.

2.3. Recruitment

Women were invited to take part by a research midwife who provided a participant information sheet, addressed any questions relating to the study and secured informed consent to participate. The sample size of 200 was based on the sample size calculation for other research questions beyond the scope of this paper, examining the association between dietary components and blood glucose levels. This was a considerably larger sample than what was required for usability testing and examining the differences in usability based on sample characteristics [23].

A pragmatic approach was adopted for interviews, using a convenience sample of women who had experienced myfood24 in the main study. Guided by other qualitative research, a minimum of 12 interviews was anticipated as sufficient to provide saturation [24]. As the aim was to interview both participants who had used the tool and those who chosen not to, different recruitment methods were used. For those who had used myfood24, their interest could be indicated via the user questionnaire, and following a substantial amendment, those who had never completed myfood24, were sent an email. Informed consent for interviews was secured separately by the interviewer (ZD).

2.4. *Study Design and Data Collection*

This was a mixed method prospective observational study. The stages of the study and the participation at each stage can be seen in Figure 1. Participants consented for relevant demographic and clinical data to be retrieved from their health records.

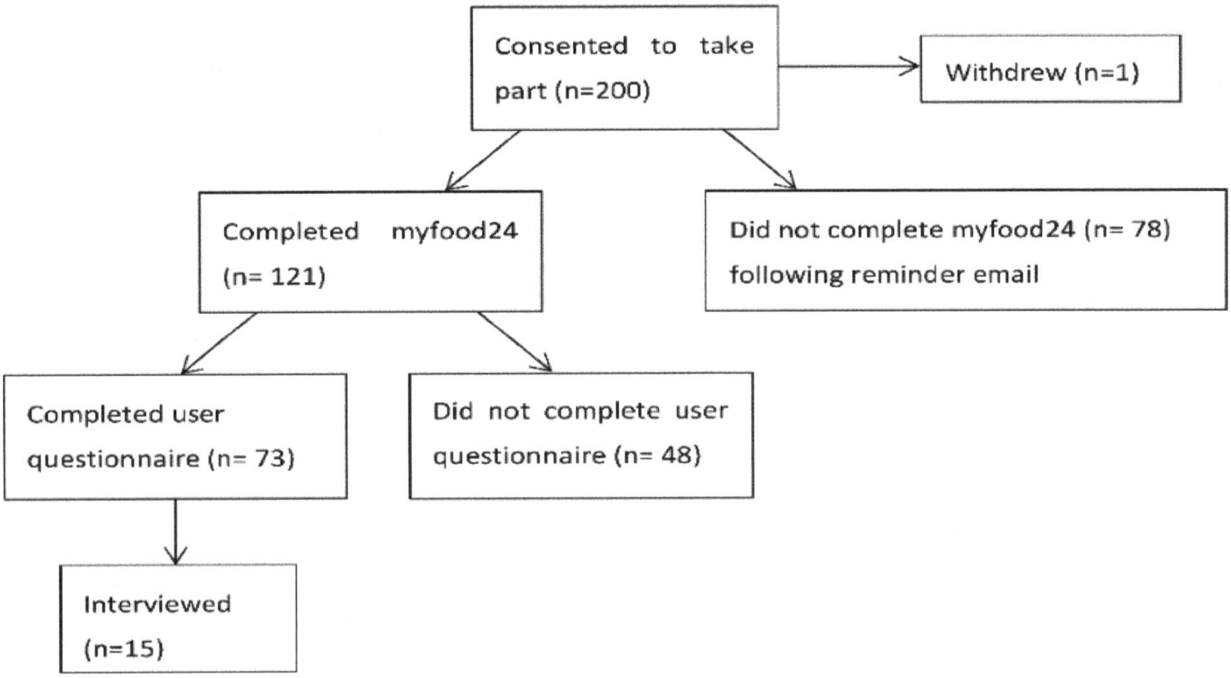

Figure 1. Study flow chart.

2.4.1. Completing a Food Record Using myfood24

Antenatal care provision followed standard care guidelines for diabetes in pregnancy, which included ongoing self-monitoring throughout the pregnancy with blood glucose monitoring seven times a day and paper food diaries. By taking part in the study, participants were also requested to complete five 24 h food records in a two-week period using myfood24. The process of accessing and completing a myfood24 food record is illustrated in Figure 2. The request for five days of records was a pragmatic decision. This would allow women to record a large proportion of their habitual intake and to become more familiar with using myfood24; thus, providing more opportunities to test out the usability and functions of the website.

The feasibility of using the tool as a food record was investigated by measuring any online submission of a myfood24 food record and the total number of submissions per participant.

2.4.2. User Questionnaire

Those who completed myfood24 on at least one occasion were emailed a link to complete the user questionnaire, administered by Bristol Online Survey [25]. The questionnaire consisted of multiple choice questions, Likert scales, yes/no responses and open-ended questions which covered demographic information, previous experience of using technology and food diaries, attitudes to technology and usability of myfood24. It included the SUS, a validated, reliable tool for measuring usability of the software [26]. This is a 10-item scale, with the users asked to rate their level of agreement with 10 usability statements (1 = strongly agree; 5 = strongly disagree) which gives a total score from 0–100. Scores below 50 are unsatisfactory with 50 to 70 are judged as marginal and above 70 considered good [27]. In practice, a SUS score above 68 is considered to be above average and anything below 68 is considered to be below average, and therefore the aim was for the SUS score to be at least 68 [28].

Usability considers user experience of the system, including the ease of understanding and ease of use of the software [29]. The SUS score from the user questionnaire, along with the interview data was the main measure used to assess usability of myfood24, when utilised as an online food record.

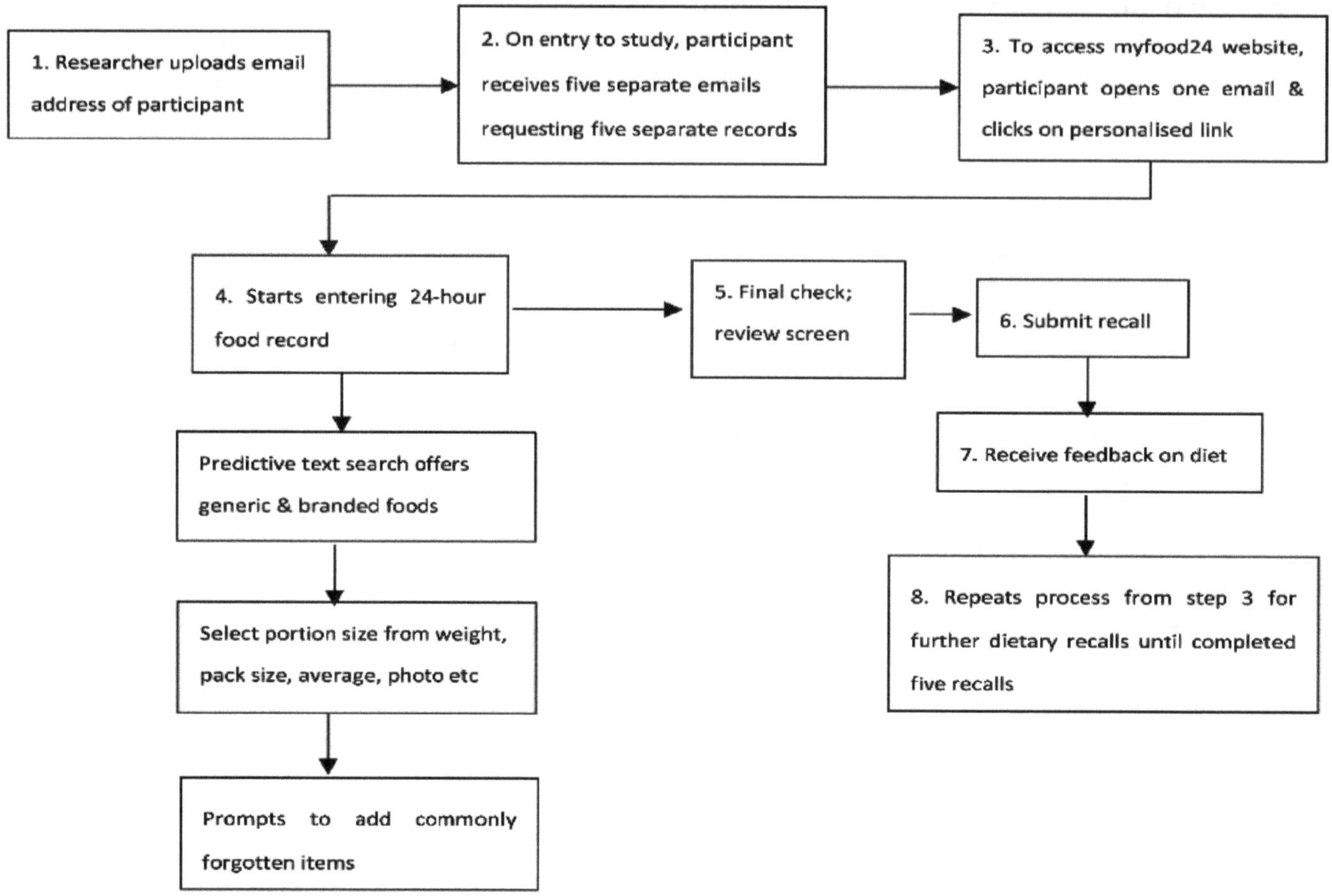

Figure 2. Process of accessing and completing an online myfood24 food record.

2.4.3. Interviews

Interviews were semi-structured and followed a pre-designed flexible topic guide, exploring women's views and experiences of using myfood24. The interviews sought to contextualise the completion rates and findings from the user questionnaire in the words of the women, exploring beyond the practical aspects relating to feasibility and usability. Women were interviewed at a time and location of their choice. All were interviewed by telephone with interviews lasting on average 35 min (range 20–54).

2.5. Data Analysis

2.5.1. Statistical Analyses

Analyses were performed using Stata IC14 statistical software. Descriptive statistics were used to define the sample characteristics. Comparisons were made using chi-squared test for categorical data and independent *t*-test for continuous data. For all inferential statistics the significance level was two-sided and set at 0.05.

Further analysis, using data from the health records of the study population along with additional data from the user questionnaire, considered the secondary aim. This was to identify specific factors that may influence the usability of myfood24, such as demographics, other participant characteristics including online literacy, and features of the tool.

2.5.2. Analysis of Interviews

Interviews were audio-recorded and transcribed verbatim in an anonymous format. Data were analysed using thematic analysis, using the principles that were outlined by Braun and Clarke [30], familiarising selfwith the data, generating initial codes, searching for potential themes, reviewing themes, defining and naming themes, and producing the report.

3. Results

3.1. Characteristics of Participants

Two hundred women consented to the study, and one of these withdrew. The mean age was 33.3 years (SD 5.0). According to health records, 76% of the women were overweight or obese at booking (first formal antenatal appointment), and the mean body mass index (BMI) was 29.7 kg/m^2 (SD 6.5). Most women were White (57%) and one-third (33%) were Asian, and 36% women were primiparous.

3.2. Completion of myfood24 Recalls

Women were asked to use myfood24 to complete and submit five online food records over a two-week period. For the full sample (n = 199), the mean number of days completed was 2.3 (SD 2.2) days; however only 61% (121/199) completed myfood24 at least once. In the 121 women who completed myfood24 at least once, the mean number days completed was 3.8 (SD 1.4); 98 (81%) completed it at least three times and 58 (48%) completed it all five times. Further details are shown in Figure 3.

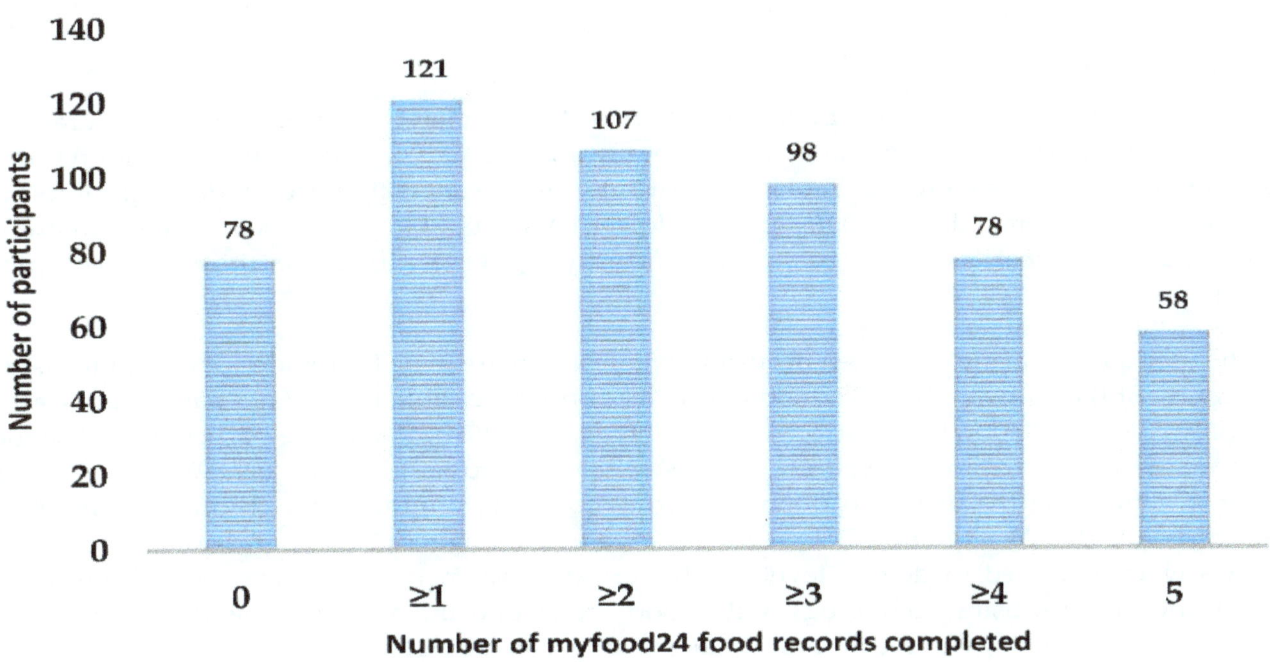

Figure 3. Number of myfood24 food records completed by participants (n = 199).

There were statistically significant demographic differences between those who did (121/199; 61%) and did not (78/199; 39%) complete myfood24 at least once, as shown in Table 1. Women who used myfood24 as a food record were statistically more likely to have lower fasting blood glucose levels ($p = 0.008$), be of White ethnicity ($p = 0.001$) and primiparous ($p = 0.02$).

Table 1. Comparison of characteristics between women who completed myfood24 at least once ($n = 121$) and those who did not ($n = 78$).

	Completed myfood24 ($n = 121$)		Not Completed myfood24 ($n = 78$)		p Value
	n	Mean	n	Mean	
Maternal Age, years (SD)	121	33.5 (4.6)	78	33.2 (5.6)	0.7
Booking body mass index (BMI), kg/m^2 (SD)	119	29.5 (6.2)	77	30.0 (7.0)	0.7
Fasting Blood Glucose, mmol/l (SD)	115	4.9 (0.6)	61	5.2 (0.8)	0.008
Ethnicity					
White (%)	79	65.3	35	44.9	0.001
Asian (%)	31	25.6	23	29.5	
* Other (%)	11	9.1	20	25.6	
Parity					
Primiparous (%)	52	43	21	26.9	0.02
Multiparous (%)	69	57	57	73.1	

* Other ethnicities included Black, Chinese and Mixed race.

Within the women who completed myfood24, no statistically significant differences in demographic characteristics were found according to the number of times that it was completed, with comparison between women who completed it one to two times ($n = 23$), versus three times or more ($n = 98$).

3.3. User Questionnaire

User questionnaires were completed by 73 of the 121 women who used myfood24, a response rate of 60%. Comparisons were made between these women ($n = 73$) and those who did not return the questionnaire ($n = 48$), as shown in Table 2. Statistically significant differences in demographics were found; responders were older ($p = 0.01$) and had lower BMI at booking ($p = 0.008$). The mean number of myfood24 food records completed was significantly higher ($p < 0.001$) in those who completed the questionnaire.

The user questionnaire contained the usability questionnaire, which provided a SUS for measuring the usability of the software [26]. Therefore, this was only accessible to 121/199 participants, and of these, only 73 completed it; hence SUS was completed by 73/199 (37%) of the participants. The mean SUS score for myfood24 in this sub-group was considered to be good at 70.9 (95% CI 67.1, 74.6). Further questions on the user questionnaire provided the following demographic details on this sub-group. Of the 73 women, 47% were employed in managerial or professional occupations, and 58% were educated to degree level or above. Most women (90%) described themselves as being confident with using technology, with good access and the ability to use the internet (97%). Previous use of technology to record food intake was reported by 45%.

Table 2. Characteristics of myfood24 users who completed the user questionnaire (n = 73) and those who did not (n = 48).

	Completed User Q		**Did Not Return User Q**		p **Value**
	n	**Mean**	n	**Mean**	
Age, Years (SD)	73	34.3 (4.3)	48	32.2 (4.7)	0.01
Pre-Pregnancy BMI, kg/m^2 (SD)	72	28.3 (5.0)	47	31.4 (7.5)	0.008
Fasting Blood Glucose, mmol/L (SD)	72	4.9 (0.7)	43	5.0 (0.5)	0.5
Ethnicity					
White (%)	52	71.2	27	56.3	0.4
Asian (%)	15	20.6	16	33.3	
Other (%)	6	8.2	5	10.4	
Parity					
Primiparous (%)	31	42.5	21	43.8	0.9
Multiparous (%)	42	57.5	27	56.2	
Number of days completed myfood24 (SD)	73	4.2 (1.1)	48	3.2 (1.6)	<0.001
System Usability Scale (SUS) score (95% CI)	73	70.9 (67.1, 74.6)	-	-	-
Occupation	68				
Managerial & professionals (%)	32	47			
Intermediate & lower supervisory	17	25	-	-	-
Semi routine & routine (%)	4	6			
Not employed (%)	15	22			
Education level	70				
Degree or above (%)	42	58.3	-	-	-
No degree (%)	30	41.7			
Had previously filled in food diary (%)	26	35.6	-	-	-
Previously used technology to record food (%)	33	45.2	-	-	-
Internet ability good to excellent (%)	71	97.3	-	-	-
Access to internet (%)	72	98.6	-	-	-
Use internet daily (%)	69	94.5	-	-	-
Confident in using technology (%)	66	90.4	-	-	-

3.4. *Interviews*

3.4.1. Characteristics of Interviewees

Despite a substantial amendment part-way through the study, to ensure that the invitation for interview was sent to those who did not complete any myfood24 food records, there were no expressions of interest to be interviewed in this group. Sixteen women who had completed myfood24 expressed an interest, resulting in 15 interviews with one declining due to time commitments. Characteristics of those interviewed were similar to the other participants who completed myfood24. The mean age was 35.1 years (SD 4.5); five were primiparous. Most women were White (13 White, two Asian). The mean BMI at booking was 28.3 (SD 4.7). All had completed myfood24 at least once, and 10 had completed it five times. The mean SUS score was 74.0 (SD 23.0).

Most women reported completing the record at the end of the day in the evenings, with a number of them using their clinic paper food records as an aid to recall that day's food intake.

3.4.2. Themes

Thematic analysis relating to usability and acceptability of using myfood24 as a food record identified the following themes: (1) ease of use, (2) impact on food choices, (3) comparisons with clinic paper records, and (4) future developments. Due to the characteristics of the interview sample, these themes represent only the views of women who had completed myfood24.

(i) Getting Acquainted: Ease of Use

Many of the women had used similar technologies before to record their diet and reported finding myfood24 to be comparable once they had become acquainted with the technology. Most found myfood24 'straightforward' and that inputting data became faster with practice, initially taking approximately 20 min.

> 'I found it quite easy ... I mean, you just typed in a word and it would bring what you wanted up and then you chose from the list' (Interview 3).

Several features were reported that helped or hindered the ease of use of myfood24. Features of the tool that were most commonly identified as being useful for input were the food photographs to help with portion estimation, and the use of reminder prompts. Some also used the recipe function and favourites list; most reported that they would use these functions on a longer-term basis. The food database received mixed feedback. Some found the food database too restrictive, whereas others found the choice overwhelming. Some reported finding food entry to be burdensome when cooking from raw ingredients, and the process was too time consuming to be feasible.

> 'Obviously you don't weigh your food ... it was nice to see actually a portion size' (interview 6)

> 'I didn't have to go back and correct anything really because it reminded me' (interview 3)

> 'For something that was quite simple, it would take actually a long time to find it' (interview 4)

> 'It was quite time consuming having to kind of search for things and put everything in in its own, you know, like all the different components that made up a meal' (interview 11).

One reported disadvantage was the need to record all food entries for the 24 h period in one go, rather than being able to add data after each meal, making myfood24 less easy to use than paper diaries. Interviews identified that accessibility was hindered by problematic initial access to the myfood24 website, offering insight into the completion rates observed. As shown in Figure 1, myfood24 uses a web link accessed from the participant's email account, with each recall requiring a separate email. Women reported that the process had been confusing and it was difficult to keep track of the multiple emails, all of which were sent on the day of entry to the study and without any indication as to which of the five days they referred to.

(ii) Feedback: Impact on Food Choices and Behaviours

On completion of a food record, myfood24 provides an instant summary of its nutritional composition, including energy, protein, fat, carbohydrate, fibre, salt, and micronutrients. This is compared to a dietary reference value.

All of the interviewees reported finding this feature useful to obtain feedback on their food intake and associated eating behaviours, although a minority questioned the accuracy. Women described how this feedback increased their knowledge of their dietary intake, how it could provide reassurance, and how it could enable women to consider what changes were required. Some women reported that the summaries were a motivating factor, influencing future choices about food types and portion sizes.

> 'I did find it frustrating, to be honest, in terms of just trying to find what matched what I was eating, I don't know how accurate it was for me' (Interview 4)

> 'a week's worth of days in front of you it does make you think about what you're eating and how much' (Interview 3)

> 'I was like ooh I shouldn't have eaten that or oh, I've had a really good day today.' (Interview 12)

Most women focused on the data relating to total carbohydrates and sugars—key to the management of GDM—but some also noted using the summaries to understand their fat and salt consumption. In addition, for some, the summary information highlighted that they had actually been too restrictive with their diet, in response to their diagnosis.

> 'Once you can see it in numbers and can see the picture of it, it's harder just to shrug off and think I'm fine...I couldn't just go on with it' (interview 11).

(iii) Comparing Online Self-Monitoring to Clinic Paper Diaries, and the Use of Real-Time Tracking

Comparing myfood24 with paper food diaries that women were required to complete as standard care, some felt myfood24 led to more accurate recording of food intake due to its use of reminders (for example prompting about snacks between meals, and the use of condiments) and recording of quantities, which had not been requested in as much detail in their paper food diaries.

> 'I thought that [myfood24] made me remember things. It was more specific. I think it was easy to forget when you're writing it down. You know because it reminded you—have you remembered to put a drink down here, have you remembered to put a snack down there.' (Interview 9)

Women felt that whilst myfood24 was more accurate than paper-based diaries, in its current format it was also less convenient than paper-based diaries, particularly given the need to track blood glucose levels alongside the dietary intake in the paper-based diaries. Hence, although women valued the myfood24 summary information highly, the utility of myfood24 was limited by being produced at the end of a 24 h period and without any connection to blood glucose readings, limiting its use as a self-monitoring tool for improving blood glucose levels.

(iv) Future Developments: Suggestions based on Experience

Several suggestions were made by women, the most common being to improve accessibility via an app so that data could be conveniently logged throughout the day using a smart phone or tablet. Other suggestions for practical aspects relating to usability and improving its acceptability as an electronic food record were a larger food database, an option to scan bar codes, and easier retrieval of favourite foods. Women made several suggestions to adapt myfood24 to develop its accessibility, and also to develop its usefulness in promoting self-management and supporting behaviour change. Of greatest priority for this clinical population was the need to record blood glucose readings alongside dietary information, in order for the information to be meaningful and to develop knowledge of the impact of different types and quantities of food on blood glucose levels.

Some also identified the need for improved visual displays of the summary nutritional information, to support behaviour change. Suggestions included the ability to track information across time and individualised targets for nutritional intake, rather than reference values. Women also emphasised their perceived additional benefit from being able to use the tool in a diary format, rather than solely as a 24 h recall. This related both to aiding recall, but also to the way in which women used feedback to guide future food choices and behaviour.

> 'I think a phone app would be a lot easier ... you'd just keep updating it as the day went along ... it'd make it more helpful like that' (Interview 12)

> 'I don't know if there was an option where you could save that information, and maybe it was something that I missed, but I would have found that useful as an ongoing thing, if you could save it ... ' (Interview 7)

> 'I thought what might be quite useful would be more like a graph ... that shows like you're here and this is what you really should be getting, aiming for.' (Interview 2)

4. Discussion

This study has demonstrated that it is feasible to use myfood24, a tool previously only used for nutritional epidemiology studies, as an electronic food record in a clinical population. Usability of the software was scored as good within a sub-group of the study population. However, the lower response rates throughout the study and the lack of sample representativeness mean that these results should be interpreted cautiously.

The study has generated a number of suggested areas for improvement which could increase the uptake of myfood24 as a dietary assessment tool in clinical populations. It is important that these are applied where possible, and their impact further evaluated. These changes, along with the ideas for improving the myfood24 software, should be considered prior to future studies examining its use as a dietary management tool to support behaviour change, in a healthcare setting.

4.1. Feasibility of Using myfood24 as An Electronic Food Record

The feasibility of using the tool as an electronic food record was investigated by measuring the total number of submissions of a completed myfood24 food record per participant.

In this study, 78/199 women (39%) did not submit any myfood24 food records. Reasons for this are not known and may extend beyond the acceptability of the tool as an electronic food record. It is noted that statistically significant differences existed between those who did and did not complete myfood24, some of which may be indicative of levels of motivation and self-management; unfortunately, further comparisons were precluded by certain data only being available for those who completed myfood24 and who went on to complete the user questionnaire.

Of those who completed the user questionnaire (n = 73), 45% of participants had used technology previously to log food, so this indicates it is common for women in this group to have similar previous experiences, potentially influencing acceptability in this is population. After participants used myfood24 at least once, the majority went on to use it again, with almost half of women completing it the five times as requested; which does suggest that it is feasible to use this tool as an electronic food record. There did not appear to be any demographic differences regarding number of times completed, however a larger sample size may be needed to determine this. Findings from the interviews suggested that there was confusion experienced with the email system. This system had remained unchanged from its application in nutritional epidemiology data collection and appeared not to suit this setting. As a consequence, this could have impacted on the uptake. In contrast, the data suggests that its perceived provision of a more complete and accurate record and the receipt of the nutritional intake summaries immediately following the diary submission, made a valuable contribution to its acceptability, and enhanced its use as a food record. This is supported in other studies [15,18]. Future work should prioritise these areas for development.

Women continued to have to complete paper-based food and blood glucose diaries as part of standard care. Some women found the paper diary more convenient, due to the ease of access and having all the data in one place, enabling links to be made between food intake and blood glucose levels. Studies in populations with diabetes and renal disease support the suggestion that being able to input foods in real time via a phone app and adding other clinical data such as blood glucose levels can improve acceptability [15,16]. The absence of this functionality may have affected completion rates, as may have the requirement to dual record data on both paper and electronic records.

myfood24 user data can be shared with both the user and the provider/health professional; hence it has the potential to promote user–provider interactions. This function was not utilised in this study. Significant benefits in diabetes outcomes have been found when patients were provided with analysis or feedback from clinicians on their data [15]. Additionally, acceptability and effectiveness of a smartphone nutritional assessment tool for healthy pregnant women, was enhanced by using a similar feature [18]. Therefore, utilisation of this function should be a priority in future studies and its impact on the uptake of the tool assessed.

4.2. Usability

Usability considers the user experience of the system, including its ease of understanding and ease of use [29]. This was measured using the SUS and interview data. The SUS score was classed as good (SUS = 70), and it was comparable to the scores obtained in the general population in other myfood24 evaluations with adults (SUS = 80) and adolescents (SUS = 74) [19,20]. However, it was only obtained in 61% of participants who used the system, and it is noted that this sub-group lacked representativeness compared to the whole study population. This lack of representativeness was also present in the group of interviewees, from whom further data on usability of myfood24 software was collected. Therefore, although this study has generated valuable insights into the usability of the software, that can be further explored and considered for future development of myfood24, no conclusions on the usability of myfood24 for this clinical population can be made at present.

4.3. *Improving Uptake of Use of the Tool and Usability of Software in the Future*

A number of suggestions were made by interviewees regarding how to improve myfood24 software. Many of these are applicable to all dietary assessment tools/ food logging applications [6,17] and include: improvements to speed up food data entry, extensions to the food database, including ethnic foods, chain restaurant meals and popular homemade recipes, and more support to estimate portion sizes. Specifically related to myfood24, women wished to input food in real time and not have to enter the entire day's food intake in one entry. They requested being able to undertake food records as frequently as they wanted, to access previous records, to be able to utilise food lists and to also make comparisons between days. Recent myfood24 developments on the visual displays of nutrient summary feedback, could be adapted for the healthcare setting to address some of these suggestions. Further thought into how the website is accessed and the setup of personal accounts for clinical rather than research purposes, is crucial to achieving this, and improving uptake. This would reduce the confusion experienced with the current email system and allow women to undertake dietary recalls as frequently as they choose to; furthermore, personal accounts could be used to promote self-monitoring during the pregnancy and beyond.

The findings highlight the importance of tailoring tools to the needs of population, illustrated here by the importance of real-time tracking for women with GDM and need for integration of dietary intake with other data; here for blood glucose, but other conditions would benefit from recording other health information (e.g., weight, other blood test results, blood pressure, activity data). Continued development by the myfood24 consortium and website developers, taking into account suggestions for further improvements from this and other studies [6] will enhance the usability further.

4.4. *Opportunities for Use of myfood24 in a Clinical Setting*

This study has established that it is feasible to use myfood24 as an electronic food record in the GDM population, and provides helpful insights into how to optimise its use in this population. There could be significant benefits of introducing myfood24 in this clinical setting. Diabetes ante-natal care includes frequent follow up at lengthy multi-professional clinic appointments and by telephone. Therefore, health apps have been developed specifically for GDM to enable health professionals to manage case-loads using remote monitoring of blood glucose levels [31]. Online food diaries could be used to share data in the same way, and these could be beneficial for a number of reasons. In diabetes care, such tools have been shown to be a more engaging and accurate way of capturing a dietary assessment [5,16] and are preferred to traditional methods [32]. Women in our study commented that they began to consider changes in their food intake from performing the recalls and receiving the feedback; this has been observed in other populations [15,17], and has been shown to improve the uptake of self-monitoring and lead to dietary changes [33]. Following initial education, women could continue to monitor their dietary intake and receive feedback from the website which could result in increased self-efficacy and self-management skills. Additionally, as demonstrated in other studies, remote monitoring and provision of feedback by the health care professional could reduce workload during clinics and enhance service provision by freeing up time for education and support [12,34]. In other chronic conditions, use of dietary assessment technologies in this way has had a beneficial effect on clinical outcomes [16,35].

The interviews highlighted the emotional aspects of living with GDM, and the breadth of behaviours that women with GDM are tasked with managing (reported in full elsewhere: [36], in preparation) indicating that if myfood24 were to be optimised for mobile devices, there would likely be other beneficial components that may support women with GDM. From diagnosis of GDM, women are expected to begin to make immediate changes to their lifestyle to meet the blood glucose target recommendations. However, there will be a wide range of levels of knowledge, skills and confidence around healthy eating. From women's feedback provided in interview, it appears that myfood24 has the potential to improve the health literacy and eating behaviours of women with GDM. This is something that would require further testing. Reducing dependence on the health care professional to advise on dietary changes, and increasing knowledge and skills, has been shown to increase an individual's sense of control. Receiving prompts as cues for action and receiving feedback on their nutritional intake alongside biofeedback through blood glucose levels are recognised behaviour change techniques that can support healthy behaviours [37]. This increased level of control over their condition and perceived treatment efficacy may additionally help to reduce the levels of distress experienced [38,39].

4.5. Strengths and Limitations of the Study

There are several strengths to this study. There was a large study population, which provided a complete data set on 73 women. The qualitative element of the study provided valuable insight into the trial of the tool in everyday life, adding depth that has been reported as lacking in other studies of this type [6].

Limitations arose from the data collection methods in the study. The user questionnaire provided valuable information on the demographics and technological skills of the women, but it was only collected from 37% of the study population. In hindsight, if this had been completed at baseline, without the SUS, this would have provided significantly more information about the women who did not respond at the different stages of the study. Furthermore, there was a lack of evaluation built into the study to routinely establish reasons for their not using myfood24 even once. This could in part reflect the methods for accessing myfood24 (i.e., through automated emails), or challenges with usability. However, other reasons should have been considered such as how the tool was introduced to women. Increasing individuals' understanding of the benefits of using myfood24, such as those highlighted in this study around accuracy and the receiving of feedback, could be important for increasing uptake, and should be built into future interventions. Additionally, it was not established how much of an impact being in the late stages of a clinical complex pregnancy affected uptake.

Another significant weakness was the lack of representativeness of the data. This included a lack of ethnic diversity, which diminished with each stage of the research. A smaller proportion of women from black and minority ethnic (BME) groups completed the user questionnaire and took part in the interviews, limiting transferability of the study findings. As GDM is more prevalent in women from BME groups, this is not representative of a typical GDM population in the UK [40], and the barriers and facilitators for using myfood24 in BME groups needs to be explored in future studies. Over-represented in the group who completed the user questionnaire were women who were well educated and who worked in professional jobs. Based on those completing the questionnaire, the study population appeared to be confident in using technology and had good access to the internet, as well as previous experience with similar technologies. Again, this limits the conclusions that can be drawn from the results.

Finally, once women had begun to use myfood24 they may have been willing to continue to use it throughout the pregnancy; however the system did not allow them to continue to access myfood24 beyond their five records. The opportunity for continued use would have provided valuable further insights into its use by participants with a health condition [16].

This study has generated a number of suggestions for the future development of myfood24 for clinical populations. Real-time data entry assisted by a phone app format, could improve acceptability and usability. Adding further features such as improving the presentation and content of the feedback, and tracking pertinent biomedical data alongside nutritional information, would increase its potential beyond dietary assessment, and are ready for testing in the context of self-management of health conditions. The feasibility of its application within the health service should be explored in a feasibility study that also captures the views of users and health professionals on its use as an alternative tool in dietetic care. Ultimately a definitive trial considering the clinical and cost-effectiveness of a refined myfood24 tool in clinical practice is recommended.

5. Conclusions

This study has demonstrated that it is feasible to use myfood24, an online 24 h dietary recall tool developed for nutritional epidemiology studies, as an electronic food record in women with GDM. Usability of the software was assessed as good by a subgroup of the women. However, a higher response rate could have potentially been possible with a more diversely representative sample; therefore, the barriers against achieving this should be explored in future research.

The findings have generated a number of suggestions to improve acceptance and to enhance the usability of such tools in clinical populations. Women were motivated to use the tool, largely due to the feedback on their nutritional intake it provided, although being able to record food intake and input clinical data (blood glucose levels) in real time using mobile-optimised technology was deemed necessary to be able to replace paper-based diaries. Issues arose from employing the tool in a different context to the one in which it had been designed for, causing practical problems which need to be addressed.

Following improvements to the tool, suggested in this study and from other research findings, myfood24 should then be further evaluated within a healthcare setting, exploring its use as a dietary management tool to enhance behaviour change.

Author Contributions: Conceptualization, N.A.A. and J.E.C.; Data curation, Z.D., M.A.M. and E.M.S.; Formal analysis, C.G., Z.D., N.A.A., R.H., L.M.G. and D.M.S.; Funding acquisition, S.A. and J.E.C.; Investigation, Z.D., M.C., M.A.M. and E.M.S.; Methodology, S.A., N.A.A. and M.A.M.; Project administration, M.C. and M.A.M.; Supervision, J.E.C.; Writing—original draft, C.G. and Z.D.; Writing—review & editing, C.G., Z.D., S.A., N.A.A., M.C., R.H., L.M.G., M.A.M., E.M.S., D.M.S. and J.E.C. All authors reviewed and approved the final version of the manuscript.

Acknowledgments: This study was funded by the Medical Research Council (ref: G1100235) and supported by the National Institute of Health Research Clinical Research Network (NIHR CRN). Research was conducted by the University of Leeds in collaboration with Leeds Teaching Hospitals NHS Trust. The qualitative data collection and transcription was supported by pump priming funds awarded by the University of Leeds School of Healthcare Research Pump Priming Fund. Funds for open access publishing were provided through the project being funded by the MRC. JC, MC, MAM and the development of myfood24 was funded by the Medical Research Council (GB) grant MRC G1100235. We acknowledge: Neil Hancock and Helen Brown for their database support for this project; Del Endersby for recruiting patients; Jayne Hutchinson for her work and advice with the data analysis and; the myfood24 consortium for contributions to development of myfood24.

References

1. NICE. *Diabetes in Pregnancy: Management from Preconception to the Postnatal Period*; NICE Guidelines [NG3]; NICE: London, UK, 2015.
2. Farrar, D.; Simmonds, M.; Bryant, M.; Sheldon, T.A.; Tuffnell, D.; Golder, S.; Lawlor, D.A. Treatments for gestational diabetes: A systematic review and meta-analysis. *BMJ Open* **2017**, *7*, e015557. [CrossRef] [PubMed]
3. Noctor, E.; Dunne, F. A practical guide to pregnancy complicated by diabetes. *Diabetes Prim. Care* **2014**, *16*, 146–153.
4. Bingham, S.; Gill, C.; Welch, A.; Day, K.; Cassidy, A.; Khaw, K.T.; Sneyd, M.J.; Key, T.J.; Roe, L.; Day, N.E. Comparison of dietary assessment methods in nutritional epidemiology: Weighed records v. 24 h recalls, food-frequency questionnaires and estimated-diet records. *Br. J. Nutr.* **1997**, *72*, 619–643. [CrossRef]

5. Illner, A.-K.; Freisling, H.; Boeing, H.; Huybrechts, I.; Crispim, S.P.; Slimani, N. Review and evaluation of innovative technologies for measuring diet in nutritional epidemiology. *Int. J. Epidemiol.* **2012**, *41*, 1187–1203. [CrossRef] [PubMed]
6. Timon, C.M.; van den Barg, R.; Blain, R.J.; Kehoe, L.; Evans, K.; Walton, J.; Flynn, A.; Gibney, E.R. A review of the design and validation of web- and computer-based 24-h dietary recall tools. *Nutr. Res. Rev.* **2016**, *29*, 268–280. [CrossRef] [PubMed]
7. Sharp, D.B.; Allman-Farinelli, M. Feasibility and validity of mobile phones to assess dietary intake. *Nutrition* **2014**, *30*, 1257–1266. [CrossRef] [PubMed]
8. Rusin, M.; Arsand, E.; Hartvigsen, G. Functionalities and input methods for recording food intake: A systematic review. *Int. J. Med. Inform.* **2013**, *82*, 653–664. [CrossRef] [PubMed]
9. Long, J.D.; Littlefield, L.A.; Estep, G.; Martin, H.; Rogers, T.J.; Boswell, C.; Shriver, B.J.; Roman-Shriver, C.R. Evidence Review of Technology and Dietary Assessment. *Worldviews Evid. Based Nurs.* **2010**, *7*, 191–204. [CrossRef] [PubMed]
10. Foster, E.; Hawkins, A.; Delve, J.; Adamson, A.J. Reducing the cost of dietary assessment: Self-completed recall and analysis of nutrtion for use with children (SCRAN24). *J. Hum. Nutr. Diet.* **2014**, *27* (Suppl. 1), 26–35. [CrossRef]
11. Thompson, F.E.; Subar, A.F.; Loria, C.M.; Reedy, J.L.; Baranowski, T. Need for technological innovation in dietary assessment. *J. Am. Diet. Assoc.* **2010**, *110*, 48–51. [CrossRef] [PubMed]
12. Probst, Y.C.; Faraji, S.; Batterham, M.; Steel, D.G.; Tapsell, L.C. Computerized dietary assessments compare well with interviewer administered diet histories for patients with type 2 diabetes mellitus in the primary healthcare setting. *Patient Educ. Couns.* **2008**, *72*, 49–55. [CrossRef] [PubMed]
13. Touvier, M.; Kesse-Guyot, E.; Mejean, C.; Pollet, C.; Malon, A.; Castetbon, K. Comparison between an interactive web-based self-administered 24 h dietary record and an interview by a dietitian for large-scale epidemiological studies. *Br. J. Nutr.* **2011**, *105*, 1055–1064. [CrossRef] [PubMed]
14. Ngo, J.; Engelen, A.; Molag, M.; Roesle, J.; García-Segovia, P.; Serra-Majem, L. A review of the use of information and communication technologies for dietary assessment. *Br. J. Nutr.* **2009**, *101* (Suppl. 2), S102–S112. [CrossRef]
15. Porter, J.; Huggins, C.E.; Truby, H.; Collins, J. The Effect of Using Mobile Technology-Based Methods That Record Food or Nutrient Intake on Diabetes Control and Nutrition Outcomes: A Systematic Review. *Nutrients* **2016**, *8*, 815. [CrossRef] [PubMed]
16. Campbell, J.; Porter, J. Dietary mobile apps and their effect on nutritional indicators in chronic renal disease: A systematic review. *Nephrology* **2015**, *20*, 744–751. [CrossRef] [PubMed]
17. Bonilla, C.; Brauer, P.; Royall, D.; Keller, H.; Hanning, R.M.; Dicenso, A. Use of electronic dietary assessment tools in primary care: An interdisciplinary perspective. *BMC Med. Inform. Decis. Mak.* **2015**, *15*, 14. [CrossRef] [PubMed]
18. Ashman, A.M.; Collins, C.E.; Brown, L.J.; Rae, K.M.; Rollo, M.E. Validation of a Smartphone Image-Based Dietary Assessment Method for Pregnant Women. *Nutrients* **2017**, *9*, E73. [CrossRef] [PubMed]
19. Carter, M.C.; Albar, S.A.; Morris, M.A.; Mulla, U.Z.; Hancock, N.; Evans, C.E.; Alwan, N.A.; Greenwood, D.C.; Hardie, L.J.; Frost, G.S.; et al. Development of a UK Online 24-h Dietary Assessment Tool: Myfood24. *Nutrients* **2015**, *7*, 4016–4032. [CrossRef] [PubMed]
20. Albar, S.A.; Carter, M.C.; Alwan, N.A.; Evans, C.E.L.; Cade, J.E. Formative evaluation of the usability and acceptability of myfood24 among adolescents: A UK online dietary assessments tool. *BMC Nutr.* **2015**, *1*, 29. [CrossRef]
21. Albar, S.; Alwan, N.; Evans, C.; Greenwood, D.; Cade, J. Agreement between an online dietary assessment tool (myfood24) and an interview-administered 24-h dietary recall in British adolescents aged 11–18 years. *Br. J. Nutr.* **2016**, *115*, 1678–1686. [CrossRef] [PubMed]
22. Wark, P.; Hardie, L.; Frost, G.; Alwan, N.; Carter, M.; Elliott, P.; Ford, H.E.; Hancock, N.; Morris, M.A.; Mulla, U.Z.; et al. Validity of an online 24-hour recall tool (myfood24) for dietary assessment in population studies: Comparison with biomarkers and standard interviews. *BMC Med.* **2018**, *16*, 136. [CrossRef] [PubMed]
23. Virzi, R.A. Streamlining the Design Process: Running Fewer Subjects. Available online: http://journals.sagepub.com/doi/abs/10.1177/154193129003400411 (accessed on 22 August 2018).
24. Guest, G.; Bunce, A.; Johnson, J. How Many Interviews Are Enough?: An Experiment with Data Saturation and Variability. *Field Methods* **2006**, *18*, 59–82. [CrossRef]

25. Bristol Online Survey. Available online: https://www.onlinesurveys.ac.uk/ (accessed on 22 August 2018).
26. Brooke, J. SUS—A Quick and Dirty Usability Scale. Available online: https://hell.meiert.org/core/pdf/sus.pdf (accessed on 22 August 2018).
27. Bangor, A.; Kortum, P.T.; Miller, J.T. An empirical evaluation of the system usability scale. *Int. J. Hum. Comput. Interact.* **2008**, *24*, 574–594. [CrossRef]
28. Bangor, A.; Kortum, P.; Miller, J. Determining what individual SUS scores mean: Adding an adjective rating scale. *J. Usability Stud.* **2009**, *4*, 114–123.
29. Petrie, H.; Bevan, N. *The Evaluation of Acceptability, Usability and User Experience*; The Universal Access Handbook; CRC Press: Boca Raton, FL, USA, 2009; pp. 10–20.
30. Braun, V.; Clarke, V. Using thematic analysis in psychology. *Qual. Res. Psychol.* **2006**, *3*, 77–101. [CrossRef]
31. NICE. Health App: GDm-Health for People with Gestational Diabetes. Available online: https://www.nice.org.uk/advice/mib131/chapter/The-technology#current-care-pathway (accessed on 22 April 2018).
32. Rollo, M.E.; Ash, S.; Lyons-Wall, P.; Russell, A.W. Evaluation of a Mobile Phone Image-Based Dietary Assessment Method in Adults with Type 2 Diabetes. *Nutrients* **2015**, *7*, 4897–4910. [CrossRef] [PubMed]
33. Lieffers, J.R.; Hanning, R.M. Dietary Assessment and Self-monitoring: With Nutrition Applications for Mobile Devices. *Can.J. Diet. Pract. Res.* **2012**, *73*, e253–e260. [CrossRef] [PubMed]
34. Probst, Y.C.; Tapsell, L.C. Computerised dietary assessment interviews: Health professionals and patients' opinions about web communications. *Nutr. Diet.* **2012**, *69*, 56–63. [CrossRef]
35. Carter, M.C.; Burley, V.; Nykjaer, C.; Cade, J. "My Meal Mate" (MMM): Validation of the diet measures captured on a smartphone application to facilitate weight loss. *Br. J. Nutr.* **2013**, *109*, 539–546. [CrossRef] [PubMed]
36. Darwin, Z.; Smith, D.; Haddrill, R.; Scott, E.; McGowan, L.; Cade, J. Women's experiences of pregnancy and the management of gestational diabetes: A qualitative interview study. *BMC Pregnancy Childbirth* **2018**. submitted.
37. Michie, S.; Ashford, S.; Sniehotta, F.F.; Dombrowski, S.U.; Bishop, A.; French, D.P. A refined taxonomy of behaviour change techniques to help people change their physical activity and healthy eating behaviours: The CALO-RE taxonomy. *Psychol. Health* **2011**, *26*, 1479–1498. [CrossRef] [PubMed]
38. Sturt, J.; Dennick, K.; Hessler, D.; Hunter, B.M.; Oliver, J.; Fisher, L. Effective interventions for reducing diabetes distress; systematic review and metaanlysis. *Int. Diabetes Nurs.* **2015**, *12*, 40–55. [CrossRef]
39. Fisher, L.; Hessler, D.; Glasgow, R.E.; Arean, P.A.; Masharani, U.; Naranjo, D.; Strycker, L.A. REDEEM: A pragmatic trial to reduce diabetes distress. *Diabetes Care* **2013**, *36*, 2551–2558. [CrossRef] [PubMed]
40. Jenum, A.K.; Mørkrid, K.; Sletner, L.; Vangen, S.; Vange, S.; Torper, J.L.; Nakstad, B.; Voldner, N.; Rognerud-Jensen, O.H.; Berntsen, S.; et al. Impact of ethnicity on gestational diabetes identified with the WHO and the modified International Association of Diabetes and Pregnancy Study Groups criteria: A population-based cohort study. *Eur. J. Endocrinol.* **2012**, *166*, 317–324. [CrossRef] [PubMed]

3

Dietary Intake and Beliefs of Pregnant Women with Gestational Diabetes in Cape Town, South Africa

Stephanie M. Krige [1], Sharmilah Booley [1], Naomi S. Levitt [2,3], Tawanda Chivese [3,4,5], Katherine Murphy [3] and Janetta Harbron [1,*]

1 Division of Human Nutrition, Department of Human Biology, Faculty of Health Sciences, University of Cape Town, Cape Town 7925, South Africa; stephkrige@hotmail.com (S.M.K.); Sharmilah.booley@uct.ac.za (S.B.)
2 Division of Diabetes and Endocrinology, Department of Medicine, Faculty of Health Sciences, University of Cape Town, Cape Town 7925, South Africa; naomi.levitt@uct.ac.za
3 Chronic Disease Initiative for Africa, Department of Medicine, Faculty of Health Sciences, University of Cape Town, Cape Town 7925, South Africa; tchivese@gmail.com (T.C.); katherine.murphy@uct.ac.za (K.M.)
4 MRC/Wits Developmental Pathways for Health Research Unit, Department of Paediatrics, Faculty of Medicine and Health Sciences, University of the Witwatersrand, Johannesburg 2000, South Africa
5 Biostats Unit, Division of Epidemiology and Biostatistics, Faculty of Medicine and Health Sciences, Stellenbosch University, Cape Town 7599, South Africa
* Correspondence: janetta.harbron@uct.ac.za

Abstract: This study investigated the dietary intake of pregnant women with gestational diabetes mellitus (GDM) and their beliefs relating to the consumption of fruits and vegetables (F&V) and sugary foods and drinks. A cross-sectional study was conducted on 239 pregnant women with GDM in Cape Town. Dietary intake was assessed using a quantified Food Frequency Questionnaire and beliefs relating to food choices were assessed using the Theory of Planned Behaviour (TPB). The mean energy intake was 7268 KJ, carbohydrate was 220 (±104.5) g, protein 60.3 (±27.5) g and fat 67.7 (±44.2) g. The macronutrient distribution was 55% carbohydrates, 14.5% protein and 30.5% fat of total energy. The majority of the sample had inadequate intakes of vitamin D (87.4%), folate (96.5%) and iron (91.3%). The median (IQR) amount of added table sugar and sugar sweetened beverages (SSBs) was 4.0 (0.00–12.5) g and 17.9 (0.0–132.8) mL per day, respectively. Only 31.4% met the recommendation (400 g per day) for F&V. Beliefs that it was not easy to exclude sugary foods/drinks and that knowing how to control cravings for sugary foods/drinks are areas to target messages on the sugar content of SSBs. In conclusion, the dietary intake of these women was not optimal and fell short of several nutritional guidelines for pregnant women with hyperglycaemia. The strongly held beliefs regarding sugary foods/drinks may contribute to poor adherence to nutritional guidelines among pregnant women with GDM in South Africa.

Keywords: hyperglycaemia first detected in pregnancy; gestational diabetes; GDM; dietary intake; beliefs; SSBs; fruits and vegetables; sugar intake; pregnancy nutrition

1. Introduction

Pregnancies complicated by hyperglycaemia are classified as pre-existing diabetes or hyperglycaemia first detected in pregnancy, which includes both gestational diabetes mellitus (GDM) and overt diabetes [1,2]. The prevalence of hyperglycaemia in pregnancy has been increasing worldwide. The estimated global prevalence is 16.2%, with the vast majority being due to GDM diagnosed in women living in low and middle-income countries [3]. Mwanri et al. [4] reported an increase in the prevalence of hyperglycaemia first detected in pregnancy in sub-Saharan Africa over the last 50 years. Recently, the prevalence of GDM in South Africa was estimated to be as high as 25.6% using the International Association of the Diabetes and Pregnancy Study Groups (IADPSG) diagnostic criteria [5]. The rise in number of women with hyperglycaemia in pregnancy is likely to be due to changes in lifestyle associated with urbanisation, including a Western style diet and sedentary lifestyle, which lead to overweight and obesity [6].

While there is no international consensus over the diagnostic criteria for GDM, it is well established that uncontrolled diabetes during pregnancy poses numerous risks for the mother and foetus [1,5]. The Hyperglycaemia and Adverse Pregnancy Outcome (HAPO) study [7] found that, outside of overt diabetes, there was an association between increasing blood glucose levels and a number of adverse pregnancy and birth outcomes such as birth weight above the 90th percentile, shoulder dystocia, neonatal hypoglycaemia, hyperbilirubinemia, preeclampsia and caesarean delivery. Although GDM usually resolves after child birth [8], it is associated with long-term health risks to the mother including postnatal depression, weight retention [9], GDM in future pregnancies and Type 2 Diabetes Mellitus in later life [10–13]. The consequences for the infant place them at risk of adiposity, impaired glucose tolerance and cardiovascular health problems in adulthood [9].

Optimal control of glycaemia is the key focus of treatment for women with GDM. Currently, guidelines for pregnant women with diabetes recommend initial diet and lifestyle intervention followed by oral hypoglycaemic agents and insulin, if diet alone does not achieve glycaemic targets [1,14,15]. After pregnancy, continuation of these healthy lifestyle practices is recommended for weight loss and reduced long-term health risks. While different associations have proposed dietary guidelines for women with hyperglycaemia in pregnancy, there is a lack of consensus on the recommended macronutrient distribution as summarized in Table 1.

Recent Cochrane reviews reported that dietary interventions have proven successful in: reducing the incidence of GDM and marginally lower fasting blood glucose levels at 32 to 36 weeks in pregnant women [9], meeting postpartum weight goals, decreasing postpartum depression and reducing the incidence of large-for-gestational age (LGA) and neonatal fat mass in pregnant women with GDM [16]. These dietary interventions have included a focus on macronutrient distribution [17], the promotion of a Mediterranean diet [18], a low glycaemic index (GI) diet [19] and increasing dietary fibre [20].

A few studies have investigated the diet of pregnant South African women [21–29]. These studies have reported high percentage of women with inadequate dietary intakes of key micronutrients such as iron, folate, vitamin A, vitamin C, calcium and zinc [22,23,26,28,29] as well as low intakes of fruits and vegetables (F&V) [26,28]. No studies to date could be traced that have investigated the diet of pregnant women with diabetes in Africa or South Africa. It is thus unknown whether they meet dietary guidelines and goals as proposed by various organizations for a healthy pregnancy and for optimal glucose control. In addition, investigating the underlying beliefs that shape dietary intake behaviours is needed to plan effective nutrition education programmes that promote lifestyle changes [30]. The primary aim of the current study was to investigate the dietary intake of pregnant women with GDM in Cape Town, South Africa and whether they adhere to established dietary recommendations in order to determine the dietary inputs needed in this population. The secondary aims of the study sought to investigate their beliefs related to sugary foods and drinks and F&V intake and the association between sociodemographic factors and dietary intake.

Table 1. Dietary recommendation in Gestational Diabetes from different associations.

Macronutrients	SEMDSA (2017) [1]	ADA (2007) [31]	Fourth International Workshop-Conference on Gestational Diabetes Mellitus, 1998 [32]	CDA (2006) [33]	FAO *(2002)/IOM * [34]
Energy		1500–2800/day +340 kcal 2nd trimester +452 kcal 3rd trimester	25 kcal/kg body weight		+85 kcal 1st trimester +285 kcal 2nd trimester +475 kcal 3rd trimester

Table 1. *Cont.*

Macronutrients	SEMDSA (2017) [1]	ADA (2007) [31]	Fourth International Workshop-Conference on Gestational Diabetes Mellitus, 1998 [32]	CDA (2006) [33]	FAO *(2002)/IOM * [34]
Carbohydrates	40% carbohydrate (complex, low-glycaemic index, high fibre)		35–45% of total calories	45–50% TE	45–65% TE At least 175 g/day
Added sugars	<5% total energy			<10%	<25% TE
Protein	20% protein		protein 20–25%		10–25% At least 71 g/day
Total Fats	40% fat (at least 50% unsaturated)		fat 35–40%	Up to 40% TE	20–35% TE

SEMDSA, Society for Endocrinology, Metabolism and Diabetes of South Africa; ADA, American Diabetes Association; CDA, Canadian Diabetes Association; FAO, Food and Agricultural Association; IOM, Institute of Medicine. * Recommendations for normal pregnancy.

2. Materials and Methods

2.1. Study Design and Participants

A cross-sectional study design with an analytical component was used. The target population was pregnant women with hyperglycaemia first diagnosed in pregnancy attending Groote Schuur Hospital (GSH) or Mowbray Maternity Hospital (MMH) in Cape Town, South Africa. GSH is a tertiary referral hospital for high risk pregnancies while MMH is a secondary hospital for lower risk pregnancies. Participants were included if they were in the third trimester, thus ≥28 weeks' gestational age and were screened for hyperglycaemia between 24–28 weeks gestational age and diagnosed by the hospital's medical doctors with hyperglycaemia for the first time during the current pregnancy.

Many international organisations have adopted the IADPSG guidelines [35] as described by the World Health Organisation (WHO) for the diagnosis of hyperglycaemia first detected in pregnancy as GDM, when fasting glucose is ≥5.1–6.9 mmol/L, 1 h ≥ 10.0 mmol/L or 2 h ≥ 8.5–11.0 mmol/L or overt diabetes when fasting glucose ≥ 7.0 mmol/L or 2 h ≥ 11.1 mmol/L [2,36]. Both GDM and overt diabetes are first recognized during pregnancy, however in overt diabetes the diagnostic criteria for diabetes in non-pregnant adults are met, while GDM is a lesser degree of hyperglycaemia that is not clearly overt diabetes and usually resolves after pregnancy [1,2]. Although SEMDSA [1] also recommends the use of the aforementioned criteria, the diagnostic criteria currently used at facility level in South Africa are not consistent and decided independently by each facility. In the Western Cape public health sector a different diagnostic criteria are used [5]. The diagnostic criteria used at GSH and MMH and therefore the inclusion criteria for the study were as follows: impaired glucose tolerance (IGT) (fasting blood glucose of 5.6–6.9 mmol/L and/or 2 h OGTT between 7.8–11.0 mmol/L) or GDM (fasting blood glucose ≥ 7.0 mmol/L and/or OGTT ≥ 11.1 mmol/L) and in line with the National Institute for Health and Care Excellence (NICE) guidelines for the diagnosis of GDM if fasting blood glucose is ≥5.6 mmol/L and/or 2 h OGTT ≥ 7.8 mmol/L [37]. As the term IGT is not used in the diagnostic criteria for pregnant women according to IADPSG, WHO, NICE and other associations and all women in our study would be classified as GDM according to the NICE diagnostic criteria we refer to the study participants as women with GDM.

Women were excluded if they were younger than 18 years, had a multiple pregnancy or were diagnosed with T1DM or T2DM before the onset of this pregnancy. Treatment received in the form of pharmacotherapy, dietary and exercise guidelines or any other were not an exclusion criterion as it was difficult to establish the amount and type of exposure received in this population. The dietary and exercise recommendations that women with hyperglycaemia in pregnancy receive in the public health sector of South Africa are not standardized across facilities and provinces. In Cape Town patients could be referred to the dietitian on diagnosis of hyperglycaemia in pregnancy, however no standardized criteria for referrals exists. Patients are either seen on the day of diagnoses or scheduled an appointment in 1–2 weeks as an outpatient depending on the availability of the dietitian.

An initial dietetic consultation is about 30 min and usually involves taking a diet history and providing recommendations to improve current dietary intake according to SEMDSA and the latest South African Food Based Dietary Guidelines [1,38]. Energy requirements, personalized meal plans, menus and diet exchanges are not calculated. The limited time for consultations and dietary inputs are due to the high number of patients requiring dietetic consultations together with the small number of dietitians employed in the public health sector. By 28 weeks, patients may or may not have seen a dietitian, it is not standard practice. Patients could also have been exposed to group nutrition talks as inpatients or as an outpatient, in the waiting room by a midwife on healthy eating during gestational diabetes pregnancy. Exercise recommendations are mostly not provided but in interspersed instances could be given if a biokineticist, physiotherapist or student interns are at the health care facilities.

2.2. Sample Size and Recruitment

According to Mostert et al. [28], in 2005, 23.9 to 26.1% of South African pregnant women had inadequate intakes of various macronutrients. Using this proportion (26.1%), a 99% confidence interval and 7.5% level of significance from an unlimited population size, a sample size of 228 was calculated using OpenEpi.

A sample of $n = 239$ pregnant women with GDM were recruited from antenatal clinics at GSH and MMH as well as in-patients at GSH using a consecutive sampling technique. The files of all patients attending the diabetic antennal clinic and the files of patients admitted in the ward were screened by fieldworkers. Patients that fitted the inclusion criteria, were provided with information on the study both verbally and by means of a written information sheet and were invited to participate in the study. At MMH and GSH, a private room was allocated for interviews to take place. Inpatients were interviewed at their bedside.

The study was approved by the University of Cape Town, Faculty of Health Sciences, Human Research Ethics Committee (HREC REF 229/2015 and 230/2015), participation was voluntary and each participant signed an informed consent form.

2.3. Questionnaire Development

An interview-administered questionnaire was developed for this study. The different sections were developed and reviewed by an expert panel of four dietitians to confirm the appropriateness of questions, coverage of core concepts and the level and comprehensibility of the questions. This ensured construct and content validity. A draft questionnaire was developed and reviewed several times before its finalization. It was then pilot tested on five people from the relevant population to check whether there was any difficulty in answering the questions and revised accordingly. All field workers were trained and standardised in the administration of the questionnaire. The completion of one questionnaire took forty to fifty minutes.

2.3.1. Demographics and Disease Related History

Sociodemographic and obstetric history data included age, race, gestational age, number of pregnancies, previous GDM and number of living children. Self-rated questions on current physical activity level and food choices were reported as well as interest in being part of a wellness program for GDM.

2.3.2. Socioeconomic Status

Socioeconomic status was assessed using the Living Standard Measurement (LSM) which was developed by the South African Advertising Research Foundation (SAARF) [39]. The LSM is a wealth measure segmentation tool to profile the South African consumer market and has been used in many different studies [40,41]. The questionnaire includes a list of 29 household items and respondents select all items they own. Each item on the LSM list has a weightage score. From the combination of household items in ownership by a participant, a LSM score is calculated using the LSM calculator [39]. Ten wealth groups have been identified based on the participants' socioeconomic status from the lowest (LSM 1) to the highest (LSM 10) [42]. The LSM gives an indication of the food cash expenditure of the participant which can be as high as 70% of their total cash expenditure, in LSM categories 1 to 3, to as low as 5% of total cash expenditure in the wealthiest consumers [40].

2.3.3. Dietary Intake Assessment

For the purpose of this study, a picture-sort [43] quantified Food Frequency Questionnaire (qFFQ) was developed to assess the usual dietary intake of the study participants after their diagnosis of GDM. The food list was compiled by an expert panel of registered dietitians using existing qFFQs that were used to assess dietary intake of educators from low socio-economic areas in the Western Cape [44] and pregnant women in Soweto, Johannesburg, [45] as well as the FFQ proposed in the Dietary Assessment and Education Kit (DAEK) [46] which was developed from extensive research to enable researchers to have a resource that was adapted to the local South African diet and available foodstuff. The FFQ included 103 food items, with some items having sub-item categories (see Supplementary file). In order to increase respondent accuracy in recalling foods consumed during the administration of the questionnaire, each food item on the FFQ list was represented by the appropriate visual card developed for the DAEK by Steyn and Senekal [46]. Study participants sorted the picture cards into 2 stacks according to foods they did and those they did not consume within the last two weeks. Using the cards from the stack of food items consumed over the last two weeks, the respondents were asked, to recall their portion size and their frequency of intake over the last two weeks. A small booklet derived from the DAEK manual, representing different portion sizes, was used to assist with portion sizes estimation. For data analyses, the household portion was converted into grams using the DAEK and then multiplied by the frequency of intake in the last two weeks and converted to daily intake. Each food item consumed on the FFQ was coded and the daily intake of energy, macro- and micronutrients were calculated for each participant using the South African food composition tables [47]. Participants who had an implausible daily energy intake of <2092 KJ (500 kcal) or >20,920 KJ (5000 kcal) [48] were excluded from data analyses (n = 9). In order to determine the adequacy of dietary intake the daily intake of protein (in grams), carbohydrates (in grams), fibre (in grams), vitamins and minerals was compared to the DRIs for pregnant women as established by the Institute of Medicine [34]. Proteins, carbohydrates and fats were computed as a percentage of total energy (TE) intake and categorized to reflect the percentage of women in our sample that consumed according to the macronutrient distribution recommendations of different international guidelines as summarized in Table 1. For instance, fat was categorized as % participants that consumed <30%, 30–34.9%, 35–40% and >40% of TE; protein was categorized as <10%, 10–15%, 15.01–20% and >20% of TE while carbohydrates were categorized as <40%, 40–44.9%, 45–50% and >50% of TE.

The daily intake of teaspoons of sugar was calculated for each participant by adding the total number of level teaspoons of sugar added to tea/coffee and used in porridge or vegetables. The daily intake of SSBs were calculated by adding the intake of squashes, fruit juice, carbonated beverages and sweetened milk drinks in millilitres. F&V intake was calculated by summing the grams of all vegetables (excluding potato which is high in carbohydrates) and all fruits (excluding avocado pear which is high in fat) eaten per day and were compared to the WHO recommendation of 400 g per day [21]. SSBs were compared to 0 mL as recommended by SEMDSA [1] and added table sugar to 0 g based on recommendation by WHO for total sugars added to foods to be <5% total energy [49]. This 5% could account for sugar added in food products such as tomato sauce, cereals and canned foods, thus recommending no added table sugar.

2.3.4. Beliefs

The theory of planned behaviour (TPB) was used in order to understand what motivates behaviour change so as to help women with GDM adopt a healthier lifestyle. The TPB suggests that intention is the immediate precursor of behaviour [50]. Further the TPB states that intention is predicted by an individual's attitude, subjective norms (the perceived social pressure to perform or not perform the behaviour) and perceived behavioural control (the perception of ease or difficulty of the particular behaviour), while each of these predictor constructs are determined or underlined by behavioural beliefs (about the consequences of performing the specific behaviour), normative beliefs (about the support/no support of specific referents of performing the specific behaviour) and control beliefs (about barriers or facilitators of the performing the specific behaviour), respectively. These beliefs are unique to each behaviour and target population [51]. It provides in-depth understanding of the behaviour within the specific population and context. To change an individual's intention and behaviour with regards to a specific behaviour, these elicited beliefs need to be addressed/or challenged in intervention (or communication).

To develop the belief statements for inclusion in our study questionnaire we followed the TPB questionnaire development guidelines outlined by Francis et al. [52]. Hence, a formative qualitative study using in depth interviews with 50 women with GDM at MMH and GSH was conducted (results not reported in this article). This was done to elicit the salient behavioural, normative and control beliefs (most commonly held beliefs that is, those that first come to mind), in relation to specific dietary behaviours (sugary foods and drinks and F&V) of the target population. The most frequent salient beliefs were identified using a process recommended by Krueger and Casey [53] for managing qualitative data and converted into incomplete sentences with bipolar endpoints (agree vs. disagree) for inclusion in our study questionnaire. By completing the sentence, the participant expresses a positive or negative evaluation of the belief statement [52]. The bipolar endpoints were expressed as a 7-point Likert scale namely, 1 = strongly disagree, 2 = disagree, 3 = disagree somewhat, 4 = neither agree nor disagree, 5 = agree somewhat, 6 = agree, 7 = strongly agree. Using the Likert scale allows the evaluation of the strength of the belief within the target population by calculating the mode of each belief.

2.4. Data Analyses

STATISTICA version 13.3 [54] and STATA 15 [55] were used to clean and analyse the data. The data were tested for normality using Shapiro Wilks tests ($p > 0.05$ = normal). Data with a normal distribution were described using means and standard deviations (SD). Medians and inter-quartile ranges (IQR) were used for data with a non-normal distribution. For ease of comparison to other studies [21–29], both median(IQR) and mean(SD) were recorded for dietary intake of energy, macronutrients and micronutrients. Categorical data were described using frequencies and percentages. Belief statements were expressed using mode values. Spearmen correlation co-efficient and their p-values were computed to test associations between beliefs and the food group intakes. Univariate logistic regression analyses were done to explore the associations between sociodemographic factors and health related perceptions with selected dietary variables (macronutrients as a percentage of TE as well as sugar, SSBs and F&V intake). To create dichotomous dietary variables to divide the group in those who met and did not met a dietary recommendation, the following cut-points were used: sugar 0 g, SSBs 0 mL and total F&V 400 g per day. Practical cut-points for macronutrient intake as a % of TE were used namely: 45% for carbohydrates, 15% for protein and 35% for fats. Variables with p-values < 0.1 at univariate analysis, were included in a forward stepwise multivariate logistic regression. If the food group had no variables that were significant at $p < 0.1$, no multivariate regression was carried out. Variables were manually added to the logistic regression, with the binary outcome of reaching recommended intake (yes/no) for each of the major food groups. Variables tested for association were socio-demographic variables, GA, perception of food choices and physical activity, self-reported reproductive health and the hospital they were treated in. A p-value of <0.05 was considered significant and 95% confidence intervals (CIs) were reported for all odds ratios (ORs).

3. Results

3.1. Socio-Demographic History and Pregnancy History

The mean (SD) age of the women was 32.2 (5.3) years and the mean gestational age was 33.0 (3.4) weeks. Table 2 shows that just more than one-third of the women had an advanced maternal age of ≥35 years. The majority, (73.6%), of the participants was recruited from GSH. Half of the sample

(58.9%) was mixed-race ancestry, 34.7% were Black and the remaining 6.5% were either White or Indian. The majority of the sample had an LSM score between 6 and 9 and 64.4% reported that their food choices are 'mostly healthy.' Most participants (97.5%) were willing to participate in a wellness program should one be available and the preferred means of communication were evenly distributed between one-on-one, group sessions and social media (Table 2).

Table 2. Sociodemographic profile and pregnancy history of sample (n = 239).

Variable	Categories	n	Percentage of Total Sample n = 239 (%)
Recruitment hospital	GSH	176	73.6
	-MMH	63	26.4
Age	<35 years	154	64.4
	≥35 years	85	35.5
Gestational Age	<33 weeks	108	45.2
	≥33 weeks	131	54.8
Race	Black	83	34.7
	White	3	1.3
	Indian	6	2.5
	Mixed-race ancestry *	141	58.9
	Other	6	2.5
Living Standard Measurement	LSM ≤ 4	6	2.5
	LSM 5–7	95	39.8
	LSM 8–10	138	57.8
Number of children	0	55	23.0
	1	67	28.0
	2	68	28.4
	3–6	49	20.5
Parity	1st	39	16.3
	2nd	62	25.9
	3rd	78	32.6
	4th	35	14.6
	5th to 10th	25	10.6
GDM in previous pregnancy	Yes	50	20.9
	No	150	62.7
	N/a if 1st pregnancy	39	16.3
What do you think of the food choices you make most of the time? (4 or more times per week)	Most very healthy	9	3.7
	Mostly healthy	154	64.4
	Mostly unhealthy	66	27.6
	Mostly very unhealthy	10	4.1
If a wellness program was available for pregnant women, would you enrol?	Yes	233	97.5
	No	6	2.5
What is the preferred way in which you like to receive information on health and nutrition?	One-on-one	64	26.7
	Group session	71	29.7
	Print material	38	15.9
	Social media	60	25.1

GSH: Groote Schuur Hospital, MMH: Mowbray Maternity Hospital, LSM: living standards measure, GDM: gestational diabetes mellitus. * Mixed-race ancestry: this population group in South Africa are also referred to as the Cape Coloureds in Cape Town and has a mixed ancestry with genetic material mainly from Khoisan, Bantu African, Northern European, South Asia and South-East Asia origins.

3.2. Dietary Intake

The mean daily energy intake was 7268 KJ (Table 3). As for fibre intake, 80.9% consumed below the recommended 28 g/day. For the micronutrients, a high percentage of the sample had inadequate intakes of vitamin D (87.4%), folate (96.5%) and iron (91.3%), which are particularly important micronutrients in pregnancy.

Table 3. Mean and adequacy of macronutrients, vitamins and mineral intake per day by the sample (n = 230).

Energy and Nutrients	Mean (SD)	Median (IQR)	Guideline (Cut Point)	Percentage of Sample That Fell below Cut Point (%)
Total energy (KJ)	7268.0 (3527.5)	6437.9 (4863.3–8687.7)		
Protein (g) (%TE)	60.3 (27.5) 14.7 (3.4)	55.0 (41.4–70.8) 14.6 (12.5–16.9)	71 g/day [a*] 20% TE [b]	77.4 93.5
Total fat (g) (%TE)	67.7 (44.2) 33.1 (7.9)	58.2(38.8–82.1) 31.8 (28.0–37.9)	40% TE [b]	80.4
MUFA (g) (%TE)	23.9 (16.6) 11.0 (3.4)	19.9 (13.2–27.5) 10.6 (8.5–13.1)	≤20% TE [c]	97.8
PUFA (g) (%TE)	17.6 (14.6) 8.0 (3.8)	13.4 (8.5–21.4) 7.1 (5.7–9.7)	≤10% TE [c]	78.2
Saturated fat (g) (%TE)	20.1 (14.1) 9.8 (3.0)	17.2 (11.1–24.0) 9.6 (7.9–11.5)	<7% TE [c]	14.7
Cholesterol (g)	265.6 (243.2)	194.9 (121.3–310.1)	<200 mg [c]	52.1
Carbohydrates (g) (% TE)	220.0 (104.5) 53.0 (8.6)	197.4 (142.9–270.4) 53.6 (47.4–58.7)	135 g/day [a] 40% TE [b]	21.7 7.8
Fibre (g)	21.7 (11.3)	20.0 (14.8–26.4)	28 g [a]	80.9
Alcohol (g)	0.019 (0.2)	0.00 (0.00–0.00)		
		FAT SOLUBLE VITAMINS		
Vitamin A (mcg)	1058.2 (645.4)	877.3 (598.7–1396.5)	550 mcg/day [a]	20.4
Vitamin D (ug)	5.5 (5.1)	4.0 (2.4–6.6)	10 ug/day [a]	87.4
Vitamin E (mg)	13.4 (10.0)	10.9 (7.0–16.1)	12 mg/day [a]	60.0
		WATER SOLUBLE VITAMINS		
Thiamin (mg)	1.3 (0.7)	1.2 (0.9–1.6)	1.2 mg/day [a]	30.9
Riboflavin (mg)	2.0 (1.5)	1.5 (1.0–2.4)	1.2 mg/day [a]	25.2
Niacin (mg)	21.7 (11.4)	19.2 (14.9–26.9)	14 mg/day [a]	30.4
Vitamin B6 (mg)	2.9 (1.6)	2.7 (1.8–3.7)	1.6 mg/day [a]	6.5
Vitamin B12 (mcg)	4.5 (4.2)	3.1 (2.1–5.2)	2.2 mcg/day [a]	21.7
Pantothenate (mg)	4.5 (2.3)	4.0 (2.9–5.7)	6 mg/day [a]	80.0
Biotin (mcg)	34.7 (19.4)	30.9 (22.9–42.1)	30 mcg/day [a]	47.8
Folate (ug)	244.8 (149.8)	218.2 (154.2–291.5)	520 ug/day [a]	96.5
Vitamin C (mg)	97.4 (124.7)	61.5 (36.2–124.7)	70 mg/day [a]	56.5
		MINERALS		
Calcium (mg)	651.9 (402.7)	561.1 (379.2–789.7)	800 mg/day [a]	75.6
Iron (mg)	13.4 (8.0)	11.6 (9.0–15.7)	22 mg/day [a]	91.3
Magnesium (mg)	251.5 (128.3)	231.2 (177.8–296.2)	290 (19–30 y) 300 (31–50 y) mg/day [a]	74.3
Phosphorus (mg)	1005.8 (491.7)	902.7 (672.6–1198.1)	580 mg/day [a]	16.1
Potassium (g)	2038.2 (945.1)	1881.1 (1400.4–2376.7)	4.7 g/day [a]	98.3
Sodium (mg)	1741.5 (944.0)	1531.8 (1138.8–2079.2)	1500 mg/day [a]	48.3
Zinc (mg)	10.3 (4.5)	9.7 (7.3–12.2)	9.5 mg/day [a]	42.6
Copper (ug)	1.1 (0.6)	1.0 (0.7–1.3)	800 ug/day [a]	32.6
Manganese (mg)	2.2 (1.3)	1.9 (1.3–2.9)	2.0 mg/day [a]	53.9

* excludes dietary data< 2092 KJ and >20,920 KJ. Data was non-normally distributed, thus Median (IQR) applies. Mean (SD) was included to compared with results from previous studies. [a] EAR or AI (when EAR is not available), [a*] RDA (of the DRI) [56], [b] SEMDSA 2017 [1]. [c] TLC guidelines by National Heart, Lung and Blood Institute [57]. TE: total energy, MUFA: mono-unsaturated fatty acids, PUFA: poly-unsaturated fatty acids, EAR: estimated average requirements, AI: adequate intakes, DRIs: dietary reference intakes, TLC: Therapeutic Lifestyle Changes.

Table 4 shows the macronutrients as a percentage of total energy and sugar, SSBs and F&V intake. The median (IQR) amount of added sugar and SSBs was 4.0 g (0.00–12.5) and 17.9 mL (0.00–132.8) per day, respectively. A quarter (25.1%) consumed more than one small glass of SSBs per day, one third (33.5%) had more than two teaspoons of sugar per day and only 31.4% of the sample consumed the recommended 400 g or more of F&V daily.

Table 4. Breakdown of the macronutrient distribution of the sample and the percentage of participants' macronutrients intake as percent of total energy and intake of table sugar, sugar sweetened beverages (SSBs) and fruits and vegetables (F&V).

Macronutrients as a % of TE and Food Categories	Percentage of Total Group (n = 230) (%)
Carbohydrates (% Total energy)	
<40	7.8
40–44.9	12.1
45–50	13.9
>50	66.0
Protein (% Total energy)	
<10	7.4
10–15	47.8
15.1–20	38.3
>20	6.5
Fat (% Total energy)	
<30	35.2
30–34.9	25.2
35–40	20.0
>40	19.5
Teaspoons sugar *	
0 tsp	34.7
less than or equal 2 tsp	31.8
more than 2 tsp	33.5
SSBs (small glasses) **	
Up to $\frac{1}{2}$ small glass	63.6
$\frac{1}{2}$ to 1 small glass	11.3
More than 1 small glass	25.1
Fruits and Vegetables	
Less than 200 g	28.9
Between 200 g and 400 g	39.3
400 g and more	31.4

* level teaspoons sugar (5 g) added to tea/coffee, breakfast cereals/porridge ** 1 small glass = 125 mL.

3.3. Beliefs Relating to the Intake of Sugary Foods and Drinks and Fruits and Vegetables

For all the behavioural, control and normative belief statements relating to F&V intake the mode was 6 indicating that the participants agree with the statements (Table 5). Agreement with behavioural beliefs indicated that participants were aware of the health benefits of eating more F&V such as feeling better physically and assisting weight loss. Agreement with the normative beliefs shows that participants believed they had support from family or peers to consume more F&V. Agreement with the control beliefs indicated the participants' perceived ease/difficulty in consuming more F&V.

Beliefs relating to sugar intake had a mode of 6, except that participants disagree (mode = 2) with the statement that "low sugar/sugar-free foods taste good or are tasty," indicating a perceived difficulty to consuming low sugar/sugar-free foods.

Table 5. Beliefs associated with the intake of Fruits and Vegetables and Sugar.

Beliefs Related to Fruit and Vegetable	Belief Type	Mode	Frequency of Mode (%)	Correlation of Belief with F&V Intake * (rho, *p*-Value)	
Eating fruits and vegetables every day will make me feel better physically.	Behavioural	6.0	49.8	0.159 (0.017)	
Eating fruits and vegetables every day will help control my weight.	Behavioural	6.0	53.9	0.081 (0.2212)	
Eating less fruit will help control my blood sugar levels (i.e., to reduce the risk of diabetes).	Behavioural	6.0	37.6	−0.036 (0.582)	
Vegetables do not take a long time to prepare.	Control	6.0	34.3	0.019 (0.765)	
Fruits and vegetables are affordable.	Control	6.0	45.6	0.029 (0.661)	
Fruits and vegetables are easy to find in the stores/shops nearby.	Control	6.0	54.8	0.151 (0.022)	
I am confident that I can eat the recommended amount of fruits and vegetables every day.	Control	6.0	44.7	0.101 (0.124)	
Most people who are important to me eat fruits and vegetables every day.	Normative	6.0	38.9	0.052 (0.431)	
Beliefs related to sugar	**Belief type**	**Mode**	**Frequency of mode (%)**	**Correlation of belief with sugar intake * (rho, *p*-value)**	**Correlation of belief with SSB intake * (rho, *p*-value)**
Eating less sugary foods/snacks/drinks will help reduce the risk of diseases e.g., diabetes.	Behavioural	6.0	51.5	−0.184 (0.005)	−0.109 (0.098)
It is also important to limit my intake of sugary foods/snacks/drinks after the pregnancy.	Behavioural	6.0	60.7	−0.175 (0.007)	0.028 (0.672)
Decreasing the amount of sugary foods/snacks/drinks I eat will help control my weight.	Behavioural	6.0	54.0	−0.004 (0.945)	−0.064 (0.337)
Increasing the amount sugary foods/snacks/drinks I eat and drink make me feel unwell (tired, headache, dizzy, signs of hyper glycaemia, etc.).	Behavioural	6.0	44.4	−0.021 (0.743)	0.063 (0.335)
I want to reduce the amount of sugary foods/snacks/drinks I eat and drink to prevent pregnancy/birth complications.	Behavioural/Control	6.0	53.6	−0.055 (0.406)	−0.016 (0.805)
It is easy to exclude sugary foods/snacks/drinks from my daily diet.	Control	6.0	33.2	−0.259 (<0.001)	−0.246 (<0.001)

Table 5. *Cont.*

Beliefs Related to Fruit and Vegetable	Belief Type	Mode	Frequency of Mode (%)	Correlation of Belief with F&V Intake * (rho, p-Value)	
Foods/snacks/drinks that are low sugar/sugar free are easy to find in my surroundings.	Control	6.0	39.9	−0.022 (0.736)	−0.069 (0.292)
Eating/drinking less sugary foods/snacks/drinks is up to me.	Control	6.0	56.1	−0.149 (0.023)	−0.128 (0.052)
Knowing how to control my cravings for sugary foods/snacks/drinks during pregnancy will make it easier for me to eat less of these foods.	Control	6.0	54.6	−0.153 (0.021)	−0.152 (0.021)
Low sugar/sugar-free foods/snacks/drinks are expensive.	Control	6.0	42.3	0.011 (0.859)	−0.002 (0.975)
Low sugar/sugar-free foods taste good/are tasty.	Control	2.0	27.3	−0.271 (<0.001)	−0.129 (0.049)
People around me eat/serve sugary foods/snacks/drinks at most events/functions (social, religious, or work events)	Normative	6.0	46.9	−0.031 (0.641)	0.061 (0.356)

* Spearman Rank Order Correlation; Behavioural beliefs: are the perceived consequences (positive or negative) of the behaviour; Control beliefs: are factors that facilitate or hinder the behaviour; Normative beliefs: extent to which other people are important to them think they should or should not perform a certain behaviour [50].

There were significant positive correlations, albeit weak, between dietary intake of F&V and the beliefs that F&V make you feel better physically ($r = 0.16$, $p = 0.0176$) as well as F&V are easy to find in shops nearby ($r = 0.15$, $p = 0.0221$), (Table 5). Significant negative correlations were found between dietary intake of sugar or SSBs and the beliefs that it was easy to exclude sugary foods/snack/drinks in 'their' daily diet (sugar: $r = -0.259$, $p < 0.001$; SSBs: $r = -0.246$, $p < 0.001$), knowing how to control cravings would make it easier to eat less sugary foods/snacks/drinks (sugar $r = -0.153$ $p = 0.0205$; SSBs $r = -0.152$ $p = 0.0209$) and low sugar/sugar-free foods/snacks/drinks taste good (sugar $r = -0.271$ $p < 0.001$; SSBs $r = -0.129$ $p = 0.0498$). Significant negative correlations were also evident between dietary intake of sugar but not SSBs and the beliefs that eating less sugary foods/snacks/drinks will help reduce the risk of disease such as diabetes ($r = -0.184$, $p = 0.0049$) and eating/drinking less sugary foods/snacks/drinks is up to themselves ($r = -0.149$ $p = 0.02$).

3.4. Univariate Association Analyses

Table 6 shows the results of univariate logistic regression analysis for associations between dietary intake variables (sugar, SSB and protein as a % of TE) and sociodemographic or health related variables. Each yearly increase in age of participants significantly increased the likelihood of them meeting the recommendation for SSBs (0 mL) by 6% (OR, 1.06, 95% CI, 1.01–1.11, $p = 0.029$) and meeting a lower intake of protein (≤15% of TE) by 9% (OR, 1.09, 95% CI, 1.03–1.14, $p = 0.002$). Participants from MMH were 77% (OR, 0.33, 95% CI 0.17–0.64, $p = 0.001$), 91% (OR, 0.09, 95% CI, 0.03–0.25, $p < 0.001$) and 61% (OR, 0.39, 95% CI, 0.20–0.73, $p = 0.003$) less likely to meet the recommended amount of SSBs (0 mL), sugar (0 g) and lower intake of protein (≤15% of TE) respectively compared to those from GSH. Participants who self-rated their food choices as 'mostly unhealthy' were 86% ($p = 0.024$), 84% ($p = 0.027$) and 93% ($p = 0.015$) less likely to meet the recommended amount of SSBs (0 mL) and sugar (0 g) and lower intake of protein (≤15% of TE) respectively compared to those who self-reported their food choices as 'mostly very healthy' (Table 6). Each additional child that a participant had increased their likelihood of meeting the recommendation for SSBs (0 mL) by 29% (OR 1.29, 95% CI, 1.04–1.59, $p = 0.020$).

Table 6. The Univariate association between sociodemographic factors and the proportion of participants consuming the recommended intakes of SSBs, added sugar and Protein.

Variables	SSBs			Added Sugar			% Protein		
Recommendation	0 mL			0 g			15% of Total Energy		
	OR	95% CI	*p*-value *	OR	95% CI	*p*-value *	OR	95% CI	*p*-value *
Age	1.06	1.01–1.11	0.029	1.02	0.97–1.08	0.353	1.09	1.03–1.14	0.002
Gestational age	0.88	0.52–1.49	0.598	0.98	0.90–1.06	0.553	0.95	0.87-1.02	0.164
Hospital GSH versus MMH	0.33	0.17–0.64	0.001	0.09	0.03–0.25	0.000	0.39	0.20–0.73	0.003
GDM in previous pregnancy	0.68	0.43–1.06	0.085	0.51	0.27–1.0	0.049	0.61	0.32-1.17	0.138
Race									
Black versus									
White	3.4	0.29–39.1	0.326	0.73	0.06–8.35	0.798	0.46	0.04–5.32	0.528
Indian	0.85	0.15–4.92	0.856	0.29	0.03–2.61	0.270	0.46	0.08–2.68	0.391
Coloured **	1.46	0.83–2.57	0.186	0.69	0.39–1.22	0.199	0.67	0.38–1.16	0.152
LSM	0.99	0.90–1.09	0.921	0.95	0.56–1.05	0.310	1.03	0.94–1.14	0.531
Self-reported food choice									
"Mostly very healthy" versus									
Mostly healthy	0.36	0.07–1.94	0.236	0.51	0.11–2.35	0.387	0.16	0.02–1.36	0.094
Mostly unhealthy	0.14	0.02–0.77	0.024	0.16	0.03–0.81	0.027	0.07	0.01–0.59	0.015
Mostly very unhealthy	0.2	0.23–1.71	0.142	0.6	0.08–4.40	0.615	0.21	0.02–2.52	0.217
Self-reported physical activity level									
"very inactive" versus									
Inactive	1.07	0.38–3.01	0.896	0.54	0.18–1.57	0.263	1.15	0.40–3.12	0.790
Active	1.04	0.39–2.72	0.936	0.88	0.33–2.31	0.797	1.61	0.60–4.30	0.341
Very active	1.25	0.36–4.26	0.721	0.85	0.24–2.98	0.809	2.68	0.76–9.37	0.122
No of children	1.29	1.04–1.59	0.020	1.14	0.92–1.41	0.224	1.14	0.92–1.40	0.225
Wellness program—Yes versus									
no	2.87	0.51–15.9	0.229	3.89	0.69–21.7	0.121	1		

* Manual logistic regression, with the binary outcome of reaching recommended intake (yes/no) for each of the major food groups. Variables with *p*-values less than 0.1 at univariate analysis, were included in the multivariate regression (forward stepwise). If the food group had no variables that were significant at $p < 0.1$, no multivariate regression was carried out. ** mixed-race ancestry: this population group in South Africa are also referred to as the Cape Coloureds in Cape Town and has a mixed ancestry with genetic material mainly from Khoisan, Bantu African, Northern European, South Asia and South-East Asia origins. CI: Confidence interval; OR: Odds Ratio.

Race, gestational age, LSM score and parity were not associated with meeting recommended intake of table sugar, SSBs and 15% protein of TE. There were no significant associations between other dietary intake variables (F&V, 35% fat and 50% carbohydrates of TE) and the sociodemographic or health related variables (results not reported in Table 6).

3.5. Multivariate Association Analyses

The univariate associations between SSBs and age or number of children were not significant in the multivariate logistic regression (Table 7), while being treated at GSH versus MMH (OR 0.41, 95% CI 0.19–0.86, p = 0.013) and having the perception of consuming a "mostly very healthy diet" compared to those indicating "mostly unhealthy" diet (OR 0.16, 95% CI 0.03–0.98, p = 0.048) remained significant predictors of meeting the recommended 0 mL SSBs per day. In the multivariate analyses for meeting the cut-point of protein intake as a % of TE, the treatment hospital was the only variable that remained significant (Table 7), while no significant associations in the multivariate analyses were found for meeting the recommended sugar intake (0 g) (results not included in the table).

Table 7. Multivariate logistic regression analyses between sociodemographic factors and the proportion of participants consuming the recommended intake of SSBs (0 mL) and a Protein intake ≤ 15% of TE.

Variables	SSBs			% Protein		
	OR	95% CI	*p*-Value *	OR	95% CI	*p*-Value *
Age	1.03	0.97–1.10	0.312	1.05	0.99–1.11	0.068
Hospital GSH versus MMH	0.41	0.19–0.86	0.019	0.36	0.18–0.74	0.005
GDMin previous pregnancy	0.67	0.32–1.39	0.279	-	-	-
Self-reported food choice "Mostly very healthy" versus						
Mostly healthy	0.34	0.06–1.97	0.230	0.37	0.06–2.17	0.277
Mostly unhealthy	0.16	0.03–0.98	0.048	0.17	0.03–1.06	0.058
Mostly very unhealthy	0.19	0.02–1.80	0.149	0.20	0.02–1.89	0.162
No of children	1.22	0.92–1.62	0.161	-	-	-

* Forward stepwise multivariate logistic regression analyses with the binary outcome of reaching recommended intake (yes/no) for SSBs of 0 mL and the cut-point for protein of 15% of TE.

4. Discussion

The dietary intake of the pregnant women with GDM in this study was not optimal and fell short of several nutritional guidelines. The total energy intake (7268 kJ) was lower than the 11,844 kJ (2830 kcal) recommended by the Institute of Medicine (IOM) of the United States (US) [34] for a normal weight female in third trimester of pregnancy. However, energy requirements during pregnancy remain controversial and are influenced by several factors, including pre-gestational weight status, gestational weight gain and fat deposition [58]. The IOM recommendation is based on healthy active Americans and Canadians at the reference height and weight and does not necessarily reflect the energy requirements of the woman in our sample. The most recent guidelines of the American Diabetes Association [15] indicate that the optimal energy requirements of women with GDM are unknown and no research could be traced that investigated whether their energy requirements are different to a pregnancy without GDM. Javonovic [59] reported that the energy requirements for obese women with GDM may be much lower, as preliminary studies indicated that diets between 6300 kJ (1500 kcal) and 7560 kJ (1800 kcal) resulted in improved fasting and mean daily glucose levels, without the development of ketonemia. As national surveys indicated that 64% [60] and 62.2% [61] of South African women aged 15 and older are overweight or obese, it is possible that such lower energy requirements reflect the needs of the majority of women in our sample. With a dearth of comparable studies on GDM women, our energy intake was slightly lower than the energy intakes of 7677.2 kJ (1834 kcal) [24] 8425.7 kJ (2013.6 kcal) [26] and 9123 kJ (2180 kcal) [29] previously reported for non-diabetic pregnant South African women. Women with hyperglycaemia in pregnancy at MMH and GSH are referred to the hospital dietitian for a one-on-one counselling session and/or they receive dietary information from the diabetes educator or nurse. At the time of administering the questionnaire, most participants had previous dietary counselling. It is possible that they might have changed their diet after counselling, or they might have been inclined to report more favourably on their intake. As energy requirement are not calculated during consultations, portion control of energy-dense foods would remain an essential strategy during dietary counselling sessions.

The macronutrient distribution as a % of TE was not optimal if evaluated against the 2017 SEMDSA guidelines [1] that recommend carbohydrates to be up to 40% of TE, 40% of TE from fats and 20% TE from protein as well as the other international associations recommending carbohydrates < 50% of TE for GDM women (Table 1). In a country where food insecurity is high and carbohydrate rich foods such as maize meal, white rice and bread are the staple diet [62], the macronutrient distribution of the women in this study (55% for carbohydrates and 14.5% for protein) could be expected. Research in the form of RCTs is needed to establish whether this type of macronutrient distribution is problematic for optimal glycaemic control in women with GDM in South Africa. There was however no significant association found between carbohydrate or protein intake and LSM.

When comparing the actual grams of carbohydrate, protein and fat to other studies that were conducted on non-GDM pregnant women in South Africa, it is noted that the mean carbohydrate intake of our participants (220 g $\pm$ 104.5 g) was similar to the 230 g (SD $\pm$ 57.5) reported by Cormick et al. [24] but slightly less than the 292.45 $\pm$ 72.2 g by Kesa and Oldewage-Theron [26] and 334.7 g reported for pregnant adolescents by Tshitaudzi [29]. The protein intake (60.3 $\pm$ 27.5 g) was in line with the other South African studies namely, 54.7 $\pm$ 7.8 g by Cormick et al. [24], 60.9 g by Tshitaudzi [29] and 73.2 $\pm$ 23 g by Kesa and Oldewage-Theron [26]. However, total fat intake of 67.7 g ($\pm$44.2 g) was slightly higher than previous studies namely 59.1 $\pm$ 6.4 g [24], 62.3 $\pm$ 23.7 g [26] and 48.4 g in Tshitaudzi [29]. For optimal blood glucose control and general health purposes during pregnancy, it is important to consider the type of carbohydrates consumed. It is recommended that carbohydrate intake should consist mostly of vegetables, legumes, fruits, dairy and whole grains [15] and consuming adequate amounts of these foods will result in sufficient intake of dietary fibre. In our sample 80% of participants were below the recommended 28 g of fibre per day, similar to the findings of Tshitaudzi [29] and Mostert et al. [28] in pregnant South African women. Fibre is an important dietary component during pregnancy as it is beneficial to prevent constipation and haemorrhoids and assists in stabilizing blood glucose levels. Louie [19] reported that a high fibre diet in women with GDM was significantly associated with a lower prevalence of LGA, macrosomia and emergency caesarean section compared to a low glycaemic index diet.

F&V are an essential source of dietary fibre but only 31.4% of participants met the WHO/FAO [21] recommendation of 400 g or more per day. The low F&V intake could possibly be due to the lack of affordable options in close vicinity of the households [63]. In line with this, our participants who had higher F&V intakes strongly held the belief that these items are easy to find in shops close to them and that they make you feel better physically. However, none of the sociodemographic factors tested, including LSM, were associated with the consumption of F&V. It is possible that the LSM were not sensitive enough to discriminate between SES of participants or that participants might not be aware of the WHO/FAO recommendation of 400 g of F&V and how to incorporate it in their daily diet. This may be an area to address in dietary intervention in this population. Participants agreed that F&V are affordable and do not take a long time to prepare, therefore it is likely that unavailability is hindering intake. Interventions aiming at increasing F&V consumption in this population could encourage consuming seasonal F&V and planting their own vegetables at home or developing community gardens.

SSBs are a source of high glycaemic carbohydrates. The intake of refined carbohydrates in the form of SSBs is strongly discouraged for optimal blood glucose control [15]. In our sample of pregnant women, 63% reported drinking up to half a small glass (125 mL) of SSBs daily. A higher intake of SSBs was found in younger women and those who self-reported that their diet consists mostly of 'unhealthy food choices.' Those who consumed more SSBs believed that it was not easy to exclude sugary foods/drinks from their diet and that low sugar/sugar free food/drinks do not taste good. Therefore, focus is required on addressing healthy alternatives to SSBs which taste good and satisfy cravings. Practical ideas may include fruit infused water or recipes for homemade ice tea and awareness of the equivalent number of spoons of table sugar present in SSBs.

Another source of glycaemic carbohydrates is table sugar. Only 34.7% of our participants reported not adding sugar to hot beverages or porridge. A higher consumption of table sugar was significantly associated with women attending MMH and those who self-reported that their diet consists of 'mostly unhealthy' food choices. As women with high risk pregnancies and poorly controlled blood glucose levels are treated at GSH, it is possible that more emphasis has been placed on the role of diet on blood glucose levels in women receiving care there than with women attending the secondary community based hospital (MMH). This could be due to receiving a higher number of inputs on changes required from various health professionals when treated at a tertiary hospital. Mothers having had GDM in a previous pregnancy may have been more cautious and have applied their knowledge from previous experience. There were more significant associations between beliefs and table sugar intake, than with the intake of SSBs. For instance, a lower sugar intake was significantly associated with agreement with five beliefs including eating less sugar will reduce their risk of disease such as diabetes, eating less sugary foods/snacks/drink is easy, low sugar foods/snacks/drinks are tasty and that eating less sugar was up to them. This may indicate that there is a stronger awareness of or emphasis on the impact of added table sugar in glycaemic control than with SSBs. The participants also believed that knowing to control 'their' cravings for sugary foods/snacks/drinks during pregnancy will make it easier for them to eat less of these foods. Sweet cravings have been reported to appear in late GDM pregnancy [64]. Different theories exist to explain food cravings in pregnancy, one of which is 'nutrient deficits' [65].

Many participants' micronutrient intake fell short of the recommendations in pregnancy, in keeping with findings of poor micronutrient intakes in pregnant women in South Africa [22,24,28]. The majority of the GDM participants fell below the recommendations for iron, calcium and folic acid which are essential micronutrients in pregnancy. However, if participants were underreporting, as found in South African population [66] it is likely that the reported micronutrient levels are not a true reflection of the participants' actual micronutrient intake. On the other hand, with the intake of energy-dense, nutrient poor foods such as SSBs and added table sugar and a low intake of F&V, the finding that the micronutrient intake was inadequate may be plausible. Several micronutrients are especially important for GDM women. For example: iron plays an important role in pregnancy and blood glucose metabolism [67] and calcium plays a critical role in muscle contraction and in glucose uptake by cells [68]. Vitamin D deficiency is common during pregnancy even in countries with sunny climates, as South Africa and is associated with an increased risk of developing pre-eclampsia [69] and GDM [70]. Dairy products and dark green leafy vegetables can be encouraged as a source of calcium and vitamin D. The mean dietary folate intake of the participants (excluding supplements) was 244.8 micrograms, which fall well below the recommended 600 micrograms. However, all pregnant women in the public-sector health service are given a folic acid supplement of 5 mg a day, which far exceeds the increased requirements of 600 micrograms during pregnancy. While supplementation of folate in pregnancy is given to reduce the chances of neural tube defects, a recent study by Zhu [71] illustrated that this daily supplementation may increase the risk of. This is therefore a possible cause for concern and the policy in South Africa and elsewhere may need reviewing. However, further evidence of the potential adverse effects of excess folate in pregnancy is still needed and for now the benefits of folate supplementation during pregnancy outweigh the potential risks of excess folate during pregnancy.

This study may serve as evidence to plan effective nutrition education programmes that promote lifestyle changes in pregnant women with hyperglycaemia first detected in pregnancy. With 97.5%

of participants responding positively to participating in a wellness programme, it indicates that this population has a desire to receive information and support to change their lifestyle habits. These women would be good candidates for a lifestyle intervention that could be delivered using a combination of methods such as one-on-one counselling, groups session, printed materials and social media platforms.

This study is limited by the fact that all variables were self-reported, which may not necessarily reflect the true situation. We aimed to improve the validity of these outcome measures by going through rigorous processes to ensure a well-developed questionnaire. We did not use an objective method to verify energy and nutrient intake nor another dietary intake method such as a 24-h recall to validate the FFQ results. It may be likely that participants under-reported their dietary intake to impress the fieldworker by not admitting 'unhealthy foods' or due to memory gaps common when recalling items over the last 2 weeks. Underreporting is common in obese populations [72,73], however this has not been investigated in GDM. Current body weight was not measured; however, pre-pregnancy weight and BMI classification would be the ideal measures for the estimation of caloric requirements. The picture-sort method used with the FFQ, improves ease and accuracy of response in diet recall [74]. As the number of participants that were classified in some categories of sociodemographic variables were small, the sample size restricted statistical power of univariate and multivariate analyses.

5. Conclusions

This study found that the macronutrient distribution in pregnant women with GDM in Cape Town did not meet the dietary guidelines of local and international associations as carbohydrate intake are high and protein and fat intakes are low. Inadequate amounts of dietary fibre, F&V and key micronutrients important for pregnancy were consumed and the intake of added table sugar and SSBs were too high in our population. We recommend that interventions be developed and tested for women with GDM in Cape Town to: (1) establish the macronutrient distribution required for optimal glucose control, (2) meet the recommendations of 400 g/d for F&V and 28 g/d for fibre, (3) limit intake of added table sugar and SSBs and (4) improve the nutrient density of the diet so that adequate intakes of micronutrients are ensured. This study contributes to new knowledge as it investigated the diet of GDM women in Cape Town, which had not previously been done. The study reveals beliefs underlying the dietary intake of F&V, table sugar and SSB. The strongly held beliefs regarding sugary foods/drinks may contribute to poor adherence to nutritional guidelines.

Author Contributions: Conceptualization, J.H., S.B., K.M. and N.S.L.; Methodology, all; Formal Analysis, S.M.K. and T.C.; Data Curation, S.M.K., S.B., N.S.L., T.C., K.M., J.H.; Writing-Original Draft Preparation, S.M.K.; Writing-Review & Editing, J.H., S.B., N.S.L., K.M. and T.C.; Supervision, J.H. and S.B.; Project Administration, J.H.; Funding Acquisition, N.S.L. and J.H. (UCT internal funding).

Acknowledgments: We thank the following dietitians for collecting data on this study: Sonja Mostert, Rosanne Lombard, Ashley Hillary and Ntokoso Ngubane. Thank you to the South African Heart and Stroke foundation for providing recipe booklets for each participant.

References

1. SEMDSA. SEMDSA 2017 guidelines for the management of type 2 diabetes mellitus. *J. Endocrinol. Metab. Diabetes S. Afr.* **2017**, *22*, S1–S196.
2. World Health Organisation. *Diagnostic Criteria and Classification of Hyperglycaemia First Detected in Pregnancy*; World Health Organisation: Geneva, Switzerland, 2013.
3. International Diabetes Federation. *IDF Diabetes Atlas*, 8th ed.; International Diabetes Federation: Brussels, Belgium, 2017; Available online: https://www.idf.org/our-activities/care-prevention/gdm (accessed on 2 August 2018).
4. Mwanri, A.W.; Kinabo, J.; Ramaiya, K.; Feskens, E.J. Gestational diabetes mellitus in sub-Saharan Africa: Systematic review and metaregression on prevalence and risk factors. *Trop. Med. Int. Health* **2015**, *20*, 983–1002. [CrossRef] [PubMed]

5. Adam, S.; Rheeder, P. Screening for gestational diabetes mellitus in a South African population: Prevalence, comparison of diagnostic criteria and the role of risk factors. *SAMJ* **2017**, *107*, 523–527. [CrossRef] [PubMed]
6. Macaulay, S.; Dunger, D.B.; Norris, S.A. Gestational diabetes mellitus in Africa: A systematic review. *PLoS ONE* **2014**, *9*, e97871. [CrossRef] [PubMed]
7. HAPO Study Cooperative Research Group. Hyperglycemia and adverse pregnancy outcomes. *N. Engl. J. Med.* **2008**, *358*, 1991–2002. [CrossRef] [PubMed]
8. Buchanan, T.A.; Xiang, A.H.; Peters, R.K.; Kjos, S.L.; Marroquin, A.; Goico, J.; Ochoa, C.; Tan, S.; Berkowitz, K.; Hodis, H.N.; et al. Preservation of pancreatic β-cell function and prevention of type 2 diabetes by pharmacological treatment of insulin resistance in high-risk Hispanic women. *Diabetes* **2002**, *51*, 2796–2803. [CrossRef] [PubMed]
9. Tieu, J.; Shepherd, E.; Middleton, P.; Crowther, C.A. Dietary advice interventions in pregnancy for preventing gestational diabetes mellitus. *Cochrane Database Syst. Rev.* **2017**, *1*, CD006674. [CrossRef] [PubMed]
10. Bellamy, L.; Casas, J.-P.; Hingorani, A.D.; Williams, D. Type 2 diabetes mellitus after gestational diabetes: A systematic review and meta-analysis. *Lancet* **2009**, *373*, 1773–1779. [CrossRef]
11. Kim, C. Maternal outcomes and follow-up after gestational diabetes mellitus. *Diabet. Med.* **2014**, *31*, 292–301. [CrossRef] [PubMed]
12. Minooee, S.; Tehrani, F.R.; Rahmati, M.; Mansournia, M.A.; Azizi, F. Diabetes incidence and influencing factors in women with and without gestational diabetes mellitus: A 15 year population-based follow-up cohort study. *Diabetes Res. Clin. Pract.* **2017**, *128*, 24–31. [CrossRef] [PubMed]
13. Zhu, Y.; Zhang, C. Prevalence of gestational diabetes and risk of progression to type 2 diabetes: A global perspective. *Curr. Diabetes Rep.* **2016**, *16*, 7. [CrossRef] [PubMed]
14. Cheng, A. Canadian Diabetes Association 2013 clinical practice guidelines for the prevention and management of diabetes in Canada. Introduction. *Can. J. Diabetes* **2013**, *37*, S1–S3. [CrossRef] [PubMed]
15. American Diabetes Association. 13. Management of Diabetes in Pregnancy: Standards of Medical Care in Diabetes—2018. *Diabetes Care* **2018**, *41*, S137–S143. [CrossRef] [PubMed]
16. Brown, S.; Brown, J.; Alwan, N.; West, J.; McKinlay, C.J.; Farrar, D.; Crowther, C.A. Lifestyle interventions for the treatment of women with gestational diabetes. *Cochrane Database Syst. Rev.* **2017**, *5*, CD011970. [CrossRef] [PubMed]
17. Goodarzi-Khoigani, M.; Mahmoodabad, S.S.M.; Moghadam, M.H.B.; Nadjarzadeh, A.; Mardanian, F.; Fallahzadeh, H.; Dadkhah-Tirani, A. Prevention of insulin resistance by dietary intervention among pregnant mothers: A randomized controlled trial. *Int. J. Prev. Med.* **2017**, *8*, 85. [PubMed]
18. Assaf-Balut, C.; de la Torre, N.G.; Durán, A.; Fuentes, M.; Bordiú, E.; del Valle, L.; Familiar, C.; Ortolá, A.; Jiménez, I.; Herraiz, M.A.; et al. A Mediterranean diet with additional extra virgin olive oil and pistachios reduces the incidence of gestational diabetes mellitus (GDM): A randomized controlled trial: The St. Carlos GDM prevention study. *PLoS ONE* **2017**, *12*, e0185873. [CrossRef] [PubMed]
19. Louie, J.C.Y.; Markovic, T.P.; Perera, N.; Foote, D.; Petocz, P.; Ross, G.P.; Brand-Miller, J.C. A Randomized Controlled Trial Investigating the Effects of a Low-Glycemic Index Diet on Pregnancy Outcomes in Gestational Diabetes Mellitus. *Diabetes Care* **2011**, *34*, 2341–2346. [CrossRef] [PubMed]
20. Zhang, C.; Liu, S.; Solomon, C.G.; Hu, F.B. Dietary fiber intake, dietary glycemic load, and the risk for gestational diabetes mellitus. *Diabetes Care* **2006**, *29*, 2223–2230. [CrossRef] [PubMed]
21. Food and Agriculture Organization; World Health Organisation. *Fruit and Vegetables for Health: Report of a Joint FAO/WHO Workshop, 1–3 September 2004, Kobe, Japan*; World Health Organisation: Geneva, Switzerland, 2005.
22. Bopape, M.M.; Mbhenyane, X.; Alberts, M. The prevalence of anaemia and selected micronutrient status in pregnant teenagers of Polokwane Municipality in the Limpopo Province. *S. Afr. J. Clin. Nutr.* **2008**, *21*, 332–336. [CrossRef]
23. Cape, W.; Mamabolo, R.; Alberts, M.; Steyn, N.; de Waal, H.D.; Nthangeni, N.; Levitt, N. Evaluation of the effectiveness of iron and folate supplementation during pregnancy in a rural area of Limpopo province. *S. Afr. J. Clin. Nutr.* **2004**, *17*, 15–21. [CrossRef]
24. Cormick, G.; Betrán, A.P.; Harbron, J.; Purnat, T.D.; Parker, C.; Hall, D.; Seuc, A.H.; Roberts, J.M.; Belizán, J.M.; Hofmeyr, G.J. Are women with history of pre-eclampsia starting a new pregnancy in good nutritional status in South Africa and Zimbabwe? *BMC Pregnancy Childbirth* **2018**, *18*, 236. [CrossRef] [PubMed]

25. Jaffer, S. An Assessment of the Dietary Intake of Pregnant Women in the West Coast/Winelands Region, Western Cape Province: Relation to Low Birth Weight. Master's Thesis, University of Western Cape, Cape Town, South Africa, 2008.
26. Kesa, H.; Oldewage-Theron, W. Anthropometric indications and nutritional intake of women in the Vaal Triangle, South Africa. *Public Health* **2005**, *119*, 294–300. [CrossRef] [PubMed]
27. Klinger, I. The Nutritional Status of Pregnant Women in Relation to Alcohol Consumption during Pregnancy, and Pregnancy Outcome. Master's Thesis, University of Stellenbosch, Stellenbosch, South Africa, 2004.
28. Mostert, D.; Steyn, N.P.; Temple, N.J.; Olwagen, R. Dietary intake of pregnant women and their infants in a poor black community in South Africa. *Curationis* **2005**, *28*, 12–19. [CrossRef] [PubMed]
29. Tshitaudzi, G.T. Nutritional Status of Pregnant Women (under 20 Years of Age) with Special Emphasis on Iron and Folic Acid Status. Master's Thesis, University of Stellenbosch, Stellenbosch, South Africa, 2003.
30. Newson, R.S.; Lion, R.; Crawford, R.J.; Curtis, V.; Elmadfa, I.; Feunekes, G.I.; Hicks, C.; Van Liere, M.; Lowe, C.F.; Meijer, G.W.; et al. Behaviour change for better health: Nutrition, hygiene and sustainability. *BMC Public Health* **2013**, *13*, S1. [CrossRef] [PubMed]
31. Reader, D.M. Medical nutrition therapy and lifestyle interventions. *Diabetes Care* **2007**, *30*, S188–S193. [CrossRef] [PubMed]
32. Metzger, B.E.; Coustan, D.R. The Organizing Committee. Summary and recommendations of the fourth international workshop-conference on gestational diabetes mellitus. *Diabetes Care* **1998**, *21*, B161. [PubMed]
33. Canadian Diabetes Association. Recommendations for Nutrition Best Practice: In the Management of Gestational Diabetes Mellitus. *Can. J. Diet. Pract. Res.* **2006**, *67*, 206. [CrossRef] [PubMed]
34. Trumbo, P.; Schlicker, S.; Yates, A.; Poos, M. Food and Nutrition Board of the Institute of Medicine, The National Academies. Dietary reference intakes for energy, carbohydrate, fiber, fat, fatty acids, cholesterol, protein and amino acids. *J. Am. Diet. Assoc.* **2002**, *102*, 1621–1630. [CrossRef]
35. International Association of Diabetes in Pregnancy Study Group (IADPSG) Working Group on Outcome Definitions; Feig, D.S.; Corcoy, R.; Jensen, D.M.; Kautzky-Willer, A.; Nolan, C.J.; Oats, J.J.; Sacks, D.A.; Caimari, F.; McIntyre, H.D. Diabetes in pregnancy outcomes: A systematic review and proposed codification of definitions. *Diabetes Metab. Res. Rev.* **2015**, *31*, 680–690. [PubMed]
36. Rani, P.R.; Begum, J. Screening and diagnosis of gestational diabetes mellitus, where do we stand. *J. Clin. Diagn. Res.* **2016**, *10*, QE01. [CrossRef] [PubMed]
37. National Institute for Health and Care Excellence. *NICE Guideline Diabetes in Pregnancy: Management from Preconception to Postnatal Period*; National Institute for Health and Care Excellence: London, UK, 2015.
38. Vorster, H.H.; Badham, J.; Venter, C. An introduction to the revised food-based dietary guidelines for South Africa. *S. Afr. J. Clin. Nutr.* **2013**, *26*, S5–S12.
39. SAARF. Available online: http://www.eighty20.co.za (accessed on 7 June 2018).
40. Martins, J. Household cash expenditure by living standards measure group. *J. Fam. Ecol. Consum. Sci.* **2006**, *34*, 1–9. [CrossRef]
41. Schonfeldt, H.C.; Gibson, N.; Vermeulen, H. The Possible Impact of Inflation on Nutritionally Vulnerable Households in a Developing Country with South Africa as the Case Study. *Ann. Nutr. Metab.* **2009**, *55*, 663.
42. Haupt, P. The SAARF Universal Living Standards Measure (SU-LSM): 12 Years of Continuous Development. 2006. Available online: http://www.saarf.co.za/LSM/lsm-article.asp (accessed on 20 August 2018).
43. Kumanyika, S.K.; Tell, G.S.; Shemanski, L.; Martel, J.; Chinchilli, V.M. Dietary assessment using a picture-sort approach. *Am. J. Clin. Nutr.* **1997**, *65*, 1123S–1129S. [CrossRef] [PubMed]
44. Seme, Z. Formative Assessment of Teachers of Grade Four to Six Learners to Advise the Development of the Teacher Focus of a Multi-Component Primary School-Based Intervention Programme for the Prevention of Non-Communicable Diseases. Master's Thesis, University of Cape Town, Cape Town, South Africa, 2013.
45. Wrottesley, S.V.; Pisa, P.T.; Norris, S.A. The Influence of Maternal Dietary Patterns on Body Mass Index and Gestational Weight Gain in Urban Black South African Women. *Nutrients* **2017**, *9*, 732. [CrossRef] [PubMed]
46. Steyn, N.P.; Senekal, M. *A Guide for the Use of the Dietary Assessment and Education Kit (DAEK)*; Medical Research Council: Cape Town, South Africa, 2004.
47. Wolmarans, P.; Danster, N.; Dalton, A.; Rossouw, K.; Schönfeldt, H. *Condensed Food Composition Tables for South Africa*; Medical Research Council: Cape Town, South Africa 2010.

48. Cheng, Y.; Dibley, M.J.; Zhang, X.; Zeng, L.; Yan, H. Assessment of dietary intake among pregnant women in a rural area of western China. *BMC Public Health* **2009**, *9*, 222. [CrossRef] [PubMed]
49. World Health Organization. *Guideline: Sugars Intake for Adults and Children*; World Health Organization: Geneva, Switzerland, 2015.
50. Ajzen, I. The theory of planned behavior. *Org. Behav. Hum. Decis. Process.* **1991**, *50*, 179–211. [CrossRef]
51. Fishbein, M.; Yzer, M.C. Using theory to design effective health behavior interventions. *Commun. Theory* **2003**, *13*, 164–183. [CrossRef]
52. Francis, J.; Eccles, M.P.; Johnston, M.; Walker, A.; Grimshaw, J.M.; Foy, R.; Kaner, E.F.; Smith, L.; Bonetti, D. *Constructing Questionnaires Based on the Theory of Planned Behaviour: A Manual for Health Services Researchers*; University of Newcastle: Newcastle, Australia, 2004.
53. Krueger, R.; Casey, M. *Focus Groups: A Practical Guide for Applied Research*, 4th ed.; Sage Publications, Inc.: Thousand Oaks, CA, USA, 2009.
54. TIBCO Software Incorporated, Palo Alto, CA 94304, USA. 2017. Available online: http://tibco.com (accessed on 25 August 2018).
55. Stata Corporation. Stata Press: College Station, TX, USA, 2016. Available online: http://www.stata-press.com (accessed on 25 August 2018).
56. Ross, A.C.; Manson, J.E.; Abrams, S.A.; Aloia, J.F.; Brannon, P.M.; Clinton, S.K.; Durazo-Arvizu, R.A.; Gallagher, J.C.; Gallo, R.L.; Jones, G. The 2011 report on dietary reference intakes for calcium and vitamin D from the Institute of Medicine: What clinicians need to know. *J. Clin. Endocrinol. Metab.* **2011**, *96*, 53–58. [CrossRef] [PubMed]
57. Lung, N.H.; Blood Institute. *Your Guide to Lowering Your Cholesterol with TLC (Therapeutic Lifestyle Changes)*; National Institutes of Health, US Department of Health and Human Services: Bethesda, MD, USA, 2006.
58. Butte, N.F.; Wong, W.W.; Treuth, M.S.; Ellis, K.J.; Smith, E.O. Energy requirements during pregnancy based on total energy expenditure and energy deposition. *Am. J. Clin. Nutr.* **2004**, *79*, 1078–1087. [CrossRef] [PubMed]
59. Jovanovic, L. Medical Nutritional Therapy for Pre-gestational and Gestational Diabetes Mellitus. *J. Health Sci.* **2018**, *6*, 79–90.
60. Shisana, O.; Labadarios, D.; Rehle, T.; Simbayi, L.; Zuma, K.; Dhansay, A.; Reddy, P.; Parker, W.; Hoosain, E.; Naidoo, P. *The South African National Health and Nutrition Examination Survey, 2012: SANHANES-1: The Health and Nutritional Status of the Nation*; HSRC Press: Cape Town, South Africa, 2014.
61. Statistics South Africa. *South Africa Demographic and Health Survey 2016: Key Indicator Report*; Statistics South Africa: Pretoria, South Africa, 2016.
62. MacIntyre, U.; Kruger, H.; Venter, C.; Vorster, H. Dietary intakes of an African population in different stages of transition in the North West Province, South Africa: The THUSA study. *Nutr. Res.* **2002**, *22*, 239–256. [CrossRef]
63. Temple, N.J.; Steyn, N.P. The cost of a healthy diet: A South African perspective. *Nutrition* **2011**, *27*, 505–508. [CrossRef] [PubMed]
64. Belzer, L.M.; Smulian, J.C.; Lu, S.-E.; Tepper, B.J. Food cravings and intake of sweet foods in healthy pregnancy and mild gestational diabetes mellitus. A prospective study. *Appetite* **2010**, *55*, 609–615. [CrossRef] [PubMed]
65. Orloff, N.C.; Hormes, J.M. Pickles and ice cream! Food cravings in pregnancy: Hypotheses, preliminary evidence, and directions for future research. *Front. Psychol.* **2014**, *5*, 1076. [CrossRef] [PubMed]
66. Orcholski, L.; Luke, A.; Plange-Rhule, J.; Bovet, P.; Forrester, T.E.; Lambert, E.V.; Dugas, L.R.; Kettmann, E.; Durazo-Arvizu, R.A.; Cooper, R.S. Under-reporting of dietary energy intake in five populations of the African diaspora. *Br. J. Nutr.* **2015**, *113*, 464–472. [CrossRef] [PubMed]
67. Rajpathak, S.N.; Crandall, J.P.; Wylie-Rosett, J.; Kabat, G.C.; Rohan, T.E.; Hu, F.B. The role of iron in type 2 diabetes in humans. *Biochim. Biophys. Acta* **2009**, *1790*, 671–681. [CrossRef] [PubMed]
68. Richter, E.A.; Hargreaves, M. Exercise, GLUT4, and skeletal muscle glucose uptake. *Physiol. Rev.* **2013**, *93*, 993–1017. [CrossRef] [PubMed]
69. De-Regil, L.M.; Palacios, C.; Lombardo, L.K.; Peña-Rosas, J.P. Vitamin D supplementation for women during pregnancy. *São Paulo Med. J.* **2016**, *134*, 274–275. [CrossRef] [PubMed]

70. Zhang, M.-X.; Pan, G.-T.; Guo, J.-F.; Li, B.-Y.; Qin, L.-Q.; Zhang, Z.-L. Vitamin D deficiency increases the risk of gestational diabetes mellitus: A meta-analysis of observational studies. *Nutrients* **2015**, *7*, 8366–8375. [CrossRef] [PubMed]
71. Zhu, B.; Ge, X.; Huang, K.; Mao, L.; Yan, S.; Xu, Y.; Huang, S.; Hao, J.; Zhu, P.; Niu, Y. Folic acid supplement intake in early pregnancy increases risk of gestational diabetes mellitus: Evidence from a prospective cohort study. *Diabetes Care* **2016**, *39*, e36–e37. [CrossRef] [PubMed]
72. Meng, X.; Kerr, D.A.; Zhu, K.; Devine, A.; Solah, V.; Wright, J.; Binns, C.; Prince, R. Under-reporting of energy intake in elderly Australian women is associated with a higher body mass index. *J. Nutr. Health Aging* **2013**, *17*, 112–118. [CrossRef] [PubMed]
73. Scagliusi, F.B.; Ferriolli, E.; Pfrimer, K.; Laureano, C.; Cunha, C.; Gualano, B.; Lourenco, B.; Lancha, A., Jr. Characteristics of women who frequently under report their energy intake: A doubly labelled water study. *Eur. J. Clin. Nutr.* **2009**, *63*, 1192. [CrossRef] [PubMed]
74. Wengreen, H.J.; Munger, R.G.; Wong, S.S.; West, N.A.; Cutler, R. Comparison of a picture-sort food-frequency questionnaire with 24-hour dietary recalls in an elderly Utah population. *Public Health Nutr.* **2001**, *4*, 961–970. [CrossRef] [PubMed]

4

Gestational Diabetes Mellitus: The Impact of Carbohydrate Quality in Diet

Tiziana Filardi [1], Francesca Panimolle [1], Clara Crescioli [2], Andrea Lenzi [1] and Susanna Morano [1,*]

1 Department of Experimental Medicine, "Sapienza" University, Viale del Policlinico 155, 00161 Rome, Italy
2 Department of Movement, Human and Health Sciences, Section of Health Sciences, Unit of Endocrinology, Università degli Studi di Roma "Foro Italico", 00135 Rome, Italy
* Correspondence: susanna.morano@uniroma1.it

Abstract: Gestational diabetes mellitus (GDM) is defined as "glucose intolerance that is first diagnosed during pregnancy". Mothers with GDM and their infants may experience both short and long term complications. Dietary intervention is the first therapeutic strategy. If good glycaemic control is not achieved, insulin therapy is recommended. There is no consensus on which nutritional approach should be used in GDM. In the last few years, there has been growing evidence of the benefits of a low glycaemic index (LGI) diet on diabetes and cardiovascular disease. The effect of a LGI diet on GDM incidence has been investigated as well. Several studies observed a lower incidence of GDM in LGI diet arms, without adverse maternal and fetal outcomes. The main positive effect of the LGI diet was the reduction of 2-h post-prandial glucose (PPG). Several studies have also evaluated the effect of the LGI diet in GDM treatment. Overall, the LGI diet might have beneficial effects on certain outcomes, such as 2-h PPG, fasting plasma glucose and lipid profile in patients with GDM. Indeed, most studies observed a significant reduction in insulin requirement. Overall, according to current evidence, the LGI nutritional approach is safe and it might therefore be considered in clinical care for GDM.

Keywords: gestational diabetes mellitus; GDM; low glycaemic index; low glycaemic load; low glycaemic index diet; low-GI diet; LGI diet; incidence of GDM; GDM outcomes

1. Introduction

Gestational diabetes mellitus (GDM) is defined as "diabetes diagnosed in the second or third trimester of pregnancy that was not clearly overt diabetes prior to gestation" [1]. Contextually with the dramatic spread of obesity and type 2 diabetes (T2D), the prevalence of GDM has significantly increased over the last few years. The prevalence of this condition depends largely on ethnicity and it is also related to the criteria employed for diagnosis [2].

Physiologically, during pregnancy insulin sensitivity progressively decreases until the second trimester, declining by 50%–60% compared with pre-pregnancy values [3]. Insulin sensitivity is influenced by the increase in adipose tissue, and by the release of hormones, such as estrogens and progesterone, or placental factors, such as human placental lactogen (hPL) [3]. In particular, hPL has a lipolytic effect, leading to the rise in circulating fatty acids. Consequently, maternal metabolism is shifted towards a greater use of lipids rather than glucose as an energy source, which is necessary to give the fetus an adequate glucose reserve [3]. Insulin resistance develops as a consequence of high maternal circulating fatty acids [3]. Contextually, insulin secretion is implemented to balance peripheral insulin resistance. However, if the increase in pancreatic β-cell secretion is not able to compensate insulin resistance, diabetes occurs [4]. Moreover, physiological pregnancy is characterized by low grade inflammation, which is exacerbated in GDM. Thus, insulin resistance might develop from this pro-inflammatory state [5].

The main risk factors for GDM are pre-pregnancy body mass index (BMI) in the range of overweight or obesity, high maternal age, and first degree family history of T2D [6,7].

GDM may lead to several adverse pregnancy outcomes. Indeed, mothers affected by GDM have a high prevalence of gestational hypertension and preeclampsia. The incidence of caesarean section in GDM patients is considerably higher than in normal pregnancies, as well as the occurrence of obstetrical complications, such as preterm delivery, dystocia, acute respiratory distress syndrome, neonatal jaundice, and neonatal hypoglycemia [8,9]. Besides short-term complications, women with previous GDM are at increased risk for GDM recurrence, T2D, cardiovascular disease (CVD), and hypertension. Furthermore, it has been observed that even the offspring of mothers with GDM has increased risk of obesity, insulin resistance, and T2D later in life [10].

As for diagnosis, a single-step approach has been proposed by the International Association of the Diabetes and Pregnancy Study Groups (IADPSG), which consists of performing an oral glucose tolerance test (OGTT) with 75-g of glucose and assessing fasting, 1 h and 2 h glycaemia. A single value higher than the cut-off value at any time of the OGTT is sufficient to establish the diagnosis [11]. The IADPSG criteria have been developed after the results of the Hyperglycemia and Adverse Pregnancy Outcome (HAPO) study, a multinational prospective study of 25,000 pregnant women, which observed that high glucose levels were significantly associated with increased risk of maternal and fetal complications [12].

The treatment of GDM is aimed to achieve normal levels of fasting plasma glucose (FPG) and post-prandial glycaemia (PPG) in order to prevent complications. Indeed, high glucose levels, especially postprandial elevations, are linked to negative pregnancy outcomes [13]. The first therapeutic approach consists of dietary and lifestyle education. However, insulin therapy is mandatory unless good glycaemic control is achieved [14]. Medical nutritional therapy should provide adequate nutrients for normal fetal growth, but it should not induce maternal weight gain or loss [15]. Gestational weight gain is largely due to excessive energy intake and fuel requirements usually increase from 10 to 30 weeks of gestation [16]. Caloric restriction is not recommended during pregnancy, even in GDM, because it may have adverse effects on birth weight. Advice for energy intake, as well as for weight gain, should take into account pre-pregnancy BMI [16,17]. As yet, there is no consensus on which specific nutritional approach should be used in GDM, in terms of total energy intake and macronutrient distribution [18].

This paper provides a brief overview on medical nutritional therapy in GDM, with a specific focus on the low glycaemic index (LGI) diet approach. To date, although several studies and meta-analyses have been performed, their results are not univocal and the LGI diet is still a debated topic in GDM. The most recent findings on this issue have been discussed and compared. In addition, the main limits of the latest studies and meta-analyses have been indicated.

2. Carbohydrates, Glycaemic Index, and Glycaemic Load

Carbohydrates (CHOs) are an important source of energy, but they increase PPG more than other macronutrients [19]. Since a proportion higher than 55% of CHO in diet is associated with elevations in PPG [20], moderation of CHO intake is reasonable in GDM. However, restriction of CHO is not mandatory to reduce PPG. The decrease in the rate of CHO digestion and absorption is effective in preventing PPG abnormal elevations. Not only is blood glucose influenced by the total amount of CHOs, but it is also affected by the type of CHO. CHO polymer length influences digestion and absorption, and consequently might prevent the elevations of glycaemia after meals.

Glycaemic response (GR), glycaemic index (GI), and glycaemic load (GL) are measures of the effect of different foods on glycaemia [21]. When a food containing CHO is ingested, the PPG variation induced is the GR [21]. "Available CHO" is the amount of CHO that goes through digestion, absorption, and metabolism. The GR induced by a portion of food containing 50 g of available CHO is the GI, which represents a percentage of the GR induced by 50 g of the reference CHO (generally glucose or white wheat bread) [21,22]. For instance, rice and potatoes are considered high GI foods, as they induce a rapid increase in glycaemia, which subsequently drops sharply. On the contrary, fruits and dairy are considered LGI foods, since they contain CHOs which are digested slowly and induce lower PPG elevations [16,21,22]. High GI foods have a GI ≥70 on the glucose scale and contain CHOs which are digested, absorbed and metabolized sharply. Whereas LGI foods have a GI ≤55 and are digested, absorbed and metabolized slowly. Thus, GI is a standardized measure of GR, defined by a standardized amount of CHO and it is relative to a reference food. It can also be considered as an indicator of the quality of CHO. The GL is a measure of both the quality and the amount of CHOs. It is calculated by multiplying the GI by the quantity of available CHO in a given amount of food ("GL = GI x available CHO/given amount of food") [21]. The glycaemic effect of whole diets, meals, and foods can be easily compared on the basis of their GL [21,23].

The GI was defined for the first time many years ago by Jenkins et al. [24]. The International Organization for Standardization has developed the reference method, which is still valid [21,25], and international tables indicating the GI of foods are available [26]. Besides the adoption of GI for single foods classification and comparison, the use of GI has spread to mixed meals and entire diets as well. Indeed, meal and dietary GI employed in clinical trials and in clinical setting are obtained by calculating the weighted mean of the GI of each food, considering the proportion of CHO contained in them [27].

In addition, the content of dietary fibers (DF), plant-based CHO that are not digestible, is another important indicator of the quality of diets. DF contained in fruits, vegetables, and legumes are soluble. Soluble DF slow digestion, reduce PPG, and cholesterol absorption. Insoluble DF are contained in nuts, wholegrain bread, and cereals. Cooked potato and rice contain resistant starch [16]. Insoluble DF and resistant starch have limited metabolic actions [23].

3. LGI Diets and Risk of GDM

In the last 30 years there has been growing evidence of the benefits of the LGI diet not only on weight reduction and body composition but also on diabetes, CVD, and cancer. LGI food produces lower PPG increase, prevents the excessive rise in post-prandial insulin, and it might also induce satiety. All these effects may contribute to weight loss [28].

Besides weight reduction, in epidemiological studies the LGI diet was associated with a lower risk of T2D, CVD, and cancer, mainly breast and colorectal neoplasms [29–31]. Furthermore, in clinical studies, the LGI diet had positive effects on glycaemic control in diabetes, lipid profile, and other CV risk factors [31–34]. The mechanisms behind these beneficial effects remain not completely understood, but they might include slow absorption of CHOs and improvement even in novel cardiovascular risk factors, such as chronic inflammation.

A growing amount of research has focused on the effects of the LGI diet on the incidence of GDM as well. The ROLO study ("randomized control trial of low glycaemic index diet versus no dietary intervention to prevent recurrence of fetal macrosomia") enrolled 800 women with previous macrosomia (infant >4 kg). In this study, women in the LGI diet group experienced significantly lower weight increase during pregnancy than women in the control group. Although the incidence of large for gestational age (LGA) infants was not influenced by the intervention diet, the incidence of glucose intolerance was lower in the LGI arm. Indeed, a lower percentage of mothers had fasting glycaemia ≥92 mg/dL or 1-h glucose at OGTT ≥140 mg/dL [35]. Later, the same authors performed a secondary analysis of 621 participants. A lower increase in circulating levels of insulin was observed from the beginning of pregnancy to 28 weeks of gestation, in women in the intervention group, although no differences were found between the two groups in maternal and fetal adipokines and inflammation markers (tumor necrosis factor α, interleukin 6, leptin) [36]. A further analysis of 542 mothers and babies previously involved in the ROLO study indicated a positive association between neonatal central adiposity and the LGI group [37].

In the GI Baby 3 Randomized Controlled Trial (RCT), Markovic et al. enrolled 139 women at high risk for GDM, between 14 and 20 weeks of pregnancy. The treatment arms were either an LGI diet with a target GI around 50 (72 women), or a conventional moderate-GI high DF diet, with a target GI around 60 (67 women). At 36 weeks, no differences in glycosylated hemoglobin (HbA1c) as well as in lipids, birth weight, percentage of fat of infants, and incidence of GDM were observed. In a subsequent prospective study, including a selection of 59 mothers and infant pairs (30 from the LGI group and 29 from the high-fiber group), infants had lower birth weight and length in the LGI group than in the high-fiber group. However, growth curves and fat mass from birth to 1 year of age were not significantly different. Notably, in the LGI group, babies had a significantly lower aortic intima-media thickness than in the high-fiber group. Even though subjects involved in the follow-up study were different from those initially assigned to the study, and although the follow-up study was under-powered in detecting differences in fat mass, these results suggest that GI might have an effect on the offspring vascular health [38].

A meta-analysis of 11 randomized controlled trials (1985 women) showed a significant reduction in FPG, 2-h PPG, and in the percentage of LGA in the LGI diet arm than in the control arm. Birth weight and weight increase during pregnancy were lower in the LGI arm, but not significantly, and the heterogeneity was high in gestational weight gain and birth weight analyses, probably due to different methods of intervention and control treatment, characteristics of participants, criteria for diagnosis of GDM. However, these data show that the LGI diet may improve several maternal metabolic outcomes, without negative effects on the infant [39].

Interestingly, total CHO intake in diet seems to be less important than CHO quality (DF content, GI, GL) in prevention of GDM. The Australian Longitudinal Study on Women's Health aimed to investigate the relationship between the amount and the quality of pre-pregnancy CHOs in diet and the risk of developing GDM [40]. A total of 3607 women (25–30 years) were enrolled and followed up for a 10-year period. The low CHO diet score referred to high fat, high protein, and low CHO relative content. Paradoxically, this score and the risk of GDM were found to be positively correlated. However, the risk of GDM was reduced by 33% in women with the highest DF intake. The amount of fruits was negatively associated with GDM as well, whilst a high cereal content was a risk factor for GDM. Thus, it is crucial to take into account not only the quantity but also the source of CHO in diet, in terms of fiber content, GI, and GL.

Overall, it seems that clinical phenotypes with increased insulin resistance and therefore with high post-prandial insulin, higher BMI, or waist circumference, especially in the presence of diabetes, might benefit the most from the LGI diet. Several studies have indicated a lower incidence of GDM in pregnant women in LGI diet arms, without adverse maternal and fetal outcomes. The main positive effect of the LGI diet was found to be the reduction of 2-h PPG. Nevertheless, considering the high heterogeneity between studies in population characteristics, outcomes, intervention, and control treatment, and the relative limited number of studies considered in meta-analyses, further research should confirm these findings. Finally, the exact effect of DF content in the LGI diet in preventing GDM has not been elucidated so far.

4. LGI Diet and Pregnancy Outcomes in GDM

The efficacy of the LGI diet in GDM has been evaluated in several RCT and meta-analyses. Moses et al. performed an RCT, involving 63 GDM women. The treatment arms were either an LGI diet (31) or a standard high-fiber diet, with higher GI (32), and patients were followed from 28–32 weeks of pregnancy until delivery. A significantly lower percentage of patients required insulin treatment in the LGI diet arm than in the high-GI diet arm (29% vs. 59% respectively, $p = 0.023$). However, among the women needing insulin, a proportion of 47% avoided it by shifting to an LGI intervention. Obstetric and fetal outcomes, such as type of delivery, birth weight, length, cranial circumference, and Apgar index did not differ between the two groups. Notably, fiber intake, which may act as a confounding factor in evaluating the potential advantages of the LGI diet, was similar in both groups [41].

Hu et al. performed an RCT, randomizing 140 women with GDM to either the LGI diet (66) or normal diabetic control diet (74). In the LGI diet group rice was replaced by an LGI food in the principal meals. Remarkably, PPG levels were significantly lower in the LGI group than in the control group, although the two arms had similar total energy and CHO content [42].

Similarly, the LGI diet induced a decrease in FPG and 2-h PPG in an RCT involving 95 Chinese patients with GDM, assigned either to general dietary intervention or intensive LGL intervention, from 24–26 weeks of pregnancy until delivery. Total cholesterol, triglycerides, and HDL-cholesterol significantly improved in the LGI arm. No significant differences in other outcomes emerged between the two groups. However, since the DF intake was significantly greater in the intervention arm, the effects of the LGI and the high DF could not be differentiated [43].

In another RCT, 99 women with GDM were randomized to either an LGI diet (50) or a high fiber moderate GI diet (49) and followed up from 20–32 weeks of pregnancy until delivery. In contrast to the results of other studies, there were no significant differences in insulin treatment requirement or other maternal and fetal outcomes [44]. A subgroup of 58 pregnant women assigned either to the LGI diet (33) or to the high-fiber diet (25) was followed up further. Three months after delivery there were no significant differences in glucose levels after a 75-g OGTT and in blood lipids [45]. It should be noted that the latter results might be explained by a very modest difference in GI in diets between the two arms (target GI: Around 50 in the LGI arm and around 60 in high-fiber moderate-GI arm).

A meta-analysis of RCTs of dietary intervention in GDM showed that in the LGI group (4 RCT, 257 patients diet) the use of insulin was less frequent and the birth weight was lower than in the control group [46]. The energy intake did not differ between the groups and the mean value of GI score in the LGI dietary intervention was 48.9, whereas in the control group was 53.5. Remarkably, the LGI diet did not increase the number of small for gestational age (SGA) infants. As regarding macrosomia, no significant differences were observed, probably due to the relatively low incidence of this condition both in the intervention and in the control groups.

In another meta-analysis of 5 RCTs (302 patients with GDM) [47] the risk of insulin usage was reduced by 33% in the LGI diet, although not significantly. Since fiber content was considerably higher in LGI diets than in the control diets in two of the selected studies, in subgroup analyses the authors investigated the effect of this confounder on the specific outcome insulin usage. Considering the 3 studies in which the fiber intake was similar between the two groups, the risk of insulin requirement was significantly lower in LGI diets (−31%, $p = 0.01$). However, the increase in the content of DF in the LGI diet did not lead to a further reduction in the risk of insulin requirement. Besides this, the risk of macrosomia was significantly lower in the LGI groups than in the control groups and the risk of SGA was not statistically different between the two groups. Interestingly, the addition of DF to LGI diets further reduced the risk of macrosomia, compared with LGI diets without added fiber.

Recently, in a meta-analysis of 6 RCTs, including 532 patients with GDM (270 treated with the LGI diet vs. 262 treated with control-diet), the LGI diet lead to a significant reduction in 2 h PPG, without any influence on FPG, HbA1c, insulin requirement, birth weight, and macrosomia [48].

It is known that previous GDM increases the risk of T2D. In an RCT, 77 Asian women with previous GDM were assigned to either a standard healthy diet, which consisted of receiving advice on energy restriction, fat and simple sugar reduction, fiber content increase, or an LGI diet, with the addition of instructions for lowering the GI. After 6 months, body weight, BMI, waist-to-hip ratio, and 2 h PPG significantly reduced only in the LGI group. Notably, although caloric intake was similar between groups, fiber content was higher in the LGI diet group than in the control group (17 ± 4 vs. 13 ± 4 g, $p < 0.001$) [49]. The same authors investigated the effects of LGI by grouping patients according to fasting insulin levels at baseline. Considering the subjects with low levels of insulin, no significant differences in outcomes between the diet groups were observed. After 12 months, FPG and triglycerides reduced in normal or high insulin subjects in the LGI group, whereas in the conventional healthy dietary recommendation group an increase was observed [50]. These findings might indicate that clinical phenotypes with increased insulin resistance could take more advantage from LGI diets.

Several reasons may explain the main differences in the results between the above-mentioned studies. Firstly, different diagnostic criteria for GDM have been adopted. The variation in patient characteristics (age, ethnicity, weeks of gestation, BMI) and in the methods of intervention/control diets should be taken into consideration. Moreover, different or not standardized outcomes were evaluated. Furthermore, most studies were limited by the lack of assessment of adherence to diet. The relatively small number of some studies included in the meta-analyses ($n < 100$) is another important limitation. A further explanation for the contrasting findings between studies is the different amount and type of DF intake in treatment arms, which may act as a confounder.

5. Conclusions

Overall, a considerable body of research suggests that the LGI diet might have positive effects on certain metabolic outcomes, such as 2 h PPG, FPG, and likely, lipid profile in patients with GDM. Indeed, most clinical studies observed a significant reduction in insulin requirement. By contrast, the LGI diet has not shown to have a marked influence on other obstetric maternal or fetal outcomes (body weight gain, birth weight, proportion of LGA, and macrosomia) so far. Interestingly, current evidence suggests that an LGI nutritional approach is reasonably safe in GDM, since it was not associated to adverse fetal-maternal outcomes in clinical trials. In clinical care, giving LGI advice in pregnancy complicated by GDM might therefore be considered, especially in women with uncontrolled PPG or FPG, before starting insulin treatment. As yet, evidence about clear reduction in GDM incidence with the LGI diet is still insufficient. Similarly, further studies should focus on long term complications of GDM as well, such as the incidence of T2D and CVD in mothers and infants.

Author Contributions: Conceptualization, S.M.; data curation, T.F. and F.P.; writing—review and editing, T.F., F.P., S.M. and C.C.; visualization, A.L..; supervision, S.M., C.C. and A.L.

References

1. American Diabetes Association. 2. Classification and Diagnosis of Diabetes: Standards of Medical Care in Diabetes—2019. *Diabetes Care* **2019**, *42*, S13–S28. [CrossRef] [PubMed]
2. Zhu, Y.; Zhang, C. Prevalence of Gestational Diabetes and Risk of Progression to Type 2 Diabetes: A Global Perspective. *Curr. Diabetes Rep.* **2016**, *16*, 7. [CrossRef] [PubMed]
3. Baz, B.; Riveline, J.P.; Gautier, J.F. Endocrinology of Pregnancy: Gestational diabetes mellitus: Definition, aetiological and clinical aspects. *Eur. J. Endocrinol.* **2016**, *174*, R43–R51. [CrossRef] [PubMed]
4. Catalano, P.M.; Tyzbir, E.D.; Wolfe, R.R.; Calles, J.; Roman, N.M.; Amini, S.B.; Sims, E.A. Carbohydrate metabolism during pregnancy in control subjects and women with gestational diabetes. *Am. J. Physiol.* **1993**, *264*, E60–E67. [CrossRef] [PubMed]
5. Lowe, L.P.; Metzger, B.E.; Lowe, W.L., Jr.; Dyer, A.R.; McDade, T.W.; McIntyre, H.D.; HAPO Study Cooperative Research Group. Inflammatory mediators and glucose in pregnancy: Results from a subset of the Hyperglycemia and Adverse Pregnancy Outcome (HAPO) Study. *J. Clin. Endocrinol. Metab.* **2010**, *95*, 5427–5434. [CrossRef] [PubMed]
6. Hedderson, M.; Ehrlich, S.; Sridhar, S.; Darbinian, J.; Moore, S.; Ferrara, A. Racial/ethnic disparities in the prevalence of gestational diabetes mellitus by BMI. *Diabetes Care* **2012**, *35*, 1492–1498. [CrossRef] [PubMed]
7. Filardi, T.; Tavaglione, F.; Di Stasio, M.; Fazio, V.; Lenzi, A.; Morano, S. Impact of risk factors for gestational diabetes (GDM) on pregnancy outcomes in women with GDM. *J. Endocrinol. Investig.* **2018**, *41*, 671–676. [CrossRef] [PubMed]
8. Pintaudi, B.; Fresa, R.; Dalfra, M.; Dodesini, A.R.; Vitacolonna, E.; Tumminia, A.; Sciacca, L.; Lencioni, C.; Marcone, T.; Lucisano, G.; et al. The risk stratification of adverse neonatal outcomes in women with gestational diabetes (STRONG) study. *Acta Diabetol.* **2018**, *55*, 1261–1273. [CrossRef] [PubMed]
9. Xiang, A.H.; Li, B.H.; Black, M.H.; Sacks, D.A.; Buchanan, T.A.; Jacobsen, S.J.; Lawrence, J.M. Racial and ethnic disparities in diabetes risk after gestational diabetes mellitus. *Diabetologia* **2011**, *54*, 3016–3021. [CrossRef] [PubMed]

10. Kelstrup, L.; Damm, P.; Mathiesen, E.R.; Hansen, T.; Vaag, A.A.; Pedersen, O.; Clausen, T.D. Insulin resistance and impaired pancreatic beta-cell function in adult offspring of women with diabetes in pregnancy. *J. Clin. Endocrinol. Metab.* **2013**, *98*, 3793–3801. [CrossRef]
11. International Association of Diabetes; Pregnancy Study Groups Consensus; Metzger, B.E.; Gabbe, S.G.; Persson, B.; Buchanan, T.A.; Catalano, P.A.; Damm, P.; Dyer, A.R.; Leiva, A.; et al. International association of diabetes and pregnancy study groups recommendations on the diagnosis and classification of hyperglycemia in pregnancy. *Diabetes Care* **2010**, *33*, 676–682. [CrossRef] [PubMed]
12. Group, H.S.C.R.; Metzger, B.E.; Lowe, L.P.; Dyer, A.R.; Trimble, E.R.; Chaovarindr, U.; Coustan, D.R.; Hadden, D.R.; McCance, D.R.; Hod, M.; et al. Hyperglycemia and adverse pregnancy outcomes. *N. Engl. J. Med.* **2008**, *358*, 1991–2002. [CrossRef]
13. Crowther, C.A.; Alsweiler, J.M.; Hughes, R.; Brown, J.; Target Study, G. Tight or less tight glycaemic targets for women with gestational diabetes mellitus for reducing maternal and perinatal morbidity? (TARGET): Study protocol for a stepped wedge randomised trial. *BMC Pregnancy Childbirth* **2018**, *18*, 425. [CrossRef] [PubMed]
14. American Diabetes Association. 14. Management of Diabetes in Pregnancy: Standards of Medical Care in Diabetes—2019. *Diabetes Care* **2019**, *42*, S165–S172. [CrossRef] [PubMed]
15. Santangelo, C.; Zicari, A.; Mandosi, E.; Scazzocchio, B.; Mari, E.; Morano, S.; Masella, R. Could gestational diabetes mellitus be managed through dietary bioactive compounds? Current knowledge and future perspectives. *Br. J. Nutr.* **2016**, *115*, 1129–1144. [CrossRef] [PubMed]
16. Mousa, A.; Naqash, A.; Lim, S. Macronutrient and Micronutrient Intake during Pregnancy: An Overview of Recent Evidence. *Nutrients* **2019**, *11*, 443. [CrossRef] [PubMed]
17. Kramer, M.S.; Kakuma, R. Energy and protein intake in pregnancy. *Cochrane Database Syst. Rev.* **2003**. [CrossRef]
18. Cheung, N.W. The management of gestational diabetes. *Vasc. Health Risk Manag.* **2009**, *5*, 153–164. [CrossRef]
19. Reader, D.M. Medical nutrition therapy and lifestyle interventions. *Diabetes Care* **2007**, *30* (Suppl. 2), S188–S193. [CrossRef]
20. Jovanovic-Peterson, L.; Peterson, C.M. Dietary manipulation as a primary treatment strategy for pregnancies complicated by diabetes. *J. Am. Coll. Nutr.* **1990**, *9*, 320–325. [CrossRef]
21. Augustin, L.S.; Kendall, C.W.; Jenkins, D.J.; Willett, W.C.; Astrup, A.; Barclay, A.W.; Bjorck, I.; Brand-Miller, J.C.; Brighenti, F.; Buyken, A.E.; et al. Glycemic index, glycemic load and glycemic response: An International Scientific Consensus Summit from the International Carbohydrate Quality Consortium (ICQC). *Nutr. Metab. Cardiovasc. Dis.* **2015**, *25*, 795–815. [CrossRef] [PubMed]
22. Brouns, F.; Bjorck, I.; Frayn, K.N.; Gibbs, A.L.; Lang, V.; Slama, G.; Wolever, T.M. Glycaemic index methodology. *Nutr. Res. Rev.* **2005**, *18*, 145–171. [CrossRef] [PubMed]
23. Ludwig, D.S.; Hu, F.B.; Tappy, L.; Brand-Miller, J. Dietary carbohydrates: Role of quality and quantity in chronic disease. *BMJ* **2018**, *361*, k2340. [CrossRef] [PubMed]
24. Jenkins, D.J.; Wolever, T.M.; Taylor, R.H.; Barker, H.; Fielden, H.; Baldwin, J.M.; Bowling, A.C.; Newman, H.C.; Jenkins, A.L.; Goff, D.V. Glycemic index of foods: A physiological basis for carbohydrate exchange. *Am. J. Clin. Nutr.* **1981**, *34*, 362–366. [CrossRef] [PubMed]
25. International Organization for Standardization. Food Products—Determination of the Glycaemic Index (GI) and Recommendation for Food Classification: ISO 26642. Available online: https://www.iso.org/standard/43633.html (accessed on 25 June 2019).
26. Atkinson, F.S.; Foster-Powell, K.; Brand-Miller, J.C. International tables of glycemic index and glycemic load values: 2008. *Diabetes Care* **2008**, *31*, 2281–2283. [CrossRef] [PubMed]
27. Aziz, A. The glycemic index: Methodological aspects related to the interpretation of health effects and to regulatory labeling. *J. AOAC Int.* **2009**, *92*, 879–887. [PubMed]
28. Slabber, M.; Barnard, H.C.; Kuyl, J.M.; Dannhauser, A.; Schall, R. Effects of a low-insulin-response, energy-restricted diet on weight loss and plasma insulin concentrations in hyperinsulinemic obese females. *Am. J. Clin. Nutr.* **1994**, *60*, 48–53. [CrossRef]

29. Barclay, A.W.; Petocz, P.; McMillan-Price, J.; Flood, V.M.; Prvan, T.; Mitchell, P.; Brand-Miller, J.C. Glycemic index, glycemic load, and chronic disease risk—A meta-analysis of observational studies. *Am. J. Clin. Nutr.* **2008**, *87*, 627–637. [CrossRef]
30. Choi, Y.; Giovannucci, E.; Lee, J.E. Glycaemic index and glycaemic load in relation to risk of diabetes-related cancers: A meta-analysis. *Br. J. Nutr.* **2012**, *108*, 1934–1947. [CrossRef]
31. Ma, X.Y.; Liu, J.P.; Song, Z.Y. Glycemic load, glycemic index and risk of cardiovascular diseases: Meta-analyses of prospective studies. *Atherosclerosis* **2012**, *223*, 491–496. [CrossRef]
32. Brand-Miller, J.; Hayne, S.; Petocz, P.; Colagiuri, S. Low-glycemic index diets in the management of diabetes: A meta-analysis of randomized controlled trials. *Diabetes Care* **2003**, *26*, 2261–2267. [CrossRef] [PubMed]
33. Goff, L.M.; Cowland, D.E.; Hooper, L.; Frost, G.S. Low glycaemic index diets and blood lipids: A systematic review and meta-analysis of randomised controlled trials. *Nutr. Metab. Cardiovasc. Dis.* **2013**, *23*, 1–10. [CrossRef] [PubMed]
34. Jenkins, D.J.; Kendall, C.W.; McKeown-Eyssen, G.; Josse, R.G.; Silverberg, J.; Booth, G.L.; Vidgen, E.; Josse, A.R.; Nguyen, T.H.; Corrigan, S.; et al. Effect of a low-glycemic index or a high-cereal fiber diet on type 2 diabetes: A randomized trial. *JAMA* **2008**, *300*, 2742–2753. [CrossRef] [PubMed]
35. Walsh, J.M.; McGowan, C.A.; Mahony, R.; Foley, M.E.; McAuliffe, F.M. Low glycaemic index diet in pregnancy to prevent macrosomia (ROLO study): Randomised control trial. *BMJ* **2012**, *345*, e5605. [CrossRef] [PubMed]
36. Walsh, J.M.; Mahony, R.M.; Culliton, M.; Foley, M.E.; McAuliffe, F.M. Impact of a low glycemic index diet in pregnancy on markers of maternal and fetal metabolism and inflammation. *Reprod. Sci.* **2014**, *21*, 1378–1381. [CrossRef] [PubMed]
37. Horan, M.K.; McGowan, C.A.; Gibney, E.R.; Donnelly, J.M.; McAuliffe, F.M. Maternal low glycaemic index diet, fat intake and postprandial glucose influences neonatal adiposity—Secondary analysis from the ROLO study. *Nutr. J.* **2014**, *13*, 78. [CrossRef] [PubMed]
38. Kizirian, N.V.; Kong, Y.; Muirhead, R.; Brodie, S.; Garnett, S.P.; Petocz, P.; Sim, K.A.; Celermajer, D.S.; Louie, J.C.; Markovic, T.P.; et al. Effects of a low-glycemic index diet during pregnancy on offspring growth, body composition, and vascular health: A pilot randomized controlled trial. *Am. J. Clin. Nutr.* **2016**, *103*, 1073–1082. [CrossRef] [PubMed]
39. Zhang, R.; Han, S.; Chen, G.C.; Li, Z.N.; Silva-Zolezzi, I.; Pares, G.V.; Wang, Y.; Qin, L.Q. Effects of low-glycemic-index diets in pregnancy on maternal and newborn outcomes in pregnant women: A meta-analysis of randomized controlled trials. *Eur. J. Nutr.* **2018**, *57*, 167–177. [CrossRef]
40. Looman, M.; Schoenaker, D.; Soedamah-Muthu, S.S.; Geelen, A.; Feskens, E.J.M.; Mishra, G.D. Pre-pregnancy dietary carbohydrate quantity and quality, and risk of developing gestational diabetes: The Australian Longitudinal Study on Women's Health. *Br. J. Nutr.* **2018**, *120*, 435–444. [CrossRef]
41. Moses, R.G.; Barker, M.; Winter, M.; Petocz, P.; Brand-Miller, J.C. Can a low-glycemic index diet reduce the need for insulin in gestational diabetes mellitus? A randomized trial. *Diabetes Care* **2009**, *32*, 996–1000. [CrossRef]
42. Hu, Z.G.; Tan, R.S.; Jin, D.; Li, W.; Zhou, X.Y. A low glycemic index staple diet reduces postprandial glucose values in Asian women with gestational diabetes mellitus. *J. Investig. Med.* **2014**, *62*, 975–979. [CrossRef] [PubMed]
43. Ma, W.J.; Huang, Z.H.; Huang, B.X.; Qi, B.H.; Zhang, Y.J.; Xiao, B.X.; Li, Y.H.; Chen, L.; Zhu, H.L. Intensive low-glycaemic-load dietary intervention for the management of glycaemia and serum lipids among women with gestational diabetes: A randomized control trial. *Public Health Nutr.* **2015**, *18*, 1506–1513. [CrossRef] [PubMed]
44. Louie, J.C.; Markovic, T.P.; Perera, N.; Foote, D.; Petocz, P.; Ross, G.P.; Brand-Miller, J.C. A randomized controlled trial investigating the effects of a low-glycemic index diet on pregnancy outcomes in gestational diabetes mellitus. *Diabetes Care* **2011**, *34*, 2341–2346. [CrossRef] [PubMed]
45. Louie, J.C.; Markovic, T.P.; Ross, G.P.; Foote, D.; Brand-Miller, J.C. Effect of a low glycaemic index diet in gestational diabetes mellitus on post-natal outcomes after 3 months of birth: A pilot follow-up study. *Matern. Child Nutr.* **2015**, *11*, 409–414. [CrossRef] [PubMed]

46. Viana, L.V.; Gross, J.L.; Azevedo, M.J. Dietary intervention in patients with gestational diabetes mellitus: A systematic review and meta-analysis of randomized clinical trials on maternal and newborn outcomes. *Diabetes Care* **2014**, *37*, 3345–3355. [CrossRef] [PubMed]
47. Wei, J.; Heng, W.; Gao, J. Effects of Low Glycemic Index Diets on Gestational Diabetes Mellitus: A Meta-Analysis of Randomized Controlled Clinical Trials. *Medicine* **2016**, *95*, e3792. [CrossRef] [PubMed]
48. Xu, J.; Ye, S. Influence of low-glycemic index diet for gestational diabetes: A meta-analysis of randomized controlled trials. *J. Matern. Fetal Neonatal Med.* **2018**, *31*, 1–6. [CrossRef]
49. Shyam, S.; Arshad, F.; Abdul Ghani, R.; Wahab, N.A.; Safii, N.S.; Nisak, M.Y.; Chinna, K.; Kamaruddin, N.A. Low glycaemic index diets improve glucose tolerance and body weight in women with previous history of gestational diabetes: A six months randomized trial. *Nutr. J.* **2013**, *12*, 68. [CrossRef]
50. Ghani, R.A.; Shyam, S.; Arshad, F.; Wahab, N.A.; Chinna, K.; Safii, N.S.; Nisak, M.Y.; Kamaruddin, N.A. The influence of fasting insulin level in post-gestational diabetes mellitus women receiving low-glycaemic-index diets. *Nutr. Diabetes* **2014**, *4*, e107. [CrossRef]

5

The Role of Dietary Carbohydrates in Gestational Diabetes

Vikkie A. Mustad [1], Dieu T.T. Huynh [2], José M. López-Pedrosa [3], Cristina Campoy [4,5] and Ricardo Rueda [3,*]

1 R&D Department, Abbott Nutrition, Columbus, OH 43219, USA; vikkie.mustad@abbott.com
2 R&D Department, Abbott Nutrition, Singapore 138668, Singapore; dieu.huynh@abbott.com
3 R&D Department, Abbott Nutrition, 18004 Granada, Spain; jose.m.lopez@abbott.com
4 Department of Paediatrics, University of Granada, 18071 Granada, Spain; ccampoy@ugr.es
5 EURISTIKOS Excellence Centre for Paediatric Research, University of Granada, 18071 Granada, Spain
* Correspondence: ricardo.rueda@abbott.com

Abstract: Gestational diabetes (GDM) is hyperglycemia that is recognized for the first time during pregnancy. GDM is associated with a wide range of short- and long-term adverse health consequences for both mother and offspring. It is a complex disease with a multifactorial etiology, with disturbances in glucose, lipid, inflammation and gut microbiota. Consequently, its management is complex, requiring patients to self-manage their diet, lifestyle and self-care behaviors in combination with use of insulin. In addition to nutritional recommendations for all pregnant women, special attention to dietary carbohydrate (CHO) amount and type on glucose levels is especially important in GDM. Dietary CHO are diverse, ranging from simple sugars to longer-chain oligo- and poly- saccharides which have diverse effects on blood glucose, microbial fermentation and bowel function. Studies have established that dietary CHO amount and type can impact maternal glucose and nutritional recommendations advise women with GDM to limit total intake or choose complex and low glycemic CHO. However, robust maternal and infant benefits are not consistently shown. Novel approaches which help women with GDM adhere to dietary recommendations such as diabetes-specific meal replacements (which provide a defined and complete nutritional composition with slowly-digested CHO) and continuous glucose monitors (which provide unlimited monitoring of maternal glycemic fluctuations) have shown benefits on both maternal and neonatal outcomes. Continued research is needed to understand and develop tools to facilitate patient adherence to treatment goals, individualize interventions and improve outcomes.

Keywords: gestational diabetes mellitus; pregnancy; dietary carbohydrates; diabetes-specific formula; continuous glucose monitoring

1. Introduction

Gestational diabetes (GDM) is one of the most common adverse medical conditions of pregnancy, and its prevalence is rising as part of the global diabetes pandemic, both in developed and developing countries. GDM is complex and multifactorial, with several aspects contributing to explain its pathophysiology, although this is not fully clarified yet.

Nutrition in general and some particular nutritional compounds, such as carbohydrates (CHO) and fiber, contribute to regulate glycemic index and glycemic response, and consequently can influence establishment and evolution of gestational diabetes during pregnancy as well as risk of clinical outcomes both in the mother and the infant. Consequently, nutrition may be a key tool for prevention and management of gestational diabetes.

After a brief overview of the prevalence, short- and long-term health consequences and pathophysiology of GDM, this review will focus on what is known about the role of dietary carbohydrates in its prevention and treatment. Nutrition recommendations from professional health groups will be summarized, with a focus on the specific research on dietary carbohydrate quantity and quality that informs the basis for carbohydrate recommendations. Finally, the use of novel approaches such as specialized nutritional supplements and continuous glucose monitoring to help patients adhere to treatment goals will be discussed.

2. Background

2.1. *Prevalence Worldwide and the Trends over the Past Decade*

Gestational diabetes (GDM) is hyperglycemia that is recognized for the first time during pregnancy. It encompasses undiagnosed type 2 diabetes and hyperglycemia which develops later in pregnancy [1]. It is one of the most common adverse medical conditions of pregnancy, and its prevalence is rising as part of the global diabetes pandemic. It is estimated that GDM affects around 21.3 million or one in six live births in 2017 [2]. Studies have shown that GDM increases with a faster rate in lower- and middle-income countries than high-income countries, especially over the past decade [1–3]. Yan et al. reported the GDM prevalence increased from 15.5% to 19.9% from 2012 to 2017 in Xiamen, China [1]. Lavery et al. reported about 5.5% increase in GDM prevalence in the USA over a 20-year period from 1990 to 2010 [3]. A study in Spain examining the trend of GDM prevalence showed an increase of 4.8% over a period of 9 years from 2006 to 2015 [4]. According to the International Diabetes Federation, South East Asia had the highest prevalence of GDM with 26.6% followed by Middle East/North Africa (18%), Europe (14%) and Africa (9.5%) [2]. Because of significant health and economic burdens, the increasing prevalence of GDM in most populations has become a global health challenge, especially in low- and middle-income countries.

2.2. *Short- and Long-Term Health Consequences for Mothers and Offspring*

In the short-term, GDM increases pregnancy and birth complications. Women with GDM are more likely to develop gestational hypertension and preeclampsia. A population-based retrospective cohort including 426,296 deliveries over a 10-year period reported a 90% higher risk of preeclampsia in women with GDM than those without GDM [5]. Pre-pregnancy obesity, excessive gestational weight gain and poor glycemic control are linked with greater risk of gestational hypertension and pre-eclampsia in women with GDM [6]. GDM is considered an independent risk factor for newborn large for gestational age (LGA) and macrosomia. A meta-analysis reported the pooled odds ratio of macrosomia was 5.5 folds higher in women with GDM than those without GDM [7]. Additionally, the risk for LGA increases as fasting and two-hour post-oral glucose tolerance test (OGTT) glucose increase during pregnancy. Farrar et al. studied the association between blood glucose and perinatal outcomes in a meta-analysis involving up to 207,172 women [8]. They found that the odds ratios for LGA per 18 mg/dL increase in fasting and two-hour post-OGTT glucose concentrations were 2.15 (95% confidence interval 1.60 to 2.91) and 1.20 (1.13 to 1.28), respectively. Infants born LGA and with macrosomia increased instrumental delivery, caesarean section, premature birth and shoulder dystocia [8,9]. Such pregnancy and neonatal complications were associated with delayed initiation of breastfeeding, lower rates of breastfeeding and breastfeeding duration in women with GDM [10,11]. Because breastfeeding has been shown to be a protective factor for the development of T2DM in GDM mothers and in their offspring [12,13], suboptimal breastfeeding has an implication in future health risk for both mother and child.

Additionally, these pregnancies and neonatal complications impose substantial economic burdens. A burden-of-illness study on GDM conducted in China has shown that the cost of a pregnancy with GDM was 95% more than for a pregnancy without GDM, due to additional expenses for GDM diagnosis and management, and for mother and neonatal complications. With a number around

2.9 million pregnancies affected by GDM in 2015, the estimated annual economic burden of GDM was an international $5.59 billion from incremental direct medical costs [14].

In the long-term, GDM increases the risk—in both mother and offspring—of type 2 diabetes, metabolic syndrome and obesity. In their systematic review, Hopmans et al. [15] showed that the increased risk of type 2 diabetes and cardiovascular disease was 13 times and two times higher, respectively, in women with GDM when compared with healthy control [15]. In a recent meta-analysis, Kramer et al. investigated the association between GDM and long-term cardiovascular disease in 5,390,591 women. They found that GDM was associated with a 2.3-fold increased risk of cardiovascular events in the first decade postpartum when compared with women without GDM [16].

In children, intrauterine exposure to GDM increases the risk for overweight/obesity and abnormal glucose tolerance. A total of 26,509 children born to mothers with and without GDM were included in a meta-analysis to investigate the association of maternal hyperglycemia exposure during pregnancy with obesity and abnormal glucose tolerance in offspring [17]. The rate of obesity or overweight in children aged 2–17 years was 1.35 times higher in the offspring of GDM mothers. This increased risk was highest in the age group of 11 years and above [17]. Additionally, the children of women with GDM had higher two-hour plasma glucose through early adulthood (pooled MD: 0.43 mmol/L, 95% CI: 0.18–0.69), [17]. Another study reported a four-fold increased risk for metabolic syndrome in children from GDM mothers, with the risk increasing significantly with increasing maternal fasting and two-hour blood glucose [18]. Overwhelmingly, GDM has significant and adverse implications on the future burden of non-communicable diseases in both mother and offspring.

3. Key Aspects of GDM Pathophysiology

GDM is a complex disease with a multifactorial etiology; however, the exact mechanisms involved in its pathophysiology are not fully clarified [19]. The purpose of this section is to review the key aspects implicated in its onset and recent advances regarding GDM.

3.1. Glucose and Lipid Metabolism

During normal pregnancy, the body undergoes numerous metabolic and immunological changes that are designed to maintain maternal and fetal health. One of the major metabolic changes is related to glucose metabolism [20]. Glucose metabolism changes according to the course of pregnancy and fetal needs. At first, fasting glucose levels drop, likely due to both increased maternal blood volume and the fetal use. To adjust to this physiological change, pancreatic β cells suffer hyperplasia and hypertrophy to increase insulin secretion, maintaining maternal euglycemic state and preserving the embryo [19]. Another common change that occurs during normal pregnancy is a reduction of insulin sensitivity and an increase of insulin resistance. This is normally seen in normal pregnancies, presumably to spare the glucose for the fetus, and can be attributed to the production of placental hormones such as estrogens, progesterone, placental lactogen, placental growth hormone, leptin and cortisol and may be intensified by genetic susceptibility and/or mother's lifestyle [21].

Exacerbated peripheral insulin resistance during pregnancy and poor β-cell adaptation likely contribute to GDM. Decreased insulin-stimulated glucose disposal by 22% has been observed in GDM when compared with normal pregnancy [22]. As compared to normal pregnancy, impaired skeletal muscle glucose uptake in women with GDM is usually explained by the failure of insulin signaling, due to an additional decrease in tyrosine phosphorylation of the insulin receptor, which inhibits insulin signaling from activating GLUT4 translocation. Decreased insulin-stimulated glucose uptake can trigger failure of the β-cell and hyperglycemia in GDM [23]. Indeed, β-cell failure or insufficiency were described by Buchanan et al. [24], showing that insulin secretion increases throughout pregnancy in both women with and without GDM, but beginning at a lower starting point in women with GDM.

Along with changes in insulin resistance and the subsequent response of pancreatic β-cells, hepatic glucose production is also significantly altered in women with GDM. Basal endogenous glucose production increases in a similar way in women with and without GDM [22]. However, in late gestation the ability of insulin to suppress gluconeogenesis was lower in GDM as compared to the normal pregnant women.

Major changes in lipid metabolism also occur during pregnancy [25]. In the mother, during the early stage of pregnancy there is an increase in the fat depot accumulation as result of increased lipid synthesis and hyperphagia. During this period, these lipidic disturbances are caused by enhanced adipose insulin responsiveness that facilitates the accumulation of circulating lipids in the adipose tissue. However, in late gestation, and as consequence of the insulin resistant condition, adipose lipolytic activity is increased with a parallel reduction in the lipoprotein lipase activity and fatty acid synthesis in the adipose tissue. These changes determine the development of maternal hypertriglyceridemia in normal pregnancy [26]. In GDM, the pronounced peripheral resistance and inadequate β-cell function cause these alterations to be exacerbated, resulting in enhanced lipolysis and ketogenesis. Under these circumstances, the dyslipidemia in diabetic pregnancy compared with normal pregnancy actively contributes to the chronic maternal insulin resistance and increases the exposure of lipids to the fetus, contributing to fat accumulation, macrosomia and LGA. Enhanced levels of small size and dense LDL particles have been consistently found in GDM [27] regardless the circulating concentrations of LDL-cholesterol [28].

3.2. *Inflammation*

A tightly-regulated balance between pro- and anti-inflammatory cytokines is believed to be necessary for normal implantation, trophoblast invasion and placentation [29]. In early and late-pregnancy, elevated secretion of pro-inflammatory cytokines (TNF- α and Interleukin (IL)-6) and reduced levels of anti-inflammatory cytokines (Il-10 and IL-4) are observed in women developing GDM [30], suggesting that inflammation may be involved in the development of insulin resistance associated with GDM. Pro-inflammatory cytokines can alter the insulin signaling pathway by dampening insulin receptor (IR) tyrosine kinase activity, amplifying serine phosphorylation of IRS-1, or by altering the STAT3-SOCS3 pathway. In a study by Kirwan et al., 2002 [31] and corroborated by Catalano and coworkers, 2014 [22] they showed that plasma TNF α was the most strongly correlated factor with insulin sensitivity. Similarly, placental gene expression of TNF-α, IL-1β and their receptors have been reported to be increased in GDM. Besides that, in a study published in October 2019 [32], another pro-inflammatory cytokine (IL-34) which operates as a ligand for colony-stimulating factor-1 receptor (CSF-1R) was discovered to contribute to the apoptosis of pancreatic β cells, playing a crucial role in the development of GDM [32].

3.3. *Gut Microbiota*

The normal gut microbiota composition appears to undergo important shifts during normal pregnancy. In late pregnancy, the gut microbiota pattern resembles the disruptive gut microbiota composition to that of adults with type 2 diabetes [33]. Individuals with insulin resistance show significant changes in the *Firmicutes/Bacteroidetes* ratio, with a reduction in butyrate-producing bacteria compared to healthy individuals [34]. Fugmann et al. (2015) [35] analyzed stool microbiota both in insulin resistant women with a recent history of GDM and women after a normoglycemic pregnancy. They found that women with a *Prevotellaceae*-dominated intestinal microbiome were overrepresented in the GDM group. Similarly, Bassols et al. (2012) [36] extracted and analyzed microbial DNA and RNA from the appendix contents of eight insulin resistant and eight insulin-sensitive obese subjects. They concluded that gut RNA microbial profile varies in accordance with insulin action. Recently, Crusell et al. (2018) [33] showed that gut microbiota of women with GDM are distinct from microbiota changes of normal pregnant women, including phylum and genus levels. In this study, there was a difference in the abundance of 17 species level operational taxonomic units (OTUs) in GDM compared with the normoglycemic pregnant women. Although different studies report the link between the gut microbial profile and insulin resistance, the potential pathophysiological role of gut bacteria in GDM remains still unknown.

4. Role of Dietary Carbohydrates in GDM

Dietary carbohydrates (CHO) are an important energy source for both mother and fetus, and all pregnant women need at least 175 g of CHO, including 28 g of fiber per day [37]. However, for women with GDM, there is an additional need to pay careful attention to amount and type of CHO as it is well-established that dietary CHO have the greatest impact on blood glucose. Dietary CHO are diverse in structure with variable effects on blood glucose responses and other physiological outcomes [38]. Many dietary CHO (glucose, sucrose, cooked starches found in pastas, potatoes, white bread) are readily digested and absorbed in the small intestines, and these contribute to a rapid increase in blood glucose. Some dietary CHO have a structure that makes them resistant to digestion—or completely non-digested—and these result in a small and/or slower increase in blood glucose (e.g., low glycemic index, LGI). Components of CHO that are not digested (fiber) pass through the small and large intestine where they can provide important physiological benefits such as stimulate incretin production, serve as an energy source for colonic microbiota, and promote normal bowel movements.

Early studies established that elevated postprandial glucose responses contribute to an increased glucose transport to the fetus and hyperglycemia correlates significantly with infant size and/or adiposity [39,40]. Studies also have established that maternal glucose responses can be markedly influenced by the total amount of CHO [39,41,42] or the type of CHO [43] consumed. Evidence from preclinical studies [44,45] using animals models of gestational diabetes shows that negative effects of feeding high-GI sucrose and maltodextrin on the pathophysiology of GDM in dams and their offspring can be reversed by substituting these rapidly-metabolized CHO with more slowly-digesting CHO (i.e., isomaltulose and resistant maltodextrins). As a result, in order to improve maternal fasting and postprandial glucose during GDM, current dietary guidelines recommend either to restrict CHO intake or to replace high glycemic/rapidly-digesting (HGI) CHO with those that are more slowly digesting (Table 1).

However, as commented in numerous publications [46–49], these dietary recommendations are limited by the lack of robust evidence. Randomized nutritional intervention trials that have evaluated dietary strategies focusing on CHO in women with [50–58] or at risk of [59–62] GDM have not shown consistent benefits on maternal or infant outcomes. The details of the studies, their dietary interventions and outcomes have been critically reviewed in other recent publications [46–49]. Overall, it is widely viewed that these studies suffer from small sample size and thus are underpowered and observed benefits on LGA or other infant and maternal outcomes are not consistent across studies. The most current Cochrane analysis [63] did not show significant maternal and/or infant benefits; in contrast, Yamamoto et al. [64] focused their primary analysis on maternal glycemic outcomes and concluded that interventions that improved maternal glycemic control would improve infant birthweight outcomes. In agreement was another meta-analysis by Wan et al. [65] who focused their meta-analysis on dietary intervention strategies to include all Chinese-language studies. Their conclusion was that CHO-modified diets were associated with improved glycemic control and infant birth outcomes in ethnic Chinese women with GDM.

Table 1. Nutrition Recommendations for gestational diabetes mellitus (GDM).

Organization	General Recommendation for GDM	Carbohydrate-Specific Recommendations	Reference/Link
International Federation of Gynecology and Obstetrics	Caloric intake should be calculated based on pre-pregnancy BMI and desirable weight gain; Caloric intake may be reduced by 30%, but not below 1600–1800 kcal/d; for women with diabetic nephropathy, protein may be lowered to 0.6–0.8 g/kg ideal body weight.	Carbohydrate intake should be limited to 35%–45% of total calories, with a minimum of 175 g CHO per day, distributed in three small-to-moderate sized meals and 2–4 snacks.	*M. Hod* et al./*International Journal of Gynecology and Obstetrics 131 S3 (2015) S173–S211*
Endocrine Society	Medical nutrition therapy is recommended for all pregnant women with overt or gestational diabetes to help achieve and maintain desired glycemic control while providing essential nutrient requirements.	Carbohydrate should be limited to 35% to 45% of total calories, distributed in 3 small-to-moderate-sized meals and 2 to 4 snacks including an evening snack	Blumer I., Hadar E., Haddan DR., et al., Diabetes and Pregnancy: An Endocrine Society Clinical Practice Guideline. J Clin Endo Metab 2013:98:4227–4249.
American College of Obstetrics and Gynecologists	Eat regular meals throughout the day; three meals and two–three snacks per day. Gain healthy amount of weight.	Complex CHO are recommended over simple CHO because they are digested more slowly, are less likely to produce significant postprandial hyperglycemia, and potentially reduce insulin resistance.	Obstetrics & Gynecology. 131(2):e49–e64, FEBRUARY 2018 OI: 10.1097/AOG.0000000000002501 PMID: 29370047 Issn Print: 0029–7844 Publication Date: February 2018
National Institute for Health and Care Excellence (NICE) guidelines	Advise women to eat a healthy diet during pregnancy, refer all women with gestational diabetes to a dietitian.	Foods with a low glycemic index should replace those with a high glycemic index.	NICE National Institute for Health and Care Excellence Guideline. Diabetes in pregnancy: Management from preconception to the postnatal period. Published: 25 February 2015 www.nice.org.uk/guidance/ng3
Diabetes Canada	Meal planning for women with GDM should emphasize a healthy diet during pregnancy.	Women should consume a minimum of 175 g/day of CHO, distributed over 3 moderate-sized meals and 2 or more snacks (1 of which should be at bedtime), replacing high-GI foods with low-GI ones.	*Feig DS, Berger H., Donovan L., et al., Diabetes and Pregnancy. Diabetes Canada 2018. Clinical Practice Guidelines for the Prevention and Management of Diabetes in Canada: Pharmacologic Glycemic Management of Type 2 Diabetes in Adults. Can J Diabetes 2018;42(Suppl 1):S255–S282.*

Table 1. *Cont.*

Organization	General Recommendation for GDM	Carbohydrate-Specific Recommendations	Reference/Link
American Academy of Nutrition and Dietetics	A registered dietitian nutritionist (or international equivalent) should provide Medical Nutrition Therapy that includes an individual nutrition prescription and nutrition counseling for all women diagnosed with GDM.	All pregnant women should eat a minimum of 157 g CHO and 28 g fiber. The amount and type of CHO should be individualized based on nutrition assessment, treatment goals, blood glucose response and patient needs. Three meals and 2 or more snacks helps to distribute CHO intake and reduce postprandial blood glucose elevations.	Duarte Gardea et al., Academy of Nutrition and Dietetics Gestational Diabetes Evidence-Based Nutrition Practice Guideline Journal of the Academy of Nutrition and Dietetics. September 2018 Volume 118, Issue 9, Pages 1719–1742. https://doi.org/10.1016/j.jand.2018.03.014
American Diabetes Association	The food plan should be based on a nutrition assessment with guidance from the Dietary Reference Intakes.	All pregnant women should eat a minimum of 175 g total CHO and 28 g fiber. For women with GDM, the amount and type of CHO will impact glucose levels, especially post-meal excursions.	American Diabetes Association. 14. Management of Diabetes in Pregnancy: Standards of Medical Care in Diabetes. 2019 Diabetes Care 2019;42(Suppl. 1): S165–S172| https://doi.org/10.2337/dc19-S014

Studies have evaluated nutritional interventions for preventing GDM [59–62,66] Most have combined increasing physical activity with energy restriction through reducing on the quantity and/or changing the type of CHO to reduce or slow weight gain during early pregnancy. Studies and their findings are diverse. In the LIMIT trial [59] over 2000 pregnant overweight and obese pregnant women were randomized before 20 weeks of gestation to standard of care or an intensive lifestyle arm including advice to reduce intake of refined CHO. Babies born to women in the intensive lifestyle intervention were significantly less likely to be LGA, have respiratory distress syndrome and had shorter hospital stays. In the GI Baby 3 study of 139 women at high risk of GDM [60], those following low-GI diet advice required less insulin to maintain normoglycemia ($p = 0.007$) compared to a group following a high-GI diet. Walsh et al. [61], in the ROLO study, evaluated 800 women in their second half of pregnancy who were at high risk for GDM having previously delivered an infant weighting greater than 4 kg. Pregnant women who were randomized to receive low-GI diet advice had significantly lower gestational weight gain and less maternal glucose intolerance compared to those following standard of care. However, the incidence of LGA infants was not reduced. The UPBEAT study [0] randomized 1555 obese women to receive a standard of care or an intensive behavioral intervention to increase physical activity and improve diet quality with an emphasis on low-GI foods. Despite improvements in gestational weight gain, the intervention was not associated with additional benefits.

Most recently, Zhang et al., [67] reviewed the effects of low-GI diets in all pregnant women, both those having healthy pregnancies, at risk for GDM, and those with GDM. In a total of 11 trials involving 1985 women, low-GI diets significantly reduced fasting and two-hour postprandial glucose level. Pregnant women following low-GI diet advice had a higher risk of delivery of low for gestational age neonates; however, there were no significant benefits on maternal or newborn outcomes.

Taken together, a low-GI diet during early pregnancy can improve postprandial glucose and weight gain, at least in some studies. However, these interventions are not adequate to prevent GDM or to consistently reduce the incidence of LGA infants. Whether the type of CHO (low-GI or slowly digesting and low-GI) or additional factors are necessary to offset the rapidly changing and complex pathophysiology that occurs during pregnancy are unknown. Additional insight into the role of CHO can be gained from observational studies that have investigated nutritional intakes and/or patterns before or during pregnancy and GDM; these studies [68,69] show GDM is higher in those having higher intakes of meat and a lower intake of whole grain carbohydrates, fruits, vegetables, and fish. These studies suggest that CHO along with other dietary components are likely involved. A high intake of saturated fat can interfere with insulin signaling, and they can also induce inflammation and endothelial dysfunction, both pathogenic factors in GDM. Amino acids can act as substrates for hepatic glucose production and in hepatic lipotoxicity. Although CHO such as fructose found in fruit are lower GI, more slowly digesting CHO such as those found in whole grains can slow sugar absorption, reducing the demand on cells and insulin signaling mediators. In addition, proper intake of micronutrients and polyunsaturated fats, including those derived from fish and seafood, have anti-inflammatory properties consistently associated with a reduced risk of GDM. Another key consideration in all intervention studies is the ability of the women to adopt the intervention. In their systematic review, Lammimpaa and coauthors concluded that variability in the delivery of dietary interventions is a key factor affecting study outcomes in GDM. Thus, additional research on the benefits of dietary CHO, with or without other nutritional factors, should also pay attention to the consistency of its delivery [70].

5. Promising Approaches to Help Patients with GDM Adhere to Dietary Recommendations

GDM is a complex disease requiring patients to self-manage their diet, lifestyle, and self-care behaviors in combination with use of insulin or, in some cases, oral medications such as metformin or glyburide [71]. Trying to engage pregnant women with (or at risk of) GDM to change their diet is especially challenging; although most women are especially attuned to the health of their developing fetus, food cravings, palatability, hunger and time pressure are cited as barriers to adherence to prescribed diets [72].

Meal replacements can be helpful for people not only for being convenient, but also for providing known calorie amounts with specific macro- and micro-nutrient levels that facilitate meal planning.

When used as part of lifestyle intervention in diabetes prevention programs, meal replacements have been shown to promote weight loss and reduction in the incidence of type 2 diabetes in overweight/obese people at increased risk of developing type 2 diabetes [73,74]. There is good evidence that meal replacement as part of a lifestyle intervention is effective in promoting weight loss and improving metabolic outcomes in individuals with type 2 diabetes [75,76] The current diabetes guidelines from the American Diabetes Association [77], the Canadian Diabetes Association [78], and Diabetes UK [79] have recommended the use of meal replacements in the management of individuals with diabetes.

The role of meal replacements in preventing the development of GDM has not been well studied. Given the risk of pregnancy complications such as gestational diabetes, macrosomia and Cesarean delivery, and the risk of adverse metabolic health outcomes associated with excessive gestational weight gain (GWG), recently Phelan et al. [80] conducted an RCT involving 257 overweight and obese pregnant women (mean ± SD: 13.6 ± 1.8 weeks of gestation) to evaluate the effect of a behavioral lifestyle intervention (n = 129) with partial meal replacement in comparison of enhanced usual care (n = 128) on weekly gestational weight gain (GWG) rate, cardiovascular disease risk factors, and incidence of pregnancy complications. Participants in the enhanced usual care group received all aspects of usual care offered by their prenatal care providers. In addition, they were given the general information about healthy eating, physical activity, and the Institute of Medicine (IOM) recommendations for total gestational weight gain at the time of study randomization. The intervention group received all aspects of enhanced usual care plus a behavioral lifestyle intervention designed to prevent excessive weight gain during pregnancy. Each participant received a 20-min individual, face-to-face counseling session with a study interventionist every two weeks until 20 weeks of gestation and then monthly visits until delivery. To promote weight control, they were instructed to replace two meals with the provided meal replacement shakes or bars and to consume ≥ 1 meal of regular foods and 2–4 healthy snacks/day. The meal replacement products included organic and lactose-free drinks and bars in which 80% of the study's meal replacements purchased were for organic meal replacement products high in protein, 15% were for the bar also high in protein; and 4% were for powder meal replacement including a standard oral nutritional supplement (4%) and a diabetes-specific formula (1%). The meal plan using partial meal replacement provided a calorie intake of ~18 kcal/kg body weight at study entry in which 30%, 15%–20% and 50–55% of calories were from fat, protein, and carbohydrates, respectively. The intervention group had significantly lower weekly GWG rates compared with the control group (0.33 vs 0.39 kg/week, respectively, $p = 0.02$). In addition, 43% women in the intervention group were less likely to exceed the (IOM) recommendations for total GWG than were those in the control group (OR: 0.57; 95% CI: 0.34, 0.95; $P = 0.03$). From study entry to 35–36 weeks of gestation, when compared with the enhanced usual care, the intervention significantly reduced triglycerides ($P = 0.03$) and resulted in trend reductions in fasting glucose ($P = 0.09$) and systolic blood pressure ($P = 0.06$). Regardless of group assignment, greater increases in GWG rate were associated with increases in insulin (2.63 μU/mL; 95% CI: 1.63, 4.23 μU/mL; $P < 0.0001$), HOMA-IR (2.84; 95% CI: 1.67, 4.85; $P < 0.0001$), and C-peptide (1.52 ng/mL; 95% CI: 1.15, 2.01 ng/mL; $P < 0.0001$). There were no significant differences between groups in triglycerides, HDL cholesterol, LDL cholesterol, total cholesterol, diastolic blood pressure and systolic blood pressure. The incidence of pregnancy complications was similar between groups. The study has suggested that partial meal replacements as part of a behavioral lifestyle intervention is effective for GWG control in women who are overweight and obese. There is a need for further research on its effectiveness before it could be considered as part of the usual prenatal care for pregnant women with obesity.

5.1. Evidence for the Use of Complete and Balanced Nutritional Supplements Containing Low-Glycemic and Slowly Digested Carbohydrates on GDM Outcomes

Specialized diabetes-specific formulas (DSF) are designed using low glycemic index and slowly digested carbohydrates and monosaturated fatty acids to support glycemic control [81–83]. Systematic reviews and meta-analyses have shown that DSF as part of lifestyle interventions effectively improves glycemic control and reduces cardiometabolic risks [84,85]. The effects of DSF on blood glucose management in women with GDM were investigated in a few studies. Yu et al. [86] conducted a randomized, controlled, unblinded study to investigate the effects of a DSF on postprandial blood glucose and pregnancy outcomes in Chinese women with GDM from October 2011 to January 2012. A total of 69 women diagnosed with GDM around 26 weeks of gestation were randomized to the intervention consisting of individualized dietary recommendations using DSF ($n = 32$) or receiving individualized dietary recommendation only ($n = 31$), as the control group. The DSF was consumed twice daily to replace regular milk during breakfast and a meal. The 2-h postprandial blood glucose was measured weekly over a period of eight weeks from enrollment to the week prior to delivery. When compared with the control group, the intervention group had significantly lower 2-h postprandial blood glucose levels based on the General Linear Model Repeated Measures ($P < 0.01$) and significantly lower HbA1c (5.5% vs. 5.7%; $P < 0.05$). Pregnancy outcomes were found to be in favour of the intervention group in which the intervention had significantly lower incidences of premature rupture of membranes (9.7% vs, 34.5%; $P < 0.05$), polyhydramnios (12.9% vs. 37.9%; $P < 0.05$), and neonatal pneumonia (6.5% vs. 31.0%; $P < 0.05$), and significantly lower birth weight (3346 g vs. 3549 g; $P < 0.05$) [86].

Liu et al. [87] evaluated the effects of a DSF on fasting blood glucose, 2-h postprandial blood glucose, triglycerides and total cholesterol in a 2-week randomized, controlled trial on 40 GDM pregnant women. All participants received individualized dietary counseling in which the total calories were calculated to achieve an ideal body weight with 30–38 kcal/kg body weight. They were instructed to consume six meals a day including three normal meals plus three extra meals to achieve the target calories. For women in the intervention group ($n = 20$), a DSF was given in two extra meals at 9:00 am and 3:00 pm. The calories from two servings of a DSF account for about 25% of total daily calories. Women in the control group ($n = 10$) were instructed to select CHO such as skim milk, fruits and oatmeal as part of a diabetes meal plan. There were no significant differences in 2-h postprandial blood glucose (at 11 am) between the DSF (8.1 ± 0.9 mmol/L) and the control groups (8.4 ± 1.1 mmol/L) at baseline. Both study groups showed a significant reduction in 2-h postprandial glucose levels (at 11 am) from baseline after two weeks of intervention. However, the intervention group achieved a significantly greater improvement compared with the control (6.6 ± 1.5 mmol/L and 7.1 ± 1.3 mmol/L, respectively, between-group $P < 0.05$). Similar findings were observed for 2-h postprandial blood glucose for the extra meal in the afternoon (at 5 pm). No differences in serum triglyceride and total cholesterol concentrations were found after two weeks of intervention [87].

The effects of a DSF on blood glucose control were evaluated in another randomized, controlled trial with nine weeks of intervention involving 70 Chinese GDM pregnant women [88]. Both the intervention ($n = 34$) and the control ($n = 36$) groups received a diabetes diet in which the total daily calories were distributed as follows: 10%, 30%, 30% and 30% for breakfast, lunch, dinner and snacks, respectively. For the intervention group, a DSF was used as a snack replacement. Fasting plasma glucose levels and 2-h postprandial blood glucose levels were measured on a weekly basis over the period of nine weeks. There were some differences in fasting plasma glucose levels and 2-h postprandial blood glucose levels between the groups over a 9-week period. However, it is unclear if the intervention group had better glycemic control because the results of using a statistical test to compare the differences was not mentioned [88].

Overall, there is evidence that use of a DSF as a partial meal or snack replacement in a diabetes meal plan resulted in a greater improvement in glycemic control compared with dietary counseling alone in women with GDM, suggesting it could be an effective treatment for glycemic control in

GDM. There are also preliminary findings suggesting its benefits in reducing pregnancy and birth complications. Further studies are needed to confirm this.

5.2. Application of Continuous Glucose Monitoring to Facilitate Close Monitoring of Diet on Glucose Control

A treatment goal for GDM to reduce maternal and perinatal outcomes is to maintain a fasting glucose concentration of less than 90–95 mg/dL, one hour postprandial glucose level < 140 mg/dL or 2-h postprandial glucose level of < 120 mg/dL) [89]. The most popular method for daily blood glucose control is self-monitoring blood glucose (SMBG), usually by fingerstick blood sampling at defined times. Use of SMBG readings provide a limited number of measurements and insufficient information of the blood sugar level changes. Recent technology, such as continuous glucose monitoring (CGM), is a promising method for improving the glucose profile by giving a more complete view and thus improving patient treatment and quality of life [90].

CGM comprises a subcutaneous glucose-sensing device and an electrode impregnated with glucose oxidase that allows interstitial glucose levels to be measured approximately every ten seconds and an average value is stored in the monitor every five minutes [90,91]. CGM is an effective tool in the management of pregnant women with type 1 diabetes and has been shown to improve neonatal outcomes. Feig et al., 2017 [92], in the multicenter, open-label, randomized controlled trial LANCET study, examined the effectiveness CGM on maternal glucose control and obstetric and neonatal health outcomes (n = 325 women). The authors concluded that the use of CGM during pregnancy is associated with improved neonatal outcomes, which are likely to be attributed to reduced exposure to maternal hyperglycemia.

Additional benefits of CGM include the ability to improve screening protocol [90]. Importantly, the ability to understand normoglycemia and its patterns of variation in nondiabetic pregnant women across the day can allow for future individualized therapies in these patients [93]. Yu et al., 2014 [94] in a prospective cohort study evaluated the effectiveness of CGM on maternal glycemic control and pregnancy outcome in 340 patients with GDM. Patients were allocated in two groups, 190 receiving a routine care self-monitoring of blood glucose (SMBG) and other 150 following the CGM. They concluded that the use of supplementary CGM can improve the glycemic variability and pregnancy outcomes in patients with GDM.

In the last decade, some studies used the CGM technology to facilitate close monitoring of diet on glucose control. Hernandez et al., 2014 [53], in a randomized crossover study, compared two different types of diets (one higher in complex CHO/lower fat and other one lower-CHO/higher fat) using CGM for 72 h to obtain glucose profiles in 16 GDM women. These data show that a diet high in complex CHO and reduced fat still achieved glycemia below current treatment targets and lower postprandial free fat acids. Subsequently, Carreiro et al., 2016 [95] used CGM to more accurately assess the impact of dietary recommendations on women suffering from gestational diabetes and they concluded that dietary counseling was able to keep glucose levels close to those of healthy patients. In a prospective observational study with GDM patients two methods to evaluate glucose readings, CGM and self-monitor blood sugar glucose (SMBG), during Ramadan fasting were compared [96]. They concluded that CGM was effective to detect more hypoglycemia than SMBG in GDM patients.

Although limited, studies have shown that CGM systems have the potential to help the patient and their health care providers manage their day-to-day diet, lifestyle, self-care and medication decisions to achieve treatment goals. However, more research is needed to understand its full potential on both mother and infant outcomes.

6. Conclusions

Nutrition is critical to the prevention and treatment of GDM for the health and well-being of both mother and offspring. Close attention to the amount and type of dietary CHO can have important benefits on GDM pathophysiology, but interventions as currently implemented may not be adequate to prevent or treat this complex disease. Continued research is needed to develop tools to facilitate patient adherence to treatment goals, individualize interventions and improve the results.

Author Contributions: All authors (V.A.M., D.T.T.H., J.M.L.-P., C.C., and R.R.) contributed to the drafting, editing and revision of this review. All authors have approved the submitted version and agree to be personally accountable for its accuracy and integrity.

Acknowledgments: The authors thank Keith Mustafa for her help to build the final version of the manuscript.

References

1. Yan, B.; Yu, Y.; Lin, M.; Li, Z.; Wang, L.; Huang, P.; Song, H.; Shi, X.; Yang, S.; Li, S.; et al. High, but stable, trend in the prevalence of gestational diabetes mellitus: A population-based study in Xiamen, China. *J. Diabetes Investig.* **2019**, *10*, 1358–1364. [CrossRef]
2. Cho, N.H.; Shaw, J.E.; Karuranga, S.; Huang, Y.; da Rocha Fernandes, J.D.; Ohlrogge, A.W.; Malanda, B. IDF Diabetes Atlas: Global estimates of diabetes prevalence for 2017 and projections for 2045. *Diabetes Res. Clin. Pract.* **2018**, *138*, 271–281. [CrossRef]
3. Lavery, J.A.; Friedman, A.M.; Keyes, K.M.; Wright, J.D.; Ananth, C.V. Gestational diabetes in the United States: Temporal changes in prevalence rates between 1979 and 2010. *BJOG* **2017**, *124*, 804–813. [CrossRef]
4. Gortazar, L.; Flores-Le Roux, J.A.; Benaiges, D.; Sarsanedas, E.; Payà, A.; Mañé, L.; Pedro-Botet, J.; Goday, A. Trends in prevalence of gestational diabetes and perinatal outcomes in Catalonia, Spain, 2006 to 2015: The Diagestcat Study. *Diabetes Metab. Res. Rev.* **2019**, *35*, e3151. [CrossRef]
5. Nerenberg, K.A.; Johnson, J.A.; Leung, B.; Savu, A.; Ryan, E.A.; Chik, C.L.; Kaul, P. Risks of gestational diabetes and preeclampsia over the last decade in a cohort. *J. Obstet. Gynaecol. Can.* **2013**, *35*, 986–994. [CrossRef]
6. Weissgerber, T.L.; Mudd, L.M. Preeclampsia and diabetes. *Curr. Diab. Rep.* **2015**, *15*, 15–579. [CrossRef] [PubMed]
7. Tabrizi, R.; Asemi, Z.; Lankarani, K.B.; Akbari, M.; Khatibi, S.R.; Naghibzadeh-Tahami, A.; Sanjari, M.; Alizadeh, H.; Afshari, M.; Khodadost, M.; et al. Gestational diabetes mellitus in association with macrosomia in Iran: A meta-analysis. *J. Diabetes Metab. Disord.* **2019**, *18*, 41–50. [CrossRef] [PubMed]
8. Farrar, D.; Simmonds, M.; Bryant, M.; Sheldon, T.A.; Tuffnell, D.; Golder, S.; Dunne, F.; Lawlor, D.A. Hyperglycaemia and risk of adverse perinatal outcomes: Systematic review and meta-analysis. *BMJ* **2016**, *354*, i4694. [CrossRef]
9. Kamana, K.; Shakya, S.; Zhang, H. Gestational diabetes mellitus and macrosomia: A literature review. *Ann. Nutr. Metab.* **2015**, *2*, 14–20.
10. Nguyen, P.T.H.; Binns, C.W.; Nguyen, C.L.; Ha, A.V.V.; Chu, T.K.; Duong, D.V.; Do, D.V.; Lee, A.H. Gestational Diabetes Mellitus Reduces Breastfeeding Duration: A Prospective Cohort Study. *Breastfeed Med.* **2019**, *14*, 39–45. [CrossRef]
11. Much, D.; Beyerlein, A.; Roßbauer, M.; Hummel, S.; Ziegler, A.-G. Beneficial effects of breastfeeding in women with gestational diabetes mellitus. *Mol. Metab.* **2014**, *3*, 284–292. [CrossRef] [PubMed]
12. Horta, B.L.; Loret de Mola, C.; Victora, C.G. Long-term consequences of breastfeeding on cholesterol, obesity, systolic blood systematic review and meta-analysis. *Acta. Paediatr.* **2015**, *104*, 30–37. [CrossRef] [PubMed]
13. Aune, D.; Norat, T.; Romundstad, P.; Vatten, L.J. Breastfeeding and the maternal risk of type 2 diabetes: A systematic review and dose-response meta-analysis of cohort studies. *Nutr. Metab. Cardiovasc. Dis.* **2014**, *24*, 107–115. [CrossRef] [PubMed]
14. Xu, T.; Dainelli, L. The short-term health and economic burden of gestational diabetes mellitus in China. *BMJ Open* **2017**, *7*, e018893. [CrossRef]
15. Hopmans, T.E.; van Houten, C.; Kasius, A.; Kouznetsova, O.I.; Nguyen, L.A.; Rooijmans, S.V.; Voormolen, D.N.; van Vliet, E.O.; Franx, A.; Koster, M.P. Increased risk of type II diabetes mellitus and cardiovascular disease after gestational diabetes mellitus: A systematic review. *Ned. Tijdschr. Geneeskd.* **2015**, *159*, A8043.
16. Kramer, C.K.; Campbell, S.; Retnakaran, R. Gestational diabetes and the risk of cardiovascular disease in women: A systematic review and meta-analysis. *Diabetologia* **2019**, *62*, 905–914. [CrossRef]

17. Kawasaki, M.; Arata, N.; Miyazaki, C.; Mori, R.; Kikuchi, T.; Ogawa, Y.; Ota, E. Obesity and abnormal glucose tolerance in offspring of diabetic mothers: A systematic review and meta-analysis. *PLoS ONE* **2018**, *13*, e0190676. [CrossRef]
18. Clausen, T.D.; Mathiesen, E.R.; Hansen, T.; Pedersen, O.; Jensen, D.M.; Lauenborg, J.; Schmidt, L.; Damm, P. Overweight and the metabolic syndrome in adult offspring of women with diet-treated gestational diabetes mellitus or type 1 diabetes. *J. Clin. Endocrinol. Metab.* **2009**, *94*, 2464–2470. [CrossRef]
19. Plows, J.F.; Stanley, J.L.; Baker, P.N.; Clare, M.R.; Vickers, M.H. The Pathophysiology of Gestational Diabetes Mellitus. *Int. J. Mol. Sci.* **2018**, *19*, 3342. [CrossRef]
20. Di Cianni, G.; Miccoli, R.; Volpe, L.; Lencioni, C.; Del Prato, S. Intermediate metabolism in normal pregnancy and in gestational diabetes. *Diabetes Metab. Res. Rev.* **2003**, *19*, 259–270. [CrossRef]
21. Harlev, A.; Wiznitzer, A. New insights on glucose pathophysiology in gestational diabetes and insulin resistance. *Curr. Diab. Rep.* **2010**, *10*, 242–247. [CrossRef] [PubMed]
22. Catalano, P.M. Trying to understand gestational diabetes. *Diabet. Med.* **2014**, *31*, 273–281. [CrossRef] [PubMed]
23. Boden, G. Fuel metabolism in pregnancy and in gestational diabetes mellitus. *Obstet. Gynecol. Clin. N. Am.* **1996**, *23*, 1–10. [CrossRef]
24. Buchanan, T.A.; Xiang, A.; Kjos, S.L.; Watanabe, R. What is gestational diabetes? *Diabetes Care* **2007**, *30*, S105–S111. [CrossRef]
25. Butte, N.F. Carbohydrate and lipid metabolism in pregnancy: Normal compared with gestational diabetes mellitus. *Am. J. Clin. Nutr.* **2000**, *71*, 1256s–1261s. [CrossRef]
26. Herrera, E.; Desoye, G. Maternal and fetal lipid metabolism under normal and gestational diabetic conditions. *Horm. Mol. Biol. Clin. Investig.* **2016**, *26*, 109–127. [CrossRef]
27. Qiu, C.; Rudra, C.; Austin, M.A.; Williams, M.A. Association of gestational diabetes mellitus and low-density lipoprotein (LDL) particle size. *Physiol. Res.* **2007**, *56*, 571–578.
28. Ryckman, K.K.; Spracklen, C.N.; Smith, C.J.; Robinson, J.G.; Saftlas, A.F. Maternal lipid levels during pregnancy and gestational diabetes: A systematic review and meta-analysis. *BJOG* **2015**, *122*, 643–651. [CrossRef]
29. Pantham, P.; Aye, I.L.M.H.; Powell, T.L. Inflammation in maternal obesity and gestational diabetes mellitus. *Placenta* **2015**, *36*, 709–715. [CrossRef]
30. Abell, S.K.; De Courten, B.; Boyle, J.A.; Teede, H.J. Inflammatory and Other Biomarkers: Role in Pathophysiology and Prediction of Gestational Diabetes Mellitus. *Int. J. Mol. Sci.* **2015**, *16*, 13442–13473. [CrossRef]
31. Kirwan, J.P.; Hauguel-De Mouzon, S.; Lepercq, J.; Challier, J.-C.; Huston-Presley, L.; Friedman, J.E.; Kalhan, S.C.; Catalano, P.M. TNF-alpha is a predictor of insulin resistance in human pregnancy. *Diabete* **2002**, *51*, 2207–2213. [CrossRef] [PubMed]
32. Piao, C.; Wang, X.; Peng, S.; Guo, X.; Zhao, H.; He, L.; Zeng, Y.; Zhang, F.; Zhu, K.; Wang, Y. IL-34 causes inflammation and beta cell apoptosis and dysfunction in gestational diabetes mellitus. *Endocr. Connect.* **2019**, *8*, 1503–1512. [CrossRef] [PubMed]
33. Crusell, M.K.W.; Hansen, T.H.; Nielsen, T.; Allin, K.H.; Rühlemann, M.V.; Damm, P.; Vestergaard, H.; Rørbye, C.; Jørgensen, N.R.; Christiansen, O.B.; et al. Gestational diabetes is associated with change in the gut microbiota composition in third trimester of pregnancy and postpartum. *Microbiome* **2018**, *6*, 89. [CrossRef] [PubMed]
34. Serino, M.; Fernandez-Real, J.M.; Fuentes, E.G.; Queipo-Ortuño, M.; Moreno-Navarrete, J.M.; Sánchez, Á.; Burcelin, R.; Tinahones, F. The gut microbiota profile is associated with insulin action in humans. *Acta Diabetol.* **2013**, *50*, 753–761. [CrossRef]
35. Fugmann, M.; Breier, M.; Rottenkolber, M.; Banning, F.; Ferrari, U.; Sacco, V.; Grallert, H.; Parhofer, K.G.; Seissler, J.; Clavel, T.; et al. The stool microbiota of insulin resistant women with recent gestational diabetes, a high risk group for type 2 diabetes. *Sci. Rep.* **2015**, *5*, 13212. [CrossRef]
36. Bassols, J.; Serino, M.; Carreras-Badosa, G.; Burcelin, R.; Blasco-Baque, V.; Lopez-Bermejo, A.; Fernandez-Real, J.-M. Gestational diabetes is associated with changes in placental microbiota and microbiome. *Pediatr. Res.* **2016**, *80*, 777–784. [CrossRef]

37. Institute of Medicine. *Dietary Reference Intakes for Energy, Carbohydrate, Fiber, Fat, Fatty Acids, Cholesterol, Protein, and Amino Acids*; The National Academies Press: Washington, DC, USA, 2005; p. 1358.
38. Lovegrove, A.; Edwards, C.H.; De Noni, I.; Patel, H.; El, S.N.; Grassby, T.; Zielke, C.; Ulmius, M.; Nilsson, L.; Butterworth, P.J.; et al. Role of polysaccharides in food, digestion, and health. *Crit. Rev. Food Sci. Nutr.* **2017**, *57*, 237–253. [CrossRef]
39. Jovanovic-Peterson, L.; Peterson, C.M.; Reed, G.F.; Metzger, B.E.; Mills, J.L.; Knopp, R.H.; Aarons, J.H.; The National Institute of Child Health and Human Development—Diabetes in Early Pregnancy Study. Maternal postprandial glucose levels and infant birth weight: The Diabetes in Early Pregnancy Study. *Am. J. Obstet. Gynecol.* **1991**, *164 Pt 1*, 103–111. [CrossRef]
40. Combs, C.A.; Gunderson, E.; Kitzmiller, J.L.; Gavin, L.A.; Main, E.K. Relationship of fetal macrosomia to maternal postprandial glucose control during pregnancy. *Diabetes Care* **1992**, *15*, 1251–1257. [CrossRef]
41. Peterson, C.M.; Jovanovic-Peterson, L. Percentage of carbohydrate and glycemic response to breakfast, lunch, and dinner in women with gestational diabetes. *Diabetes* **1991**, *40* (Suppl. 2), 172–174. [CrossRef]
42. Clapp, J. Diet, exercise, and feto-placental growth. *Arch. Gynecol. Obstet.* **1997**, *260*, 101–108.
43. Louie, J.C.Y.; Markovic, T.P.; Ross, G.P.; Foote, D.; Brand-Miller, J.C. Timing of peak blood glucose after breakfast meals of different glycemic index in women with gestational diabetes. *Nutrients* **2012**, *5*, 1–9. [CrossRef]
44. Martin, M.J.; Manzano, M.; Bueno-Vargas, P.; Rueda, R.; Salto, R.; Giron, M.D.; Vilchez, J.D.; Cabrera, E.; Cano, A.; Castro, A.; et al. Feeding a slowly digestible carbohydrate diet during pregnancy of insulin-resistant rats prevents the excess of adipogenesis in their offspring. *J. Nutr. Biochem.* **2018**, *61*, 183–196. [CrossRef]
45. Salto, R.; Manzano, M.; Girón, M.D.; Cano, A.; Castro, A.; Vílchez, J.D.; Cabrera, E.; López-Pedrosa, J.M. A Slow-Digesting Carbohydrate Diet during Rat Pregnancy Protects Offspring from Non-Alcoholic Fatty Liver Disease Risk through the Modulation of the Carbohydrate-Response Element and Sterol Regulatory Element Binding Proteins. *Nutrients* **2019**, *11*, 844. [CrossRef]
46. Tsirou, E.; Grammatikopoulou, M.G.; Theodoridis, X.; Gkiouras, K.; Petalidou, A.; Taousani, E.; Savvaki, D.; Tsapas, A.; Goulis, D.G. Guidelines for Medical Nutrition Therapy in Gestational Diabetes Mellitus: Systematic Review and Critical Appraisal. *J. Acad. Nutr. Diet.* **2019**, *119*, 1320–1339. [CrossRef]
47. Filardi, T.; Panimolle, F.; Crescioli, C.; Lenzi, A.; Morano, S. Gestational Diabetes Mellitus: The Impact of Carbohydrate Quality in Diet. *Nutr.* **2019**, *11*, 1549. [CrossRef]
48. Mahajan, A.; Donovan, L.E.; Vallee, R.; Yamamoto, J.M. Evidenced-Based Nutrition for Gestational Diabetes Mellitus. *Curr. Diabetes Rep.* **2019**, *19*, 94. [CrossRef]
49. Hernandez, T.L.; Mande, A.; Barbour, L.A. Nutrition therapy within and beyond gestational diabetes. *Diabetes Res. Clin. Pr.* **2018**, *145*, 39–50. [CrossRef]
50. Major, C.A.; Henry, M.J.; de Veciana, M.; Morgan, M.A. The effects of carbohydrate restriction in patients with diet-controlled gestational diabetes. *Obstet. Gynecol.* **1998**, *91*, 600–604.
51. Cypryk, K.; Kamińska, P.; Kosiński, M.; Pertyńska-Marczewska, M.; Lewiński, A. A comparison of the effectiveness, tolerability and safety of high and low carbohydrate diets in women with gestational diabetes. *Endokrynol. Polska* **2007**, *58*, 314–319.
52. Moreno-Castilla, C.; Hernandez, M.; Bergua, M.; Alvarez, M.C.; Arce, M.A.; Rodriguez, K.; Martinez-Alonso, M.; Iglesias, M.; Mateu, M.; Santos, M.D.; et al. Low-carbohydrate diet for the treatment of gestational diabetes mellitus: A randomized controlled trial. *Diabetes Care* **2013**, *36*, 2233–2238. [CrossRef] [PubMed]
53. Hernandez, T.L.; Van Pelt, R.E.; Anderson, M.A.; Daniels, L.J.; West, N.A.; Donahoo, W.T.; Friedman, J.E.; Barbour, L.A. A Higher-Complex Carbohydrate Diet in Gestational Diabetes Mellitus Achieves Glucose Targets and Lowers Postprandial Lipids: A Randomized Crossover Study. *Diabetes Care* **2014**, *37*, 1254–1262. [CrossRef]
54. Ma, W.-J.; Huang, Z.-H.; Huang, B.-X.; Qi, B.-H.; Zhang, Y.-J.; Xiao, B.-X.; Li, Y.-H.; Chen, L.; Zhu, H.-L. Intensive low-glycaemic-load dietary intervention for the management of glycaemia and serum lipids among women with gestational diabetes: A randomized control trial. *Public Health Nutr.* **2014**, *18*, 1506–1513. [CrossRef]
55. Grant, S.M.; Wolever, T.M.; O'Connor, D.L.; Nisenbaum, R.; Josse, R.G. Effect of a low glycaemic index diet on blood glucose in women with gestational hyperglycaemia. *Diabetes Res. Clin. Pr.* **2011**, *91*, 15–22. [CrossRef]

56. Moses, R.G.; Barker, M.; Winter, M.; Petocz, P.; Brand-Miller, J.C. Can a low-glycemic index diet reduce the need for insulin in gestational diabetes mellitus? A randomized trial. *Diabetes Care* **2009**, *32*, 996–1000. [CrossRef] [PubMed]
57. Perichart-Perera, O.; Balas-Nakash, M.; Rodríguez-Cano, A.; Legorreta-Legorreta, J.; Parra-Covarrubias, A.; Vadillo-Ortega, F. Low Glycemic Index Carbohydrates versus All Types of Carbohydrates for Treating Diabetes in Pregnancy: A Randomized Clinical Trial to Evaluate the Effect of Glycemic Control. *Int. J. Endocrinol.* **2012**, *2012*, 1–10. [CrossRef]
58. Louie, J.C.Y.; Markovic, T.P.; Perera, N.; Foote, D.; Petocz, P.; Ross, G.P.; Brand-Miller, J.C. A Randomized Controlled Trial Investigating the Effects of a Low–Glycemic Index Diet on Pregnancy Outcomes in Gestational Diabetes Mellitus. *Diabetes Care* **2011**, *34*, 2341–2346. [CrossRef] [PubMed]
59. Dodd, J.M.; For the LIMIT Randomised Trial Group; Cramp, C.; Sui, Z.; Yelland, L.N.; Deussen, A.R.; Grivell, R.M.; Moran, L.J.; A Crowther, C.; Turnbull, D.; et al. The effects of antenatal dietary and lifestyle advice for women who are overweight or obese on maternal diet and physical activity: The LIMIT randomised trial. *BMC Med.* **2014**, *12*, 161. [CrossRef] [PubMed]
60. Markovic, T.P.; Muirhead, R.; Overs, S.; Ross, G.P.; Louie, J.C.Y.; Kizirian, N.; Denyer, G.; Petocz, P.; Hyett, J.; Brand-Miller, J.C. Randomized Controlled Trial Investigating the Effects of a Low-Glycemic Index Diet on Pregnancy Outcomes in Women at High Risk of Gestational Diabetes Mellitus: The GI Baby 3 Study. *Diabetes Care* **2016**, *39*, 31–38. [CrossRef] [PubMed]
61. Walsh, J.M.; McGowan, C.A.; Mahony, R.; Foley, M.E.; McAuliffe, F.M. Low glycaemic index diet in pregnancy to prevent macrosomia (ROLO study): Randomised control trial. *BMJ* **2012**, *345*, e5605. [CrossRef]
62. Poston, L.; Bell, R.; Croker, H.; Flynn, A.C.; Godfrey, K.M.; Goff, L.; Hayes, L.; Khazaezadeh, N.; Nelson, S.M.; Oteng-Ntim, E.; et al. Effect of a behavioural intervention in obese pregnant women (the UPBEAT study): A multicentre, randomised controlled trial. *Lancet Diabetes Endocrinol.* **2015**, *3*, 767–777. [CrossRef]
63. Han, S.; Middleton, P.; Shepherd, E.; Van Ryswyk, E.; Crowther, C.A. Different types of dietary advice for women with gestational diabetes mellitus. *Cochrane Database Syst. Rev.* **2017**, *2017*, CD009275. [CrossRef] [PubMed]
64. Yamamoto, J.M.; Kellett, J.E.; Balsells, M.; García-Patterson, A.; Hadar, E.; Sola, I.; Gich, I.; Van Der Beek, E.M.; Castañeda-Gutiérrez, E.; Heinonen, S.; et al. Gestational Diabetes Mellitus and Diet: A Systematic Review and Meta-analysis of Randomized Controlled Trials Examining the Impact of Modified Dietary Interventions on Maternal Glucose Control and Neonatal Birth Weight. *Diabetes Care* **2018**, *41*, 1346–1361. [CrossRef] [PubMed]
65. Wan, C.S.; Nankervis, A.; Teede, H.; Aroni, R. Dietary intervention strategies for ethnic Chinese women with gestational diabetes mellitus: A systematic review and meta-analysis. *Nutr. Diet.* **2019**, *76*, 211–232. [CrossRef]
66. Tieu, J.; Shepherd, E.; Middleton, P.; Crowther, C.A. Dietary advice interventions in pregnancy for preventing gestational diabetes mellitus. *Cochrane Database Syst. Rev.* **2017**, *2017*, CD006674. [CrossRef]
67. Zhang, R.; Han, S.; Chen, G.-C.; Li, Z.-N.; Silva-Zolezzi, I.; Parés, G.V.; Wang, Y.; Qin, L.Q. Effects of low-glycemic-index diets in pregnancy on maternal and newborn outcomes in pregnant women: A meta-analysis of randomized controlled trials. *Eur. J. Nutr.* **2018**, *57*, 167–177. [CrossRef]
68. Schoenaker, D.A.; Mishra, G.D.; Callaway, L.K.; Soedamah-Muthu, S.S. The Role of Energy, Nutrients, Foods, and Dietary Patterns in the Development of Gestational Diabetes Mellitus: A Systematic Review of Observational Studies. *Diabetes Care* **2016**, *39*, 16–23. [CrossRef]
69. Zhou, X.; Chen, R.; Zhong, C.; Wu, J.; Li, X.; Li, Q.; Cui, W.; Yi, N.; Xiao, M.; Yin, H.; et al. Maternal dietary pattern characterised by high protein and low carbohydrate intake in pregnancy is associated with a higher risk of gestational diabetes mellitus in Chinese women: A prospective cohort study. *Br. J. Nutr.* **2018**, *120*, 1045–1055. [CrossRef]
70. Lamminpää, R.; Vehviläinen-Julkunen, K.; Schwab, U. A systematic review of dietary interventions for gestational weight gain and gestational diabetes in overweight and obese pregnant women. *Eur. J. Nutr.* **2018**, *57*, 1721–1736. [CrossRef]
71. Mack, L.R.; Tomich, P.G. Gestational Diabetes: Diagnosis, Classification, and Clinical Care. *Obstet. Gynecol. Clin. N. Am.* **2017**, *44*, 207–217. [CrossRef]
72. Carolan, M.; Gill, G.K.; Steele, C. Women's experiences of factors that facilitate or inhibit gestational diabetes self-management. *BMC Pregnancy Childbirth* **2012**, *12*, 99. [CrossRef] [PubMed]

73. Knowler, W.C.; Barrett-Connor, E.; Fowler, S.E.; Hamman, R.F.; Lachin, J.M.; Walker, E.A.; Nathan, D.M. Diabetes Prevention Program Research Group Reduction in the incidence of type 2 diabetes with lifestyle intervention or metformin. *N. Engl. J. Med.* **2002**, *346*, 393–403. [PubMed]
74. Lindström, J.; Tuomilehto, J. The diabetes risk score: A practical tool to predict type 2 diabetes risk. *Diabetes Care* **2003**, *26*, 725–731. [CrossRef] [PubMed]
75. Hamdy, O.; Mottalib, A.; Morsi, A.; El-Sayed, N.; Goebel-Fabbri, A.; Arathuzik, G.; Shahar, J.; Kirpitch, A.; Zrebiec, J. Long-term effect of intensive lifestyle intervention on cardiovascular risk factors in patients with diabetes in real-world clinical practice: A 5-year longitudinal study. *BMJ Open Diabetes Res. Care* **2017**, *5*, e000259. [CrossRef] [PubMed]
76. Wing, R.R.; AHEAD Research Group. Long-term effects of a lifestyle intervention on weight and cardiovascular risk factors in individuals with type 2 diabetes mellitus; four year results of the look AHEAD trial. *Arch. Intern. Med.* **2010**, *170*, 1566–1575. [PubMed]
77. American Diabetes Association. Obesity management for the treatment of type 2 diabetes: Standards of Medical Care in Diabetes-2020. *Diabetes Care.* **2020**, *43* (Suppl. 1), S89–S97. [CrossRef]
78. Sievenpiper, J.L.; Chan, C.B.; Dworatzek, P.D.; Freeze, C.; Williams, S.L. Diabetes Canada Clinical Practice Guidelines Expert Committee. *Nutr. Ther. Can. J. Diabetes* **2018**, *42* (Suppl. 1), S64–S79. [CrossRef]
79. Dyson, P.A.; Twenefour, D.; Breen, C.; Duncan, A.; Elvin, E.; Goff, L.; Hill, A.; Kalsi, P.; Marsland, N.; McArdle, P.; et al. Diabetes UK evidence-based nutrition guidelines for the prevention and management of diabetes. *Diabet. Med.* **2018**, *35*, 541–547. [CrossRef]
80. Phelan, S.; Wing, R.R.; Brannen, A.; McHugh, A.; Hagobian, T.A.; Schaffner, A.; Jelalian, E.; Hart, C.N.; Scholl, T.O.; Munoz-Christian, K.; et al. Randomized controlled clinical trial of behavioral lifestyle intervention with partial meal replacement to reduce excessive gestational weight gain. *Am. J. Clin. Nutr.* **2018**, *107*, 183–194. [CrossRef]
81. Voss, A.C.; Maki, K.C.; Garvey, W.T.; Hustead, D.S.; Alish, C.; Fix, B.; Mustad, V.A. Effect of two carbohydrate-modified tube-feeding formulas on metabolic responses in patients with type 2 diabetes. *Nutrition* **2008**, *24*, 990–997. [CrossRef]
82. Devitt, A.A.; Oliver, J.S.; Hegazi, R.A.; Mustad, V.A. Glycemia Targeted Specialized Nutrition (GTSN) improves postprandial glycemia and GLP-1 with similar appetitive responses compared to a healthful whole food breakfast in persons with type 2 diabetes: A randomized, controlled trial. *J. Diabetes Res. Clin. Metab.* **2012**, *1*, 20. [CrossRef]
83. Mottalib, A.; Mohd-Yusof, B.-N.; Shehabeldin, M.; Pober, D.M.; Mitri, J.; Hamdy, O. Impact of Diabetes-Specific Nutritional Formulas versus Oatmeal on Postprandial Glucose, Insulin, GLP-1 and Postprandial Lipidemia. *Nutrients* **2016**, *8*, 443. [CrossRef] [PubMed]
84. Ojo, O.; Ojo, O.O.; Adebowale, F.; Wang, X.-H. The Effect of Dietary Glycaemic Index on Glycaemia in Patients with Type 2 Diabetes: A Systematic Review and Meta-Analysis of Randomized Controlled Trials. *Nutrients* **2018**, *10*, 373. [CrossRef] [PubMed]
85. Elia, M.; Ceriello, A.; Laube, H.; Sinclair, A.J.; Engfer, M.; Stratton, R.J. Enteral nutritional support and use of diabetes-specific formulas for patients with diabetes: A systematic review and meta-analysis. *Diabetes Care.* **2005**, *28*, 2267–2279. [CrossRef]
86. Yu, X.-Y.; Zhang, H. [Effects of a nutritional liquid supplement designed for diabetes mellitus on postprandial glucose and pregnancy outcomes in patients with gestational diabetes mellitus]. *Zhonghua Yi Xue Za Zhi* **2013**, *93*, 3450–3453.
87. Liu, J.; Zhu, W. Effects of Glucerna SR on blood glucose levels and relevant biochemical parameters in patients with gestational diabetes mellitus. *Laser J.* **2013**, *34*, 75.
88. Li, X. Effects of Abbott Glucerna SR on controlling the blood glucose levels of 34 women with gestational diabetes. *Chin. J. Trauma Disabil. Med.* **2013**, *21*, 245–246.
89. Crowther, C.A.; Hiller, J.E.; Moss, J.R.; McPhee, A.J.; Jeffries, W.S.; Robinson, J.S.; The Australian Carbohydrate Intolerance Study in Pregnant Women (ACHOIS) Trial Group. Effect of treatment of gestational diabetes mellitus on pregnancy outcomes. *N. Engl. J. Med.* **2005**, *352*, 2477–2486. [CrossRef]
90. Byrne, E.Z.; Zisser, H.C.; Jovanovic, L. Continuous glucose monitoring: Is it helpful in pregnancy? *Curr. Diabetes Rev.* **2008**, *4*, 223–226. [CrossRef]
91. Bailey, T.S.; Zisser, H.C.; Garg, S.K. Reduction in Hemoglobin A1c with Real-Time Continuous Glucose Monitoring: Results from a 12-Week Observational Study. *Diabetes Technol. Ther.* **2007**, *9*, 203–210. [CrossRef]

92. Feig, D.S.; Donovan, L.E.; Corcoy, R.; Murphy, K.E.; Amiel, S.A.; Hunt, K.F.; Asztalos, E.; Barrett, J.F.R.; Sanchez, J.J.; De Leiva, A.; et al. Continuous glucose monitoring in pregnant women with type 1 diabetes (CONCEPTT): A multicentre international randomised controlled trial. *Lancet* **2017**, *390*, 2347–2359. [CrossRef]
93. González-Quintero, V.H.; Istwan, N.B.; Rhea, D.J.; Rodriguez, L.I.; Cotter, A.; Carter, J.; Mueller, A.; Stanziano, G.J. The Impact of Glycemic Control on Neonatal Outcome in Singleton Pregnancies Complicated by Gestational Diabetes. *Diabetes Care* **2007**, *30*, 467–470. [CrossRef] [PubMed]
94. Yu, F.; Weng, J.; Lv, L.; Liang, Z.; Wang, Y.; Wen, J.; Lin, X.; Zhou, Y.; Mai, C.; Niu, J. Continuous Glucose Monitoring Effects on Maternal Glycemic Control and Pregnancy Outcomes in Patients with Gestational Diabetes Mellitus: A Prospective Cohort Study. *J. Clin. Endocrinol. Metab.* **2014**, *99*, 4674–4682. [CrossRef] [PubMed]
95. Carreiro, M.P.; Lauria, M.W.; Naves, G.N.T.; Miranda, P.A.C.; Leite, R.B.; Rajão, K.M.A.B.; De Aguiar, R.A.L.P.; Nogueira, A.I.; Ribeiro-Oliveira, A. Seventy two-hour glucose monitoring profiles in mild gestational diabetes mellitus: Differences from healthy pregnancies and influence of diet counseling. *Eur. J. Endocrinol.* **2016**, *175*, 201–209. [CrossRef]
96. Afandi, B.; Hassanein, M.; Roubi, S.; Nagelkerke, N. The value of Continuous Glucose Monitoring and Self-Monitoring of Blood Glucose in patients with Gestational Diabetes Mellitus during Ramadan fasting. *Diabetes Res. Clin. Pr.* **2019**, *151*, 260–264. [CrossRef] [PubMed]

6

Self-Reported Eating Speed and Incidence of Gestational Diabetes Mellitus: The Japan Environment and Children's Study

Jia-Yi Dong [1], Satoyo Ikehara [1], Takashi Kimura [2], Meishan Cui [1], Yoko Kawanishi [3], Tadashi Kimura [3], Kimiko Ueda [4], Hiroyasu Iso [1,5,*] and the Japan Environment and Children's Study Group [†]

1 Public Health, Department of Social Medicine, Osaka University Graduate School of Medicine, Osaka 5650871, Japan; dongjy@mail3.sysu.edu.cn (J.-Y.D.); s-ikehara@pbhel.med.osaka-u.ac.jp (S.I.); saimiyoshi@163.com (M.C.)

2 Department of Public Health, Hokkaido University Graduate School of Medicine, Sapporo 0608638, Japan; kimura@med.hokudai.ac.jp

3 Department of Obstetrics and Gynecology, Osaka University Graduate School of Medicine, Osaka 5650871, Japan; angeltears90@hotmail.co.jp (Y.K.); tadashi@gyne.med.osaka-u.ac.jp (T.K.)

4 Maternal & Child Health Information Center, Osaka Women's and Children's Hospital, Osaka 5941101, Japan; kimi-h-u@wch.opho.jp

5 Department of Public Health Medicine, Faculty of Medicine, University of Tsukuba, Tsukuba 3058575, Japan

* Correspondence: iso@pbhel.med.osaka-u.ac.jp

† Membership of the Japan Environment and Children's Study is provided in the Acknowledgments.

Abstract: There is little evidence linking eating speed to gestational diabetes mellitus (GDM) incidence. We therefore aimed to evaluate the prospective association of eating speed with GDM incidence. Overall, 97,454 pregnant women were recruited between January 2011 and March 2014. Singleton pregnant women who did not have GDM, heart disease, stroke, cancer, type 1 diabetes, and/or type 2 diabetes at the time of study enrollment were eligible. Each woman was asked about her eating speed at that time via a questionnaire. Odds ratios of GDM in relation to eating speed were obtained using logistic regression. Among the 84,811 women eligible for analysis, 1902 cases of GDM were identified in medical records. Compared with women who reported slow eating speed, the age-adjusted odds ratios (95% confidence interval) of GDM for women who reported medium, relatively fast, or very fast eating speed were 1.03 (0.90, 1.18), 1.07 (0.94, 1.23), and 1.28 (1.05, 1.58), respectively. Adjustment for demographic, lifestyle-related, and dietary factors including dietary fat, dietary fiber, and energy intakes yielded similar results. The association was attenuated and no longer significant after further adjustment for pre-pregnancy body mass index. The mediation analysis showed that being overweight accounted for 64% of the excess risk of GDM associated with eating speed. In conclusion, women who reported very fast eating speed, compared with those reporting slow eating speed, were associated with an increased incidence of GDM, which may be largely mediated by increased body fat.

Keywords: eating speed; gestational diabetes; cohort study; prevention

1. Introduction

Diet is widely known to play an essential role in promoting health and preventing disease. In addition to what we eat, the way we eat may also impact our health. In particular, the effects of eating speed on obesity, as well as obesity-related diseases, have received increasing research interest over the past decade. A number of cross-sectional studies have suggested eating quickly is associated with a higher prevalence of obesity [1]. Excess energy intake is one possible explanation for the association between faster eating and risk of weight gain and obesity [2]. Emerging evidence also indicates that eating quickly may increase the risk of metabolic syndrome [3–5] and type 2 diabetes [6].

Gestational diabetes mellitus (GDM) is a complication affecting about 7% of pregnant women and has various influences on both mothers and their offspring [7–9]. Adverse pregnancy outcomes stemming from GDM include macrosomia, cesarean section, and shoulder dystocia [10,11]. Over the long term, GDM has been shown to be associated with an elevated risk of type 2 diabetes and cardiovascular diseases in mothers [12,13], and a higher risk of obesity and insulin insensitivity in their children [14,15].

Observational studies and clinical trials have suggested diet plays an important role in preventing GDM [16,17], but whether eating speed is independently associated with GDM is largely unknown. Moreover, whether body mass index (BMI) plays a mediating role and to which extent BMI may account for the possible association between eating speed and GDM are also uncertain. In the present study we used a large Japanese national birth cohort to examine the prospective association between eating speed and GDM and to test whether BMI was a mediator of the association.

2. Research Design and Methods

The present analysis was based on the Japan Environment and Children's Study (JECS), launched by the Ministry of the Environment, Japan, which was primarily aimed at evaluating the effects of environmental factors on pregnancy and children's health. Genetic, socioeconomic, and lifestyle factors were also examined. The study design is detailed elsewhere [18,19]. In brief, about 100 thousand pregnant women (median gestational age: 12 weeks) were recruited in 15 areas across Japan, from January 2011 to March 2014. We obtained information on demographic information, socioeconomic status, disease history, lifestyles, and dietary habits of each mother at the time of study enrollment via a self-administered questionnaire.

There were 103,099 pregnancies from 97,454 women recruited. Women were recruited voluntarily at the first prenatal examination and/or when they reported their pregnancies at local government offices. In 2013, the recruitment covered about 45% of pregnancies in the study area [19]. Among the 97,454 women, those who had singleton pregnancy and were not multiple participations were considered for this analysis. Women were eligible if they did not have GDM, heart disease, stroke, Kawasaki disease, cancer, type 1 diabetes, and/or type 2 diabetes at study enrollment. Extreme body mass index (BMI) before pregnancy (i.e., <14 or >40 kg/m^2), implausible energy intake (lower or upper 2.5%), or no data on exposure, outcome, or other critical variables were criteria for exclusion. A total of 84,811 women were eligible for this analysis (Figure 1).

At the time of study enrollment, each woman was asked "how fast is your eating speed" with no specific guidance. Candidate responses were "very slow", "relatively slow", "medium", "relatively fast", or "very fast". A validation study regarding eating speed in this population has not been performed, but there was evidence that self-reported eating speed showed good agreement with that reported by a friend [20]. The first two categories ("very slow" and "relatively slow") were grouped as "slow" because of a low number of women in the "very slow" category (2.3%). Dietary assessment was performed using a semi-quantitative food frequency questionnaire that was used and validated in another cohort study [21]. Nutrient intakes were calculated based on the Japan Standard Tables of Food Composition (5th Revised Edition).

The first incidence of GDM was the outcome of interest. GDM was diagnosed when two or more values during the 75 g oral glucose tolerance test were greater than the cutoff levels: fasting plasma glucose ≥ 5.5 mmol/L (100 mg/dL), 1 h value ≥ 10.0 mmol/L (180 mg/dL), and 2 h value ≥ 8.3 mmol/L (150 mg/dL) [22]. GDM cases were identified using medical record transcripts, which were completed after delivery by physicians, research coordinators, nurses, or midwives.

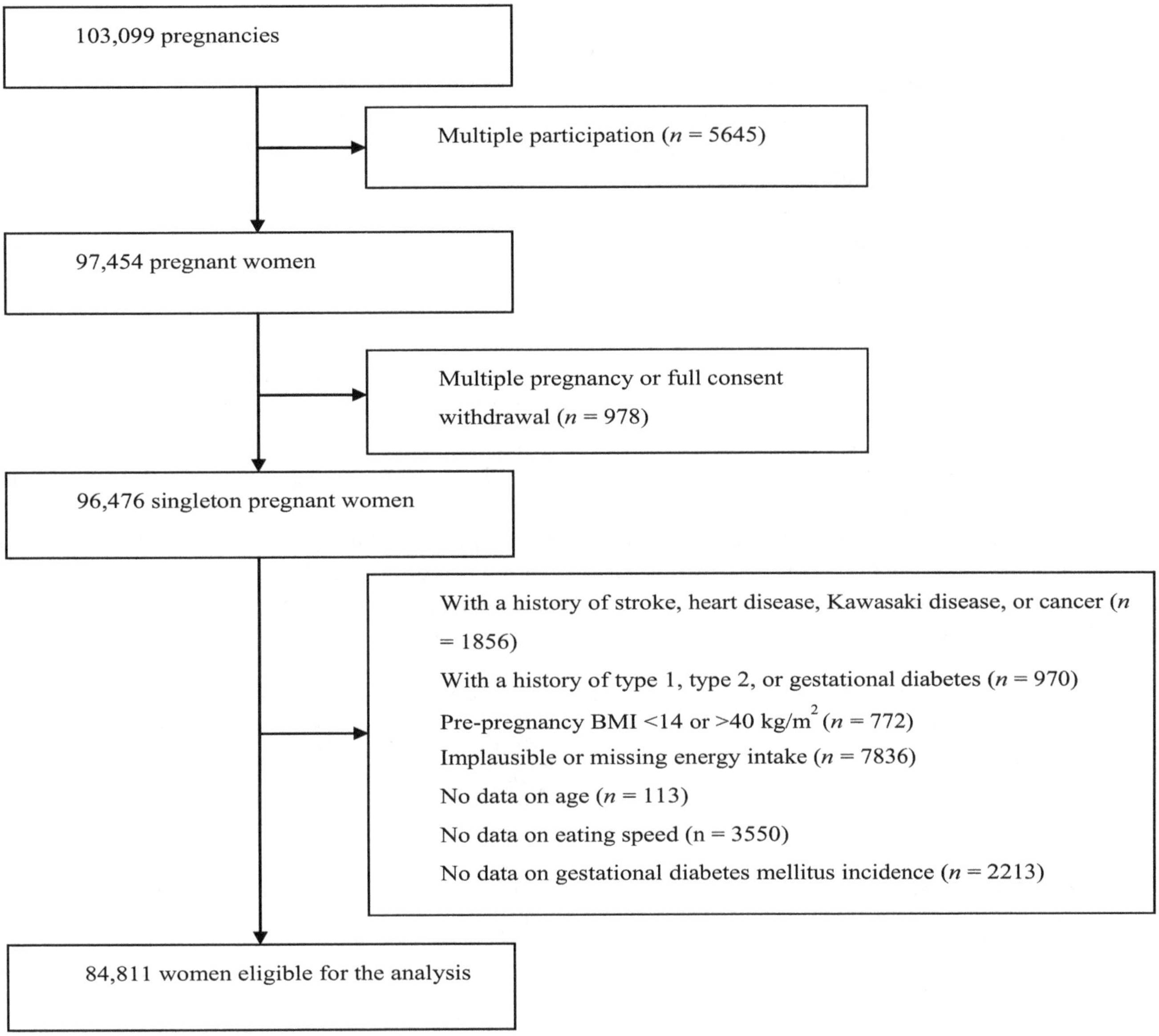

Figure 1. Flowchart for participant selection.

Age-adjusted means and proportions of the pregnant women's characteristics were calculated based on eating speed. Women who reported either very slow or relatively slow eating speed were treated as the reference group, and logistic regression was used to obtain the odds ratio (OR) and 95% confidence interval (CI) of GDM for other groups by comparing with the reference group. All ORs were age-adjusted in a basic model (model 1). We also adjusted for smoking status (never, past, or current smoker), drinking status (never, past, or current drinker), education level (middle school, high school, junior or specialized training college, or university or higher), occupation (15 categories), household income (nine categories), history of depression (yes or no), history of polycystic ovarian syndrome (yes or no), history of having macrosomia babies (yes or no), marital status (married, divorced, widowed, or other), parity (0, 1, 2, or ≥3), gestational weight gain (quintile), and physical activity (quintile) in model 2. In model 3, we further adjusted for dietary factors including white rice, seafood, meat, egg, coffee, green tea, milk, chocolate, soy isoflavones, dietary fiber, dietary magnesium, and dietary fat, and total energy intake (all quintiles). Pre-pregnancy BMI was adjusted in an additional model. To examine whether being overweight (pre-pregnancy BMI ≥25 kg/m^2) could mediate the association between eating speed and GDM, and we also conducted a mediation analysis by treating being overweight as a potential mediator. This analysis was performed to compute the proportion of excess risk of GDM that could be attributed to the mediator, i.e., overweight. The mediation analysis was adjusted for the same covariates in model 3. Additionally, we performed sensitivity analyses to test the robustness of the results by restricting the analysis in women who reported the same eating speed in a second survey during mid-late pregnancy (gestational age: quartile 1 = 24 weeks, median = 27 weeks, quartile 3 = 29 weeks). All analyses were carried out using SAS 9.4 (SAS Institute Inc., Cary, NC, USA). All *P*-values were two-sided, with $p < 0.05$ considered statistically significant.

The JECS protocol was reviewed and approved by the Ministry of the Environment's Institutional Review Board on Epidemiological Studies and by the Ethics Committees of all participating institutions (No.100406001). Written informed consent was obtained from all participants.

3. Results

We documented 1902 GDM cases from singleton pregnant women during follow-up, with the majority diagnosed during mid and late pregnancy. Table 1 shows the baseline characteristics of women by self-reported eating speed. Overall, the proportions of women who reported slow, medium, relatively fast, and very fast eating speed were 17.8%, 41.1%, 35.5%, and 5.7%, respectively. Women reporting very fast eating speed, compared with those reporting slow eating speed, were older and more likely to have a higher BMI, greater gestational weight gain, and a higher level of physical activity, but were less likely to be a housewife, nulliparous, or have never smoked. Regarding dietary factors, very fast eaters appeared to have higher intakes of total energy, white rice, meat, coffee, green tea, dietary fat, magnesium, and isoflavones, but lower intake of milk.

Table 1. Characteristics of 84,811 pregnant women according to self-reported eating speed.

	Slow	Medium	Relatively Fast	Very Fast	*p*
No. of participants	15,061	34,857	30,080	4813	
Age, years	29.8	30.7	31.0	31.5	<0.001
BMI before pregnancy, kg/m^2	20.6	21.0	21.5	21.8	<0.001
Gestational weight gain, kg	10.1	10.3	10.3	10.5	0.03
University or higher education, %	23.2	20.8	22.4	22.4	<0.001
Family income < 2 million/y, %	5.3	5.1	4.6	5.2	<0.001
Housewife, %	28.2	29.0	26.3	23.0	<0.001
Married, %	94.6	95.3	95.5	94.9	<0.001
Nulliparous, %	48.3	39.2	40.6	42.4	<0.001
History of macrosomia baby, %	0.3	0.5	0.5	0.6	0.006
Never smoker, %	61.1	59.7	56.9	52.4	<0.001
Never drinker, %	54.4	54.5	56.3	56.0	<0.001
Depression, %	3.7	2.7	2.8	3.9	<0.001
Polycystic ovarian syndrome, %	2.4	2.0	2.4	2.2	0.005
Physical activity, Met·h/day	3.6	3.9	3.9	4.6	<0.001
Total energy, kcal/day	1752	1750	1798	1880	<0.001
White rice, g/day	272.9	281.3	292.5	305.2	<0.001
Seafood, g/day	37.5	37.5	38.2	39.3	<0.001
Meat, g/day	68.9	69.8	74.2	81.0	<0.001
Egg, g/day	29.6	30.4	31.9	34.5	<0.001
Coffee, g/day	101	104	111	118	<0.001
Green tea, g/day	165	161	165	182	<0.001
Milk, g/day	135	127	123	122	0.003
Total dietary fat, g/day	58.6	58.2	60.1	63.6	<0.001
Magnesium, mg/day	233	233	238	246	<0.001
Total dietary fiber, g/day	11.0	11.0	11.2	11.5	<0.001
Chocolate, g/day	6.2	5.6	5.8	6.4	<0.001
Isoflavones, mg/day	30.6	31.2	31.6	32.8	<0.001

Values are means unless otherwise specified. *P* values were calculated using ANOVA or the chi-square test for continuous or categorical variables, respectively. BMI: body mass index.

Table 2 shows the ORs (95% CIs) of GDM by self-reported eating speed. Compared with those for women reporting slow eating speed, the age-adjusted ORs (95% CI) of GDM for women who reported medium, relatively fast, and very fast eating speed were 1.03 (0.90, 1.18), 1.07 (0.94, 1.23), and 1.28 (1.05, 1.58), respectively. Adjustment for demographic factors, lifestyle-related factors, and other risk factors (model 2) and further adjustment for dietary factors (model 3) yielded similar results. When further analyses were performed after the inclusion of pre-pregnancy BMI, the association was attenuated and became no longer significant. In the mediation analysis, we examined whether being overweight could be a mediator for the association between eating speed and GDM. After controlling for the same covariates in model 3, being overweight accounted for 64% of the excess risk of GDM associated with eating speed ($p < 0.001$), indicating that increased body fat may have largely mediated the association observed.

Table 2. Self-reported eating speed and risk of gestational diabetes mellitus among 84,811 women.

	Slow	Medium	Relatively Fast	Very Fast
No of participants	15,061	34,857	30,080	4813
No of cases	298	766	699	139
Model 1	1.00	1.03 (0.90, 1.18)	1.07 (0.94, 1.23)	1.28 (1.05, 1.58)
Model 2	1.00	1.08 (0.94, 1.24)	1.13 (0.99, 1.30)	1.35 (1.10, 1.66)
Model 3	1.00	1.08 (0.94, 1.24)	1.11 (0.97, 1.28)	1.29 (1.05, 1.59)
Model 3 + pre-pregnancy BMI	1.00	1.04 (0.90, 1.19)	1.01 (0.88, 1.16)	1.14 (0.93, 1.41)

Model 1: adjusted for age; Model 2: Model 1 and further adjusted for education, occupation, household income, smoking, drinking, history of depression, history of polycystic ovarian syndrome, history of macrosomia babies, parity, gestational weight gain, physical activity; Model 3: Model 2 and further adjusted for intakes of white rice, seafood, meat, egg, coffee, chocolate, green tea, milk, soy isoflavone, magnesium, total dietary fat, total dietary fiber, and total energy. BMI: body mass index.

Table 3 shows the ORs (95% CIs) of GDM by self-reported eating speed among 64,183 women who reported the same eating speed during early and late pregnancy. Overall, the association appeared to be somewhat stronger in this sensitivity analysis. After adjustment for all covariates including pre-pregnancy BMI, a very fast eating speed was independently associated with GDM (OR = 1.32; 95% CI: 1.03, 1.70).

Table 3. Self-reported eating speed and risk of gestational diabetes mellitus among 64,183 women who reported the same eating speed during early and mid-late pregnancy.

	Slow	Medium	Relatively Fast	Very Fast
No. of participants	10,783	26,520	23,777	3103
No. of cases	206	578	541	97
Model 1	1.00	1.07 (0.91, 1.25)	1.09 (0.93, 1.29)	1.45 (1.13, 1.85)
Model 2	1.00	1.11 (0.95, 1.31)	1.16 (0.98, 1.37)	1.55 (1.21, 1.99)
Model 3	1.00	1.17 (0.95, 1.31)	1.15 (0.97, 1.35)	1.50 (1.16, 1.92)
Model 3 + pre-pregnancy BMI	1.00	1.07 (0.91, 1.26)	1.04 (0.88, 1.23)	1.32 (1.03, 1.70)

Model 1: adjusted for age; Model 2: Model 1 and further adjusted for education, occupation, household income, smoking, drinking, history of depression, history of polycystic ovarian syndrome, history of macrosomia babies, parity, gestational weight gain, physical activity; Model 3: Model 2 and further adjusted for intakes of white rice, seafood, meat, egg, coffee, chocolate, green tea, milk, soy isoflavone, magnesium, total dietary fat, total dietary fiber, and total energy.

4. Discussion

To our knowledge, this large prospective cohort study is the first study to investigate eating speed in relation to GDM risk. Women who reported very fast eating speed at recruitment (median: 12 weeks of gestation), compared with those reporting slow eating speed, had an increased incidence of GDM, which was independent of demographic, lifestyle-related, and dietary factors. The association was attenuated and no longer significant after further adjustment for pre-pregnancy BMI. The mediation analysis showed that being overweight accounted for 64% of the excess risk of GDM associated with eating speed.

Interestingly, in our sensitivity analysis, restricting for 64,183 women (75.7%) who reported the same eating speed during early and mid-late pregnancy, the association remained significant for women reporting very fast eating speed. One explanation for this result may be that changes in eating speed during pregnancy may have biased the association in the main analysis toward the null.

The central nervous system regulates appetite [23], and eating induces production of satiety hormones including cholecystokinin, peptide YY, and glucagon-like peptide-1, which are involved in appetite regulation [24,25]. Fast eating speed has been found to be associated with a lower level of satiety hormones [26], which may result in a delayed feeling of fullness and, thus, excess energy intake. In fact, in the present study eating speed was positively associated with energy intake (Table 1). A meta-analysis of 22 randomized controlled trials examining the effect of eating speed on energy intake also provided evidence that faster eating speed was associated with higher energy intake than slower eating speed [2].

Excess energy intake over the long term could lead to weight gain, and thereby to being overweight and obesity. A meta-analysis of cross-sectional studies showed a significant difference in BMI between individuals who ate quickly and those who ate slowly (mean difference: 1.78 kg/m^2, 95% CI:1.53, 2.04) [1]. The same meta-analysis also found fast easting speed had a stronger association with higher prevalence of obesity (pooled OR 2.15, 95% CI: 1.84, 2.51) than slow eating speed. Prospective cohort studies, in which a temporal relationship can be established, also showed fast eating speed may be a risk factor for weight gain and obesity. For example, a cohort study of 1314 university students found, after 3 years of follow-up, that those who ate quickly had an increased risk of obesity compared with those who ate slowly [27].

The mechanisms underlying the association between eating speed and GDM are unclear. As mentioned above, fast eating speed was associated with excess energy intake and higher risk of obesity, leading to development of GDM. This was supported by our mediation analysis, showing that pre-pregnancy BMI was a potential mediator in the association between eating speed and GDM. Evidence also showed eating quickly was associated with insulin resistance: in a cross-sectional study of 2704 men and 761 women, eating speed was positively associated with insulin resistance, which was independent of age, energy intake, and lifestyle factors [28]. However, the association persisted only in men when BMI was further adjusted.

We are aware of one prospective cohort study examining the effect of eating speed on the incidence of type 2 diabetes. In that study of 2050 men, after 7 years of follow-up, fast eating speed was associated with an increased risk of type 2 diabetes (relative risk = 1.97 [95% CI: 1.10–3.55]) [6]. However, that association disappeared after further adjustment for baseline BMI, which was in line with our findings in the main analysis.

The main strengths of the present study include a large sample size and a prospective design. Limitations, however, should also be mentioned. First, measurement of eating speed was based on responses to a self-reported questionnaire but not based on objective measurement, such as the size of the meal and time spent on the meal. We could not rule out the risk of measurement errors, which could bias the association toward the null. Of note, a previous study in a Japanese population showed good agreement between self-reported and friend-reported eating speed [20]. Second, although we carefully controlled for known risk factors and potential confounding factors, it was uncertain to what extent residual confounding due to unmeasured factors may have influenced our results. For example, data on family history of diabetes were absent, though this factor was unlikely to be associated with the exposure (eating speed). Third, GDM incidence was relatively lower in this population compared with that in other populations. We have reported possible explanations elsewhere [29]. Briefly, it may be explained by the lower pre-pregnancy BMI in this population, by different diagnosis criteria used, and by the exclusion of about 800 women with a history or current diagnosis of GDM at the time of study enrollment. Fourth, dietary habits including eating speed may change in pregnant women.

In our sensitivity analysis, restricting for women who reported the same eating speed during early and mid-late pregnancy, the association remained significant, indicating changes in eating speed during pregnancy may have biased the association in the main analysis toward the null.

5. Conclusions

In conclusion, the present large prospective cohort study suggested that very fast eating speed was associated with increased incidence of GDM, which may be largely mediated by increased body fat. Further studies among other populations are warranted.

Author Contributions: J.-Y.D. designed the study, analyzed the data, and wrote the manuscript. T.K. (Takashi Kimura), S.I., K.U., and H.I. helped to collect the data. J.-Y.D., T.K. (Takashi Kimura), S.I., M.C., Y.K., T.K. (Tadashi Kimura), K.U., and H.I. reviewed the manuscript. All authors have read and agreed to the published version of the manuscript.

Acknowledgments: Analysis was based on the jecs-ag-20160424 dataset released in June 2016 and revised in October 2016. Members of the Japan Environment and Children's Study (JECS) as of 2019 (principal investigator, Michihiro Kamijima): Shin Yamazaki (National Institute for Environmental Studies, Tsukuba, Japan), Yukihiro Ohya (National Centre for Child Health and Development, Tokyo, Japan), Reiko Kishi (Hokkaido University, Sapporo, Japan), Nobuo Yaegashi (Tohoku University, Sendai, Japan), Koichi Hashimoto (Fukushima Medical University, Fukushima, Japan), Chisato Mori (Chiba University, Chiba, Japan), Shuichi Ito (Yokohama City University, Yokohama, Japan), Zentaro Yamagata (University of Yamanashi, Chuo, Japan), Hidekuni Inadera (University of Toyama, Toyama, Japan), Michihiro Kamijima (Nagoya City University, Nagoya, Japan), Takeo Nakayama (Kyoto University, Kyoto, Japan), Hiroyasu Iso (Osaka University, Suita, Japan), Masayuki Shima (Hyogo College of Medicine, Nishinomiya, Japan), Youichi Kurozawa (Tottori University, Yonago, Japan), Narufumi Suganuma (Kochi University, Nankoku, Japan), Koichi Kusuhara (University of Occupational and Environmental Health, Kitakyushu, Japan), and Takahiko Katoh (Kumamoto University, Kumamoto, Japan).

References

1. Ohkuma, T.; Hirakawa, Y.; Nakamura, U.; Kiyohara, Y.; Kitazono, T.; Ninomiya, T. Association between eating rate and obesity: A systematic review and meta-analysis. *Int. J. Obes.* **2015**, *39*, 1589–1596. [CrossRef] [PubMed]
2. Robinson, E.; Almiron-Roig, E.; Rutters, F.; de Graaf, C.; Forde, C.G.; Tudur Smith, C.; Nolan, S.J.; Jebb, S.A. A systematic review and meta-analysis examining the effect of eating rate on energy intake and hunger. *Am. J. Clin. Nutr.* **2014**, *100*, 123–151. [CrossRef] [PubMed]
3. Nagahama, S.; Kurotani, K.; Pham, N.M.; Nanri, A.; Kuwahara, K.; Dan, M.; Nishiwaki, Y.; Mizoue, T. Self-reported eating rate and metabolic syndrome in Japanese people: Cross-sectional study. *BMJ Open* **2014**, *4*, e005241. [CrossRef] [PubMed]
4. Shin, A.; Lim, S.Y.; Sung, J.; Shin, H.R.; Kim, J. Dietary intake, eating habits, and metabolic syndrome in Korean men. *J. Am. Diet. Assoc.* **2009**, *109*, 633–640. [CrossRef] [PubMed]
5. Zhu, B.; Haruyama, Y.; Muto, T.; Yamazaki, T. Association between eating speed and metabolic syndrome in a three-year population-based cohort study. *J. Epidemiol.* **2015**, *25*, 332–336. [CrossRef]
6. Sakurai, M.; Nakamura, K.; Miura, K.; Takamura, T.; Yoshita, K.; Nagasawa, S.Y. Self-reported speed of eating and 7-year risk of type 2 diabetes mellitus in middle-aged Japanese men. *Metab. Clin. Exp.* **2012**, *61*, 1566–1571. [CrossRef]
7. American Diabetes Association: Gestational diabetes mellitus. *Diabetes Care* **2003**, *26* (Suppl. 1), S103–S105. [CrossRef]
8. Reece, E.A.; Leguizamon, G.; Wiznitzer, A. Gestational diabetes: The need for a common ground. *Lancet* **2009**, *373*, 1789–1797. [CrossRef]
9. Morikawa, M.; Yamada, T.; Yamada, T.; Akaishi, R.; Nishida, R.; Cho, K. Change in the number of patients after the adoption of IADPSG criteria for hyperglycemia during pregnancy in Japanese women. *Diabetes Res. Clin. Pract.* **2010**, *90*, 339–342. [CrossRef]
10. Kc, K.; Shakya, S.; Zhang, H. Gestational diabetes mellitus and macrosomia: A literature review. *Ann. Nutr. Metab.* **2015**, *66* (Suppl. 2), 14–20. [CrossRef]
11. He, X.J.; Qin, F.Y.; Hu, C.L.; Zhu, M.; Tian, C.Q.; Li, L. Is gestational diabetes mellitus an independent risk factor for macrosomia: A meta-analysis? *Arch. Gynecol. Obstet.* **2015**, *291*, 729–735. [CrossRef] [PubMed]

12. Bellamy, L.; Casas, J.P.; Hingorani, A.D.; Williams, D. Type 2 diabetes mellitus after gestational diabetes: A systematic review and meta-analysis. *Lancet* **2009**, *373*, 1773–1779. [CrossRef]
13. Li, J.; Song, C.; Li, C.; Liu, P.; Sun, Z.; Yang, X. Increased risk of cardiovascular disease in women with prior gestational diabetes: A systematic review and meta-analysis. *Diabetes Res. Clin. Pract.* **2018**, *140*, 324–338. [CrossRef] [PubMed]
14. Boerschmann, H.; Pfluger, M.; Henneberger, L.; Ziegler, A.G.; Hummel, S. Prevalence and predictors of overweight and insulin resistance in offspring of mothers with gestational diabetes mellitus. *Diabetes Care* **2010**, *33*, 1845–1849. [CrossRef]
15. Maftei, O.; Whitrow, M.J.; Davies, M.J.; Giles, L.C.; Owens, J.A.; Moore, V.M. Maternal body size prior to pregnancy, gestational diabetes and weight gain: Associations with insulin resistance in children at 9–10 years. *Diabetic Med. J. Br. Diabetic Assoc.* **2015**, *32*, 174–180. [CrossRef]
16. Shepherd, E.; Gomersall, J.C.; Tieu, J.; Han, S.; Crowther, C.A.; Middleton, P. Combined diet and exercise interventions for preventing gestational diabetes mellitus. *Cochrane Database Syst. Rev.* **2017**, *11*, Cd010443. [CrossRef]
17. Zhang, C.; Rawal, S.; Chong, Y.S. Risk factors for gestational diabetes: Is prevention possible? *Diabetologia* **2016**, *59*, 1385–1390. [CrossRef]
18. Kawamoto, T.; Nitta, H.; Murata, K.; Toda, E.; Tsukamoto, N.; Hasegawa, M. Rationale and study design of the Japan environment and children's study (JECS). *BMC Public Health* **2014**, *14*, 25. [CrossRef]
19. Michikawa, T.; Nitta, H.; Nakayama, S.F.; Yamazaki, S.; Isobe, T.; Tamura, K.; Suda, E.; Ono, M.; Yonemoto, J.; Iwai-Shimada, M.; et al. Baseline Profile of Participants in the Japan Environment and Children's Study (JECS). *J. Epidemiol.* **2018**, *28*, 99–104. [CrossRef]
20. Maruyama, K.; Sato, S.; Ohira, T.; Maeda, K.; Noda, H.; Kubota, Y.; Nishimura, S.; Kitamura, A.; Kiyama, M.; Okada, T.; et al. The joint impact on being overweight of self reported behaviours of eating quickly and eating until full: Cross sectional survey. *BMJ* **2008**, *337*, a2002.
21. Yokoyama, Y.; Takachi, R.; Ishihara, J.; Ishii, Y.; Sasazuki, S.; Sawada, N. Validity of Short and Long Self-Administered Food Frequency Questionnaires in Ranking Dietary Intake in Middle-Aged and Elderly Japanese in the Japan Public Health Center-Based Prospective Study for the Next Generation (JPHC-NEXT) Protocol Area. *J. Epidemiol.* **2016**, *26*, 420–432. [CrossRef] [PubMed]
22. Minakami, H.; Hiramatsu, Y.; Koresawa, M.; Fujii, T.; Hamada, H.; Iitsuka, Y.; Ikeda, T.; Ishikawa, H.; Ishimoto, H.; Itoh, H.; et al. Guidelines for obstetrical practice in Japan: Japan Society of Obstetrics and Gynecology (JSOG) and Japan Association of Obstetricians and Gynecologists (JAOG) 2011 edition. *J. Obstet. Gynaecol. Res.* **2011**, *37*, 1174–1197. [CrossRef] [PubMed]
23. Murphy, K.G.; Bloom, S.R. Gut hormones and the regulation of energy homeostasis. *Nature.* **2006**, *444*, 854–859. [CrossRef] [PubMed]
24. Wren, A.M.; Bloom, S.R. Gut hormones and appetite control. *Gastroenterology* **2007**, *132*, 2116–2130. [CrossRef]
25. Yu, J.H.; Kim, M.S. Molecular mechanisms of appetite regulation. *Diabetes Metab. J.* **2012**, *36*, 391–398. [CrossRef]
26. Kokkinos, A.; le Roux, C.W.; Alexiadou, K.; Tentolouris, N.; Vincent, R.P.; Kyriaki, D. Eating slowly increases the postprandial response of the anorexigenic gut hormones, peptide YY and glucagon-like peptide-1. *J. Clin. Endocrinol. Metab.* **2010**, *95*, 333–337. [CrossRef]
27. Yamane, M.; Ekuni, D.; Mizutani, S.; Kataoka, K.; Sakumoto-Kataoka, M.; Kawabata, Y.; Sakumoto-Kataoka, M.; Kawabata, Y.; Omori, C.; Azuma, T.; et al. Relationships between eating quickly and weight gain in Japanese university students: A longitudinal study. *Obesity* **2014**, *22*, 2262–2266. [CrossRef]
28. Otsuka, R.; Tamakoshi, K.; Yatsuya, H.; Wada, K.; Matsushita, K.; OuYang, P.; Hotta, Y.; Takefuji, S.; Mitsuhashi, H.; Sugiura, K.; et al. Eating fast leads to insulin resistance: Findings in middle-aged Japanese men and women. *Prev. Med.* **2008**, *46*, 154–159. [CrossRef]
29. Dong, J.Y.; Ikehara, S.; Kimura, T.; Cui, M.; Kawanishi, Y.; Kimura, T. Skipping breakfast before and during early pregnancy and incidence of gestational diabetes mellitus: The Japan Environment and Children's Study. *Am. J. Clin. Nutr.* **2020**. (Epub ahead of print). [CrossRef]

7

How Can Maternal Lifestyle Interventions Modify the Effects of Gestational Diabetes in the Neonate and the Offspring?

Delphine Mitanchez [1,2,*], Cécile Ciangura [3] and Sophie Jacqueminet [3]

1 Department of Neonatology, Bretonneau Hospital, François Rabelais University, F-37000 Tours, France
2 INSERM UMR_S 938 Centre de Recherche Saint Antoine, F-75012 Paris, France
3 Department of Diabetology, Institute of Cardiometabolism and Nutrition (ICAN), APHP, University Hospital Pitié-Salpêtrière, F-75013 Paris, France; cecile.ciangura@aphp.fr (C.C.); sophie.jacqueminet@aphp.fr (S.J.)
* Correspondence: delphine.mitanchez@univ-tours.fr

Abstract: Gestational diabetes (GDM) has deleterious effects on the offspring. Maternal obesity and excessive gestational weight gain (GWG), often associated with diabetes, also contribute to these adverse outcomes. Objectives: To assess the benefit for the offspring of maternal lifestyle interventions, including diets and physical activity, to prevent or to improve GDM and to limit excessive GWG. Method: Systematic review of meta-analyses published in English between December 2014 and November 2019. Results: Lifestyle interventions to reduce the risk of GDM reported a decreased risk of 15% to 40%, with a greater effect of exercise compared to diet. Combined lifestyle interventions specifically designed to limit GWG reduced GWG by 1.6 kg in overweight and obese women, and on average by 0.7 to 1 kg in all pregnant women. In these trials, adverse neonatal outcomes were poorly studied. Combined lifestyle interventions in women with GDM significantly reduced fetal growth. Altogether, lifestyle interventions reduced the risk of preterm birth and shoulder dystocia, but individually, diets or exercise alone had no effect on neonatal adverse outcomes. Conclusion: Specific maternal, neonatal and offspring benefits of lifestyle interventions during pregnancy to prevent or improve GDM control or to limit GWG still require clarification.

Keywords: diabetes; obesity; gestational weight gain; macrosomia; adiposity; neonate; diet; exercise

---

1. Introduction

Gestational diabetes mellitus (GDM) is defined as carbohydrate intolerance of variable severity first recognized during pregnancy. However, this definition encompasses two different entities: a glucose tolerance defect which generally occurs in the second half of pregnancy and then disappears in the post-partum period and overt diabetes in pregnancy (DIP) which is undiagnosed prior to the beginning of pregnancy, mainly as type 2 diabetes. Recently, the American Diabetes Association proposed a clearer definition of GDM: "diabetes diagnosed in the second or third trimester of pregnancy that was not clearly overt diabetes prior to gestation" [1].

A recent meta-analysis confirmed the evidence on the relationship between an increased pre-pregnancy body mass index (BMI) and the risk of GDM. It showed that the GDM risk increased 4% per unit of increase in BMI [2]. In an individual participant data meta-analysis of over 265,000 births, the risk of BMI per kg/m^2 was 1.12 (95% CI 1.12–1.13) and the highest risk was for grade 3 obesity

(BMI ≥ 40 kg/m^2) with an OR 7.59 (95% CI 6.14, 9.38). It was estimated that 42.8% of GDM cases were weight gain (GWG) was associated with increased risk of GDM (per SD increase in GWG, OR 1.14, 95% CI 1.10, 1.18) and obese mothers with high GWG were at the highest risk [3].

Maternal hyperglycemia during pregnancy has deleterious effects at all stages of fetal development. A large body of evidence support the association between pregestational diabetes and increased risk of malformations [4]. In the fetus, maternal diabetes leads to fetal hyperinsulinemia, the direct consequence of which is high birth weight and increased fat mass [5,6]. Fetal overgrowth exposes the fetus to an increased risk of a number of neonatal complications, including asphyxia, obstetrical trauma, respiratory distress and hypoglycemia. The risk of these different complications is higher in pre-gestational diabetes compared to GDM [7].

Maternal obesity and excessive GWG, often associated with diabetes, also contribute to these adverse outcomes [8]. In addition, alteration of the intrauterine environment secondary to maternal diabetes, obesity and excessive GWG contributes to the early determinism of adult diseases in offspring, including obesity, diabetes and metabolic syndrome [8,9].

Many studies have investigated the effect of lifestyle interventions, mainly including exercise and diets, on maternal glycemic and GWG control. This is a systematic review exploring data from meta-analyses in order to evaluate: (1) the benefit of lifestyle interventions to prevent GDM and limit pre-pregnancy and gestational weight gain for the offspring and (2) the effectiveness of lifestyle interventions in women with GDM to improve health outcome in the offspring.

2. Methods

The MEDLINE database was systematically reviewed for papers on human subjects published in English between December 2014 and November 2019. We used the MeSH terms diabetes, gestational, obesity, pregnancy, gestational weight gain, treatment, neonate, and offspring. For this review, we selected meta-analyses that addressed lifestyle interventions for the prevention of GDM or for the improvement of pregnancy outcomes in the case of GDM and meta-analyses that specifically addressed measures to limit GWG. We also looked at meta-analyses that addressed the effect of bariatric surgery on pregnancy outcomes. Only analyses that included more than two trials were recorded.

One hundred and eighty-eight records were identified and there were 157 records after exclusion of duplicates. Forty-three were screened and 26 full-text articles were assessed for eligibility. Two were excluded: one because it was a Cochrane analysis from 2015 updated in 2017, and the other because two records were based on the same data (Figure 1).

Macrosomia was defined as birth weight > 4000 g, unless another definition is clarified. Large-for-gestational age (LGA) was defined as birth weight > 90th percentile, based on sex and gestational age. Small-for-gestational age (SGA) was defined as birth weight < 10th percentile.

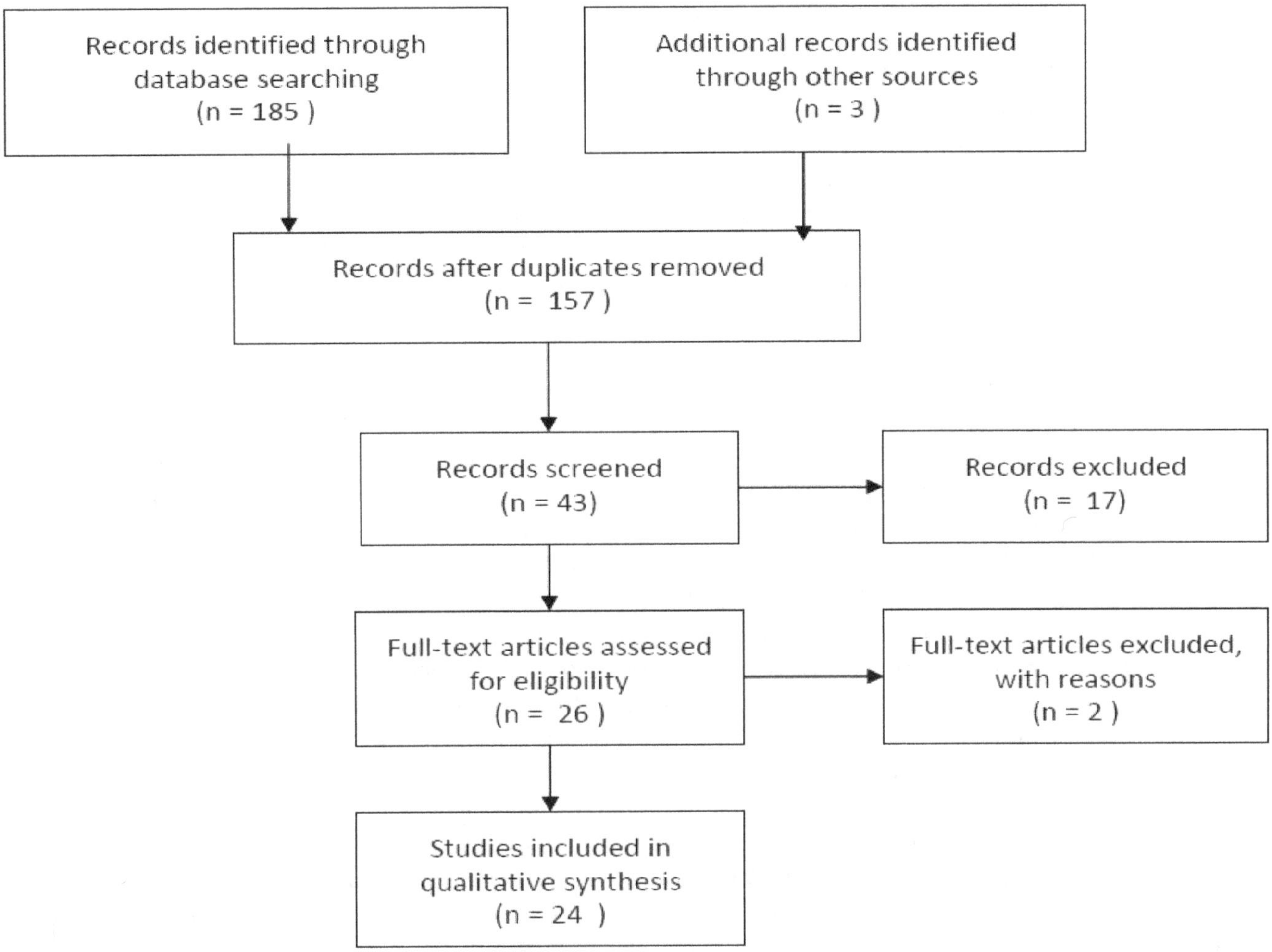

Figure 1. Flow diagram.

3. Results

3.1. Lifestyle Interventions to Prevent GDM and Maternal Weight Gain

This chapter explores the extent to which lifestyle interventions reduce the risk of GDM, or excessive maternal weight gain during pregnancy and the consequences on the health of the newborn and the child based on data from selected meta-analysis. Similarly, it explores the effects of pre-gestational weight loss observed with bariatric surgery on the health of the offspring.

3.1.1. Lifestyle Interventions to Prevent GDM (Table 1)

In a systematic review and meta-analysis of randomized clinical trials (RCT) including 11,487 pregnant women, Song et al. assessed the effect of lifestyle interventions during pregnancy, including diet and physical activity or both, on the risk of GDM. An 18% (95% confidence interval (CI) 5, to 30%; $p = 0.0091$) reduction in the risk of GDM was reported in that study. When combined diet and exercise, diet alone, and exercise alone interventions were considered separately, the observed reductions in GDM were no longer statistically significant, although the direction of effect for each type of intervention did suggest a benefit. Furthermore, subgroup analysis showed that such an intervention was effective only if initiated before the 15th gestational week (relative risk: 0.80, 95% CI 0.66, 0.97), but not among women receiving the intervention afterwards. The effect size was similar among women with pregnancy overweight or obesity (RR 0.83, 95% CI 0.69, 1.00) [10].

In an updated Cochrane review, including 23 RCTs involving almost 9000 women, Shepherd et al. compared combined diet and exercise interventions to no interventions (standard care) in pregnant women for preventing GDM. In the group with interventions, there was a reduced risk of GDM (RR 0.85, 95% CI 0.71, 1.01, $p = 0.07$), and a reduction in GWG (−0.89 kg, 95% CI −1.39, −0.40). Among infants born to mothers receiving interventions, there was no difference between groups for perinatal mortality (RR 0.82, 95% CI 0.42, 1.63), for LGA (RR 0.93 95% CI 0.81, 1.07), neonatal hypoglycemia (RR 1.42 95% CI 0.67, 2.98), or other adverse neonatal outcomes, except for macrosomia (birth weight > 4500 g) (RR 0.63, 95% CI 0.42, 0.94), preterm birth (RR 0.80, 95% CI 0.65, 0.98) and respiratory distress syndrome (RR 0.56, 95% CI 0.33, 0.97) [11]. Subgroup analyses revealed no clear differential treatment effects according to maternal BMI. In this review, the authors were unable to consider comparisons of different types of combined diet and exercise interventions. In addition, they analyzed childhood outcomes and showed that diet and exercise had no effect on weight and adiposity in infancy, nor on blood pressure, fasting glucose and insulin, HDL, triglycerides and metabolic syndrome.

Guo et al. examined the effectiveness of lifestyle interventions, including diet, exercise or both, on GDM prevention and aimed at identifying key effectiveness moderators to improve the prevention strategy. They showed that diet and exercise during pregnancy were preventive of GDM (RR 0.77, 95% CI 0.69, 0.87, $p < 10^{-3}$). Four key aspects were identified to improve the preventive effect: targeting the high-risk population, an early initiation of the intervention, the correct intensity and frequency of exercise and GWG management. In overweight or obese women, BMI failed to predict the effectiveness of an intervention. Instead, interventions were most effective in populations with high incidence of GDM rather than simply in women who are overweight or obese. Furthermore, moderate intensity exercise for 50–60 min twice a week could lead to an approximately 24% reduction in GDM [12].

Tieu et al. assessed the effects of dietary advice interventions for preventing GDM. A trend towards a reduction in GDM (RR 0.60, 95% CI 0.35, 1.04; $p = 0.07$) and lower GWG (−4.70 kg, 95% CI −8.07, −1.34) was observed for women receiving dietary advice compared with standard care. Subgroup analysis suggested a greater effect on GDM incidence for overweight and obese women receiving dietary advice (RR 0.39, 95% CI 0.19, 0.79). There were no clear differences between the dietary advice intervention and standard care groups for growth at birth, adverse neonatal outcomes and body weight, adiposity and blood pressure at six months of life [13].

Two studies assessed the effectiveness of physical exercise interventions during pregnancy to prevent GDM and excessive maternal weight gain. Sanabria-Martinez et al. found, in a sample of 2873 women, that physical exercise programs during pregnancy decreased the risk of GDM (RR = 0.69; 95% CI 0.52, 0.91; $p = 0.009$), particularly when the exercise program was performed throughout pregnancy starting from the first trimester (RR = 0.64; 95% CI 0.36, 0.98; $p = 0.038$). A decrease in maternal weight was also observed. (−1.14 kg; 95% CI −1.50, −0.78; $p < 0.001$). There was a wide variety in the type of exercises, frequency and intensity level and in most of the studies included, the adherence rate was high (>85%) [14]. Russo et al. reported a 28% reduction in the risk of GDM in the intervention group, in a meta-analysis involving 3401 participants (RR 0.72 95% CI 0.58, 0.91; $p = 0.005$). All of the interventions included at least an aerobic component (walking, land or water aerobics or both, cycling) and when reported, adherence in the intervention arm varied from 16.3% to greater than 95% [15]. In both studies, analyses were not performed according to maternal BMI and the outcome of the offspring was not studied.

Ming et al. investigated the effect of exercise during pregnancy on the occurrence of GDM among 3256 normal-weight pregnant women. The majority of the interventions adopted comprehensive exercise programs of light to moderate intensity that were performed three times per week. Exercise during pregnancy was shown to decrease the occurrence of GDM (RR = 0.58, 95% CI 0.37, 0.90; $p = 0.01$) and GWG (−1.61, 95% CI −1.99, −1.22; $p < 0.01$), but had no significant effect on gestational age at birth and birth weight [16].

In a systematic review, Davenport et al. reported that prenatal exercise-only interventions, but not exercise with co-interventions (e.g., dietary intervention), reduced the odds of GDM (n = 6934, OR 0.62, 95% CI 0.52, 0.75) [17]. One study conducted a meta-analysis of 16 cohort studies containing information on physical activity either prior to or at the commencement of pregnancy to prevent GDM. Compared to no physical activity, any pre-pregnancy or early pregnancy physical activity was associated with a 30% (OR = 0.70, 95% CI 0.57, 0.85; $p < 10^{-3}$) and a 21% (OR = 0.79, 95% CI 0.64, 0.97; $p = 0.03$) reduced risk of GDM, respectively. Engaging in >90 min/week of leisure time physical activity before pregnancy was associated with a 46% decreased risk of GDM (OR = 0.54, 95% CI 0.34, 0.87; $p = 0.01$) [18]. These two studies did not report on neonatal outcome.

The results of these studies are summarized in Table 1.

Table 1. Effect of lifestyle interventions during pregnancy on the risk of gestational diabetes (GDM), on gestational weight gain (GWG) and the risk of adverse neonatal outcomes according to meta-analyses. RDS: respiratory distress syndrome. ND: not determined.

		Risk for GDM RR or OR [95% CI]	*p*	GWG Mean [SD]	*p*	Adverse Neonatal Outcomes
Diet, exercise or both	N					
Song 2016 [10]	11,487	0.82 [0.70, 0.95]	0.033	ND		ND
Guo 2019 [12]	15,745	0.77 [0.69, 0.87]	$<10^{-4}$	ND		ND
Diet + exercise	N					
Song 2016 [10]	6047	0.85 [0.70, 1.03]	0.09	ND		ND
Shepherd 2017 [11]	8918	0.85 [0.71, 1.01]	0.07	−0.89 [−1.39, −0.40]	$<10^{-3}$	Macrosomia: 0.63 [0.42, 0.94] Preterm birth: 0.80 [0.65, 0.98] RDS: 0.56 [0.33, 0.97]
Guo 2019 [12]	7024	0.86 [0.71, 1.04]	ND	ND		ND
Diet	N					
Song 2016 [10]	1279	0.80 [0.58, 1.10]	0.17	ND		ND
Tieu 2017 [13]	1279	0.60 [0.35, 1.04]	0.07	−4.70 [−8.07, −1.34]	0.01	None
Guo 2019 [12]	2838	0.75 [0.60, 0.95]	ND	ND		ND
Exercise	N					
Sanabrina-Martinez 2015 [14]	2873	0.69 [0.52, 0.91]	0.009	−1.14 [−1.50, −0.78]	$<10^{-3}$	ND
Russo 2015 [15]	3401	0.72 [0.58, 0.91]	0.005	ND		ND
Song 2016 [10]	4161	0.77 [0.54, 1.09]	0.15	ND		ND
Davenport 2018 [17]	6934	0.62 [0.52, 0.75]	ND	ND		ND
Guo 2019 [12]	5883	0.70 [0.59, 0.84]	ND	ND		ND
Exercise in normal weight women	N					
Ming 2018 [16]	2981	0.58 [0.37, 0.90]	0.01	−1.61 [−1.99, −1.22]	$<10^{-2}$	None

3.1.2. Lifestyle Interventions to Control Pregnancy Weight Gain (Table 2)

Data from seven clinical centers that conducted separate RCT to test different lifestyle intervention strategies to modify GWG were combined to conduct an individual-participant data (IPD) meta-analysis. This included 1150 women with BMI ≥ 25 kg/m^2 randomized either to the group with interventions targeting diet, physical activity, and behavioral strategies or to the group with standard of care [19]. Mean total GWG was 1.6 kg less for the intervention group (−1.58, 95% CI −2.18, −0.99; $p < 10^{-3}$) and the percentage of women with GWG per week below Institute of Medicine (IOM) guidelines was significantly higher in the intervention group than the standard care group (20.6% vs. 14.2%; $p = 0.002$, OR 1.65, 95% CI 1.20, 2.27). There was no difference between groups for the incidence of GDM (OR 0.92, 95 CI 0.61, 1.40). Preterm birth prior to 37 and 32 weeks did not differ by group. However, preterm birth prior to 28 weeks was significantly lower in the intervention group (OR 0.46, 95% CI 0.22, 0.95; $p = 0.037$). There was no difference for growth at birth (birth weight, LGA, SGA) or for adverse neonatal outcomes (malformations, death, respiratory morbidity, hypoglycemia) [19].

In a meta-analysis of RCT including overweight and obese women, Shieh et al. found that heathy eating (specified calorie and macronutrient goals and healthy eating strategies) and/or physical activity resulted in 1.81 kg (95% CI: −3.47, −0.16, $p = 0.03$) of GWG reduction in intervention groups. Healthy eating had a larger effect size (−5.77 kg, 95% CI −9.34, −2.21, $p = 0.02$) than combined healthy eating and physical activity (−0.82 kg, 95% CI −1.28, −0.36, $p = 0.0005$) in limiting GWG. They concluded that healthy eating with calorie and macronutrient goals are especially effective in limiting excessive GWG among pregnant overweight and obese women. The outcome of the neonates was not studied [20].

One Cochrane review evaluated the effectiveness and safety of diet or exercise, or both, interventions for preventing excessive weight gain in pregnant women of any BMI [21]. Diet or exercise, or both, interventions resulted in an average reduction of excessive GWG, usually defined according to prevailing IOM guidelines, of 20% in favor of the intervention group (RR 0.80, 95% CI 0.73, 0.87). There was no difference the between intervention and control groups for preterm birth (average RR 0.91, 95% CI 0.68, 1.22), for macrosomia or LGA (respectively, RR 0.93, 95% CI 0.86, 1.02 and RR 0.92, 95% CI 0.80, 1.05). Moreover, the risk for shoulder dystocia, birth trauma, hypoglycemia and hyperbilirubinemia was not different between the groups. Neonatal respiratory distress syndrome was the only neonatal outcome with significant risk reduction in the intervention groups (RR 0.47, 95% CI 0.26, 0.85) (more than 2000 participants with diet and exercise counselling interventions conducted in overweight and obese women).

The International Weight Management in Pregnancy (i-WIP) Collaborative Group published a meta-analysis of individual participant data from RCT to synthetize the evidence on effects of interventions based on diet and physical activity during pregnancy [22]. Based on IPD meta-analysis, diet or physical activity based interventions, or a combination of both resulted in significantly less GWG compared with control (−0.70 kg, 95% CI −0.92, −0.48 kg), but the risk of GDM was not significantly reduced (OR 0.89, 95% CI 0.72 to 1.10). No strong evidence was found to suggest that interventions had an effect on preterm birth or individual adverse offspring outcomes (stillbirth, LGA, SGA and admission to a neonatal intensive care unit). These results were not different according to maternal BMI. All three individual interventions (diet, physical activity and mixed) had a similar effect on reducing GWG by an average of 0.7 kg.

Ruchat et al. examined the relationship between prenatal exercise and GWG. They showed that exercise-only interventions compared with no exercise decreased total GWG (−0.9 kg, 95% CI −1.23, −0.57 kg) and also the risk of excessive GWG by about 30% (OR 0.68, 95% CI 0.57, 0.80) [23].

None of the studies to control GWG reported strong data on long-term outcomes in offspring. The results of these studies are summarized in Table 2.

Table 2. Effects of lifestyle interventions on gestational weight gain (GWG) and the risk of gestational diabetes (GDM), and the risk of adverse neonatal outcomes according to meta-analyses. Only significant effects on adverse neonatal outcomes are reported in the table. RDS: respiratory distress syndrome. ND: not determined.

		GWG kg Mean [SD]	Risk for GDM OR or RR [95% CI]	Adverse Neonatal Outcomes OR or RR [95% CI]
All lifestyle interventions	N			
Peaceman 2018 * [19]	1150	−1.58 [−2.18, −0.99]	0.92 [0.61, 1.40]	Preterm birth < 28 wks: 0.48 [0.22, 0.95]
Diet, exercise or both	N			
Muktabhan 2015 [21]	11,444	Risk of excessive GWG RR [95% CI] 0.80 [0.73, 0.87]	ND	RDS in overweight/obese: 0.47 [0.26, 0.85]
i-WIP 2017 [22]	9320	−0.70 [−0.92, −0.48]	0.89 [0.72, 1.10]	None
Shieh 2018 * [20]	6920	−1.81 [−3.47, −0.16]	ND	ND
Diet	N			
i-WIP 2017 [22]	1168	−0.72 [−1.48, −0.04]	1.03 [0.30, 3.61]	Preterm birth: 0.28 [0.08, 0.96]
Shieh 2018 * [20]	719	−5.77 [−9.34, −2.21]	ND	ND
Exercise	N			
Sanabrina-Martinez 2015 [14]	2873	−1.14 [−1.50, −0.78]	0.69 [0.52, 0.91]	ND
i-WIP 2017 [22]	2915	−0.73 [−1.11, −0.34]	0.67 [0.46, 0.99]	None
Ruchat 2018 [23]	5819	−0.90 [−1.23, −0.57]	ND	ND
Diet + exercise	N			
i-WIP 2017 [22]	2981	−0.71 [−1.10, −0.31]	1.02 [0.79, 1.32]	None
Shieh 2018 * [20]	5853	−0.82 [−1.28, −0.36]	ND	ND

* only women with BMI ≥ 25 kg/m^2.

3.2. Pre-Pregnancy Weight Loss: Bariatric Surgery

Bariatric surgery (BS) is thought to be an effective intervention to sustain weight loss and is increasingly being used as an effective treatment for obesity. BS procedures are generally categorized into three groups. Restrictive procedures (laparoscopic adjustable gastric banding and sleeve gastrectomy) lead to weight loss by reducing gastric capacity which in turn restricts energy intake. Malabsorptive procedure (biliopancreatic diversion) leads to weight loss by restricting absorption of nutrients. Malabsorptive and restrictive procedures (Roux-en-Y gastric bypass) reduces stomach capacity, thereby causing malabsorption and a certain degree of restriction of food intake.

There are two meta-analyses under the scope of this paper that evaluated the effects of BS on pregnancy and neonatal outcomes. We also considered the meta-analysis of Galazis et al. that was published in October 2014.

Galazis et al. included 17 non-randomized cohorts or case-control studies that evaluated a total of 166,134 participants, which included 5361 women who underwent BS and 160,773 controls. They showed that compared to controls, in the BS group, there was a lower incidence of GDM (OR 0.47, 95% CI 0.40, 0.56; $p < 0.001$) and LGA (OR 0.46, 95% CI 0.34, 0.62; $p < 0.001$) and a higher incidence of SGA (OR 1.93, 95% CI 1.52, 2.44; $p < 0.001$), preterm birth (OR 1.31, 95% CI 1.08, 1.58; $p = 0.006$), and admission for neonatal intensive care (OR 1.33, 95% CI 1.02, 1.72; $p = 0.03$). There was no significant difference in the incidence of perinatal mortality [24].

Yi et al. conducted a meta-analysis of 11 cohort studies and 4178 obese women who had undergone BS and 16,016 women who had not. Among the women who had undergone BS, there was an apparent reduction in average BMI from 40–50 to 32–35 kg/m^2. BS improved pregnancy outcomes with a lower risk of GDM (OR 0.31; 95% CI 0.15, 0.65) and macrosomia (OR 0.40; 95% CI 0.24, 0.67) but a higher risk of SGA (OR 2.16; 95% CI 1.28, 3.66) [25]. The risk of preterm birth was not modified by BS in this analysis and GWG was not studied.

A larger meta-analysis, including 20 cohort studies and approximately 2.8 million subjects, 8364 of whom had BS, was published by Kwong et al. [26]. When compared with control subjects who were matched for pre-surgery BMI, patients who underwent BS showed reduced rates of GDM (OR 0.20; 95% CI 0.11, 0.37) and of LGA (OR 0.31; 95% CI 0.17, 0.59). However, there was an increased risk for SGA (OR 2.16 95% CI 1.34–3.48), and for preterm birth (1.35, 95% CI 1.02, 1.79). There was no difference in rates of malformations, neonatal death and neonatal intensive care unit admissions.

Compared with restrictive surgeries, malabsorptive surgeries resulted in a greater increase in SGA (OR 2.39; 95% CI, 1.94, 2.94 versus OR 1.38; 95% CI 0.90, 2.10; $p = 0.023$) and a greater decrease in LGA (OR 0.28; 95% CI 0.22, 0.36 versus OR 0.50; 95% CI, 0.35, 0.73; $p < 0.012$). The authors were not able to account for the amount of weight loss relative to the pre-surgical weight, nor to analyze GWG.

Data on long-term outcomes such as the effects of BS on metabolic risk in the offspring into childhood and adulthood are inconsistent [27].

3.3. Lifestyle Interventions in Mothers with GDM to Improve Neonatal Heath

3.3.1. Lifestyle Interventions: Diet, Exercise and Others

A review from Brown et al. suggested that for women diagnosed with GDM, and receiving lifestyle interventions (two or more interventions including dietary advice, physical activity, education or self-monitoring of blood glucose), there was a benefit for their neonates mainly due to reduced fetal growth. In the neonates, lifestyle interventions were associated with a decreased risk of being LGA (RR 0.60, 95% CI 0.50, 0.7), a reduction of macrosomia (RR 0.64, 95% CI 0.48, 0.87), a lower birth weight (−109.64 g, 95% CI −149.77, −69.51) and a decreased neonatal fat mass (−37.30 g, 95% CI −63.97, −10.63), compared with the control group. There was also a reduced risk of being born preterm (< 37 weeks') (RR 0.71, 95% CI 0.53, 0.96) and of shoulder dystocia (RR 0.38, 95% CI 0.21, 0.66), but no difference was found for other adverse neonatal outcomes [28]. Lifestyle interventions were also associated with a decrease in weight gain in pregnancy (−1.30 kg, 95% CI −2.26, −0.35) and an increased use of additional pharmacological therapies. In this meta-analysis, there was a wide variety of interventions including exercise, diet, self-monitoring of blood glucose and education. This makes it hard to determine which of the interventions is more effective, especially since most of the interventions included a dietary component.

Follow-up into childhood was poorly reported with only three of the 15 included trials contributing data which could not be combined in a meta-analysis [29–31]. There was no difference between groups in infancy at ages 4 to 11 years, for BMI greater or equal to the 85th percentile and no difference in dyslipidemia or blood pressure.

3.3.2. Lifestyle Intervention: Diet Alone

To date, a wide range of dietary advice interventions have been investigated in women with GDM, including low glycemic index (GI) diets, energy restricted diets, increase or decrease in carbohydrates, and modifications of fat or protein quality or quantity. Four systematic reviews analyzed the effect of the different diets on maternal and neonatal outcomes. The main results concerning the most commonly used diets are presented in Table 3 [32–35].

The energy-restricted diets may have different designs; for example, a calorie restricted diet of 35 kcal per kg ideal body weight per day or a restricted daily energy intake to 1200 kcal. The GI is used to estimate the in vivo blood glucose response to the intake of a food item, relative to that of a carbohydrate reference. The GI ranks food items on a scale of 0 to 100, with food items with higher GI values contributing to a greater increase in blood glucose. Low GI diets are based on foods with GI less than 55, producing a lower postprandial glucose elevation. Dietary Approaches to Stop Hypertension (DASH) diet is a diet rich in fruits, vegetables, whole grains and low-fat dairy products, and low in saturated fats, cholesterol, refined grains and sweets. In the low carbohydrate diet, the daily total energy intake from carbohydrates is 40% to 45% compared 55% to 60% for the control group.

When considering all diets, Yamamoto et al. showed that modified dietary interventions decreased maternal glycemic values and were significantly associated with significantly lower needs for medication treatment. This result was mainly due to low GI diets that showed a larger decrease in fasting, postprandial, and post-breakfast glucose compared with control diets [35]. The three analyses from Viana et al., Wein et al. and Han et al. reported a lower need for medication with low GI diets. The others dietary advice interventions reported in Table 3 had not effect on maternal medication need, excepted DASH diet. Only low carbohydrates and DASH diets were associated with a significant reduction in GWG in the analysis from Han et al. [34].

When considering all diets together, modified dietary interventions were significantly associated with less macrosomia and lower infant birth weight [35]. However, results concerning the effect of low GI diets on fetal growth are controversial. Viana et al. found that diet with low GI significantly reduced birth weight but not the risk of having macrosomia. Wei et al. found that low GI diets reduced the risk of macrosomia. Additionally, a subgroup analysis showed that low GI diets with increased dietary fiber reduced the risk of macrosomia beyond that of a low GI diet alone. Han et al. and Yamamoto et al. found no difference for LGA, macrosomia and birth weight with low GI diet. Energy restricted diets and low carbohydrate diets showed no benefit on fetal growth. Only DASH diet was associated with reduced relative risk of macrosomia, but not of LGA, and reduced birth weight.

None of the dietary advice interventions studied were associated with increased risk of neonatal hypoglycemia. In addition, there were significantly more neonates with hypocalcaemia born to women in the energy-restricted diet group compared with the no energy restriction group (RR 1.36, 95% CI 1.00, 1.86) [34]. None of the dietary interventions reported in Table 3 was associated with increased risk of being preterm or SGA [33,34].

Table 3. Effect of diet advice interventions in women with gestational diabetes on the risk of maternal medication use, on gestational weight gain (GWG), on the growth at birth and on the risk of neonatal hypoglycaemia according to meta-analyses. Values are in bold when the results were statistically significant; p values are indicated when they were reported in the reviews. LGA: Large for Gestational Age.

		MOTHER		NEONATE			
	N	Medication RR [95% CI]	GWG kg Mean [SD]	LGA RR [95% CI]	Macrosomia RR [95% CI]	Birth Weight g Mean [SD]	Hypoglycaemia RR [95% CI]
Viana 2014 [32]							
Low glycemic index	257	**0.77 [0.66, 0.99]** **	−0.41 [−1.84, 1.02]	ND	0.48 [0.15, 1.56]	−161.9 [−246.4, −77.4] ¶	ND
Energy restriction diet	425	ND	ND	ND	1.00 [0.65, 1.55]	ND	1.01 [0.72, 1.43]
Low carbohydrates	182	1.06 [0.15, 1.56]	ND	ND	0.35 [0.06, 1.91]	ND	ND
Wei 2016 [33]							
Low glycemic index	302	0.67 [0.44–1.00] *	ND	1.38 [0.58, 3.32]	0.27 [0.10, 0.71] §	ND	ND
Han 2017 [34]							
Low glycemic index	224	0.82 [0.39, 1.74]	−0.47 [−2.18, 1.24]	0.71 [0.22, 2.34]	0.59 [0.16, 2.26]	−56.0 [−201.9, 89.9]	ND
Energy restriction diet	437	1.05 [0.47, 2.34]	+1.88 [−1.96, 5.72]	1.17 [0.65, 2.21]	0.99 [0.64, 1.53]	−107.0 [−240.3, 26.3]	1.06 [0.48, 2.32]
Low carbohydrates	182	1.02 [0.77, 1.37]	−0.90 [−1.60, −0.20]	0.51 [0.13, 1.95]	0.20 [0.02, 1.69]	+ 22.0 [−241.1, 285.1]	0.91 [0.39, 2.12]
DASH diet	136	0.28 [0.14, 0.53] **	−2.88 [−8.48, −2.71]	ND	0.10 [0.01, 0.73]	−581.3 [−790.3, −372.2]	ND
Yamamoto 2018 [35]							
All diet	1023	0.65 [0.47, 0.88]	ND	0.96 [0.63, 1.46]	0.49 [0.27, 0.88] **	−171.6 [−333.6, −7.6] **	ND
Low glycemic index		0.80 [0.55, 1.14]	ND	1.33 [0.54, 3.31]	0.46 [0.15, 1.46]	−54.2 [−179.0, 70.5]	ND
Energy restriction diet		1.05 [0.47, 2.34]	ND	1.17 [0.65, 2.12]	1.56 [0.61, 3.94]	194.0 [−42.6, 430.6]	ND
Low carbohydrates		1.00 [0.75, 1.34]	ND	0.51 [0.13, 1.95]	0.20 [0.02, 1.69]	57.7 [−164.9, 280.4]	ND

* $p = 0.05$; ** $p < 0.05$; § $p \leq 10^{-2}$; ¶ $p \leq 10^{-3}$.

In the Cochrane review, Han et al. reported that perinatal mortality and stillbirth was studied in only one trial comparing low versus high carbohydrate diet and did not find a difference between the groups. Likewise, there were no differences between groups for shoulder dystocia and hyperbilirubinemia in trials comparing low energy-restricted diet versus no restriction [34].

None of these studies reported strong data on long-term outcome in offspring.

3.3.3. Lifestyle Intervention: Exercise-Only

In a Cochrane review, including 11 randomized trials, involving 638 women, Brown et al. specifically evaluated the effects of exercise interventions (any type of exercise program targeted at women with GDM at any stage of pregnancy) for improving maternal and fetal outcomes in women with GDM [36]. Exercise was associated with a reduced fasting and post-prandial blood glucose concentration compared with control, but there was no difference between groups for weight gain in pregnancy. There was no difference between groups for the composite outcome of mortality and morbidity (variously defined by trials, e.g., perinatal or infant death, shoulder dystocia, bone fracture or nerve palsy) (RR 0.56, 95% CI 0.12, 2.61), for being born macrosomic (RR 0.69, 95% CI 0.35, 1.35, n = 296) or for neonatal hypoglycemia (RR 2.00, 95% CI 0.20, 20.04).

In a meta-analysis involving 3670 women, Davenport et al. reported a 39% reduction in the odds of having a macrosomic baby (OR 0.61, 95% CI 0.41, 0.92) in women who exercised during the prenatal period compared with women who did not exercise, without affecting the risk of growth-restricted, preterm or low birth weight babies. Prenatal exercise was not associated with infant weight, obesity or body fat [37].

4. Discussion

4.1. Summary of the Results

Overall, trials that evaluated the effect of lifestyle interventions to reduce the risk of GDM reported a decreased risk of 15 to 40% in GDM, with a greater effect of exercise than diet. They also reported a variable decrease in GWG from 1 kg to 4 kg, when it was evaluated. The effects on adverse neonatal outcomes were poorly studied, particularly very weak effects were reported on neonatal anthropometry.

Combined lifestyle interventions specifically designed to limit GWG reduced GWG by 1.6 kg in overweight and obese women. Other lifestyle interventions to reduce GWG in all pregnant women decreased GWG on average by 0.7 to 1 kg. Diets that control calories and macronutrients had the most important effect on weight gain. Most of these interventions did not reduce the risk of GDM, excepted measures based on exercise which reduced this risk by about 35%–40%. The effects on adverse neonatal outcomes were limited. In particular, no effect was reported on growth at birth. Only two studies reported a reduced risk in preterm birth and one study reported a reduced risk of respiratory distress syndrome in infants of overweight and obese women.

BS before pregnancy decreased the risk of GDM by 70% to 80% and the risk of LGA by 60% to 70%. The risks for adverse neonatal outcomes were not modified by BS, except for a 2-fold increase in SGA and an increase of about 30% in preterm birth.

Combined lifestyle interventions in pregnant women with GDM significantly reduced fetal growth and neonatal fat mass. When all diets were considered together, they reduced the risk of macrosomia and birth weight. But, individually, specific diets had controversial or no effect on fetal growth, except the DASH diet, which reduced the risk of macrosomia and birth weight. Exercise alone during pregnancy with GDM had no effect on the risk of macrosomia, but prenatal exercise reduced it by 40%. Altogether, lifestyle interventions during pregnancy with GDM reduced the risk of preterm birth and shoulder dystocia, but individually, diets or exercise alone had no effect on neonatal adverse outcomes. Furthermore, energy restricted diet was associated with an increased risk of neonatal hypocalcaemia.

4.2. *Strengths and Limitations of the Method*

Many and various lifestyle interventions were evaluated during pregnancy and a large number of RCTs have been conducted. Individual studies have a limited ability to show effects on outcomes due to concomitant interventions and population size, and because outcomes are rare and difficult to identify. This is why we chose to work on the basis of meta-analyses which allow to pool the results of individual studies, especially since a large number of patients is required to conclude that an effect has occurred. Nonetheless, an additional limit is the heterogeneity of data. In particular, various diagnostic criteria for GDM were used in the different studies, and the outcomes evaluated were not always the same, were not uniformly standardized, or even not available. Another potential weakness is the small number of studies included in each dietary intervention category. Moreover, it was difficult to take into consideration the design of individual program intervention, the time of pregnancy when it was initiated and applied, and the compliance of patients to these interventions.

The limitation of aggregate data in meta-analysis can be addressed by meta-analyses of individual participant data, where the raw patient-level data are obtained and synthesized across trials. We have identified two such studies, but they provided limited information on the outcome of the newborn [19,22].

4.3. *Effectiveness of Interventions in Pregnant Women*

Lifestyle interventions can significantly reduce the risk of GDM with clinical relevance, but the limitation of GWG is low from a clinical standpoint. In addition, the benefits for the neonates and the offspring are limited, with a more significant impact on anthropometry of the neonates, if any. Among dietary intervention, low GI and DASH diets seem to be the most efficient.

Exercise alone or associated with diet, before or during pregnancy, significantly reduces the risk of GDM and GWG and improves fetal growth. Nevertheless, it is necessary to define precisely the type, duration and frequency of exercise that may have the greatest impact. The earlier the program is initiated during pregnancy, the better the results are.

Finally, the effects of lifestyle interventions on various groups of women based on BMI category, age, parity and risk status in pregnancy are difficult to assess or are not known.

4.4. *Why Haven Lifestyle Interventions Not Achieved Better Outcomes for the Offspring?*

Overall, the benefits of maternal lifestyle interventions are disappointing for the offspring. They do not significantly modify birth weight and have a limited impact on neonatal outcomes.

We hypothesize that the outcomes assessed are not entirely appropriate. Indeed, the measure of neonatal adiposity is probably more relevant than birth weight in assessing the effect of an intervention. In a recent RCT that included 334 neonates, counselling pregnant women with a BMI $\geq$29 kg/m^2 on both healthy eating and physical activity resulted in a significant reduction of neonatal adiposity (-63 g for fat mass, and -1.2% for fat percentage), although birth weight was not different between groups. Interestingly, these changes were not mediated by GWG alone, but a reduction in sedentary time (notably sitting time) drove the effect of the intervention on neonatal adiposity [38].

The majority of studies focus on interventions initiated after pregnancy was diagnosed. However, many physio pathological arguments demonstrate that these interventions are initiated too late to show an effect on the mother and the newborn. Indeed, Catalano et al. showed that pre-gravid women with normal glucose tolerance who developed GDM in late gestation had subclinical metabolic dysfunction prior to conception compared to women with normal glucose tolerance [39]. Their research also suggests that maternal pre-gravid and early pregnancy metabolic conditions associated with obesity, such as increased insulin resistance and inflammation, affect early placenta functions and genes expression. These alterations in placental functions occur in the first trimester of pregnancy before most intervention trials are initiated [40]. The placenta is at the interface of the maternal and fetal environment and its function plays a major role on the impact of maternal health on fetal development.

Maternal diabetes and obesity lead to modifications to substrates transport and metabolism across the placenta. This contributes to adverse fetal outcomes, the most common being macrosomia [41]. This also explains why even in pregnant women with well controlled diabetes, macrosomia remains common. All these elements argue in favor of the initiation of lifestyle interventions prior to pregnancy in order to obtain significant effects in the neonate.

BS represents an extreme model of pre-gestational intervention, with often significant weight loss in mothers before pregnancy. Compared with mothers with the same pre-gestational BMI, BS is associated with a significantly decreased risk of macrosomia, but also with an increased risk of low birth weight. In addition, BS exposes pregnant women to the risk of nutritional deficiencies with poorly known effects in the newborn and the offspring [42]. This shows that pre-gestational weight loss may have positive effects in limiting fetal growth, but that it has to be dosed reasonably to avoid adverse effects.

In addition, the benefit of lifestyle interventions on long-term outcomes was poorly studied in the meta-analyses and the few results available are inconsistent. The long-term effect of maternal diabetes on offspring outcome is controversial. Some authors claimed that there is an association between maternal diabetes and offspring diabetes and obesity [43]. Others showed that the association of maternal glucose levels during pregnancy with childhood adiposity is generally attenuated after adjusting for maternal BMI [44,45]. Recently, large cohort studies reported new evidence between the association of GDM and offspring glucose metabolism and adiposity. The HAPO Follow-up Study (HAPO FUS) followed more than 4500 children ages 10 to 14 years of age and examined the associations between maternal glucose levels during pregnancy and childhood glucose metabolism and adiposity.

It showed that GDM was significantly and independently associated with childhood impaired glucose tolerance and with childhood adiposity [46,47]. In addition, in a large population-based cohort study (2,432,000 live born offspring), during up to 40 years of follow-up, GDM was associated with increased rates of early onset cardio-vascular disease in offspring, persisting from childhood through early adulthood [48]. However, there is little evidence suggesting that the usual treatment of GDM affects long-term outcomes in the offspring. In a follow-up study of children (ages 5–10) born to women enrolled in a multicenter trial with treatment (diet therapy and insulin if required) versus no treatment of mild GDM, no reduction in childhood obesity or metabolic dysfunction in the offspring of treated women was found, except for lower fasting glucose in female offspring only. It is thus thought that the effect of lifestyle interventions will have limited effects on the long-term outcome of the offspring or that it might be difficult to demonstrate.

5. Conclusions

Specific maternal, neonatal and offspring benefits of lifestyle interventions during pregnancy to prevent or improve GDM control or to limit GWG still require clarification. While ultimately healthy lifestyle is a matter of individual behavior change, individual interventions must extend beyond individual targeted initiatives to address societal and environmental factors and enable children, adolescents and women to have a healthier lifestyle in order to prevent obesity and related complications before pregnancy [49].

Author Contributions: All the authors contributed to the acquisition, analysis, and interpretation of data, revising it critically and final approval of the version to be published. All authors have read and agreed to the published version of the manuscript.

Acknowledgments: We thank Lina Etri for the language review.

References

1. American Diabetes Association. Classification and diagnosis of diabetes: Standards of medical care in diabetes. *Diabetes Care* **2018**, *41*, S13–S27. [CrossRef]

2. Najafi, F.; Hasani, J.; Izadi, N.; Hashemi-Nazari, S.S.; Namvar, Z.; Mohammadi, S.; Sadeghi, M. The effect of prepregnancy body mass index on the risk of gestational diabetes mellitus: A systematic review and dose-response meta-analysis. *Obes. Rev.* **2019**, *20*, 472–486. [CrossRef]
3. Santos, S.; Voerman, E.; Amiano, P.; Barros, H.; Beilin, L.J.; Bergstrom, A.; Charles, M.A.; Chatzi, L.; Chevrier, C.; Chrousos, G.P.; et al. Impact of maternal body mass index and gestational weight gain on pregnancy complications: An individual participant data meta-analysis of european, north american and australian cohorts. *BJOG* **2019**, *126*, 984–995. [CrossRef]
4. Reece, E.A. Diabetes-induced birth defects: What do we know? What can we do? *Curr. Diabetes Rep.* **2012**, *12*, 24–32. [CrossRef] [PubMed]
5. Metzger, B.E.; Lowe, L.P.; Dyer, A.R.; Trimble, E.R.; Chaovarindr, U.; Coustan, D.R.; Hadden, D.R.; McCance, D.R.; Hod, M.; McIntyre, H.D.; et al. Hyperglycemia and adverse pregnancy outcomes. *N. Engl. J. Med.* **2008**, *358*, 1991–2002. [PubMed]
6. Wendland, E.M.; Torloni, M.R.; Falavigna, M.; Trujillo, J.; Dode, M.A.; Campos, M.A.; Duncan, B.B.; Schmidt, M.I. Gestational diabetes and pregnancy outcomes–A systematic review of the world health organization (who) and the international association of diabetes in pregnancy study groups (iadpsg) diagnostic criteria. *BMC Pregnancy Childbirth* **2012**, *12*, 23. [CrossRef] [PubMed]
7. Billionnet, C.; Mitanchez, D.; Weill, A.; Nizard, J.; Alla, F.; Hartemann, A.; Jacqueminet, S. Gestational diabetes and adverse perinatal outcomes from 716,152 births in france in 2012. *Diabetologia* **2017**, *60*, 636–644. [CrossRef] [PubMed]
8. Mitanchez, D.; Chavatte-Palmer, P. Review shows that maternal obesity induces serious adverse neonatal effects and is associated with childhood obesity in their offspring. *Acta Paediatr.* **2018**, *107*, 1156–1165. [CrossRef]
9. Armengaud, J.B.; Ma, R.C.W.; Siddeek, B.; Visser, G.H.A.; Simeoni, U. Offspring of mothers with hyperglycaemia in pregnancy: The short term and long-term impact. What is new? *Diabetes Res. Clin. Pract.* **2018**, *145*, 155–166. [CrossRef]
10. Song, C.; Li, J.; Leng, J.; Ma, R.C.; Yang, X. Lifestyle intervention can reduce the risk of gestational diabetes: A meta-analysis of randomized controlled trials. *Obes. Rev.* **2016**, *17*, 960–969. [CrossRef]
11. Shepherd, E.; Gomersall, J.C.; Tieu, J.; Han, S.; Crowther, C.A.; Middleton, P. Combined diet and exercise interventions for preventing gestational diabetes mellitus. *Cochrane Database Syst. Rev.* **2017**, *11*, CD010443. [CrossRef] [PubMed]
12. Guo, X.Y.; Shu, J.; Fu, X.H.; Chen, X.P.; Zhang, L.; Ji, M.X.; Liu, X.M.; Yu, T.T.; Sheng, J.Z.; Huang, H.F. Improving the effectiveness of lifestyle interventions for gestational diabetes prevention: A meta-analysis and meta-regression. *BJOG* **2019**, *126*, 311–320. [CrossRef] [PubMed]
13. Tieu, J.; Shepherd, E.; Middleton, P.; Crowther, C.A. Dietary advice interventions in pregnancy for preventing gestational diabetes mellitus. *Cochrane Database Syst. Rev.* **2017**, *1*, CD006674. [CrossRef] [PubMed]
14. Sanabria-Martinez, G.; Garcia-Hermoso, A.; Poyatos-Leon, R.; Alvarez-Bueno, C.; Sanchez-Lopez, M.; Martinez-Vizcaino, V. Effectiveness of physical activity interventions on preventing gestational diabetes mellitus and excessive maternal weight gain: A meta-analysis. *BJOG* **2015**, *122*, 1167–1174. [CrossRef] [PubMed]
15. Russo, L.M.; Nobles, C.; Ertel, K.A.; Chasan-Taber, L.; Whitcomb, B.W. Physical activity interventions in pregnancy and risk of gestational diabetes mellitus: A systematic review and meta-analysis. *Obstet. Gynecol.* **2015**, *125*, 576–582. [CrossRef] [PubMed]
16. Ming, W.K.; Ding, W.; Zhang, C.J.P.; Zhong, L.; Long, Y.; Li, Z.; Sun, C.; Wu, Y.; Chen, H.; Chen, H.; et al. The effect of exercise during pregnancy on gestational diabetes mellitus in normal-weight women: A systematic review and meta-analysis. *BMC Pregnancy Childbirth* **2018**, *18*, 440. [CrossRef]
17. Davenport, M.H.; Ruchat, S.M.; Poitras, V.J.; Jaramillo Garcia, A.; Gray, C.E.; Barrowman, N.; Skow, R.J.; Meah, V.L.; Riske, L.; Sobierajski, F.; et al. Prenatal exercise for the prevention of gestational diabetes mellitus and hypertensive disorders of pregnancy: A systematic review and meta-analysis. *Br. J. Sports Med.* **2018**, *52*, 1367–1375. [CrossRef]
18. Mijatovic-Vukas, J.; Capling, L.; Cheng, S.; Stamatakis, E.; Louie, J.; Cheung, N.W.; Markovic, T.; Ross, G.; Senior, A.; Brand-Miller, J.C.; et al. Associations of diet and physical activity with risk for gestational diabetes mellitus: A systematic review and meta-analysis. *Nutrients* **2018**, *10*, 698. [CrossRef]

19. Peaceman, A.M.; Clifton, R.G.; Phelan, S.; Gallagher, D.; Evans, M.; Redman, L.M.; Knowler, W.C.; Joshipura, K.; Haire-Joshu, D.; Yanovski, S.Z.; et al. Lifestyle interventions limit gestational weight gain in women with overweight or obesity: Life-moms prospective meta-analysis. *Obes. Silver Spring* **2018**, *26*, 1396–1404. [CrossRef]
20. Shieh, C.; Cullen, D.L.; Pike, C.; Pressler, S.J. Intervention strategies for preventing excessive gestational weight gain: Systematic review and meta-analysis. *Obes. Rev.* **2018**, *19*, 1093–1109. [CrossRef]
21. Muktabhant, B.; Lawrie, T.A.; Lumbiganon, P.; Laopaiboon, M. Diet or exercise, or both, for preventing excessive weight gain in pregnancy. *Cochrane Database Syst. Rev.* **2015**, *6*, CD007145. [CrossRef] [PubMed]
22. International Weight Management in Pregnancy Collaborative Group. Effect of diet and physical activity based interventions in pregnancy on gestational weight gain and pregnancy outcomes: Meta-analysis of individual participant data from randomised trials. *BMJ* **2017**, *358*, j3119.
23. Ruchat, S.M.; Mottola, M.F.; Skow, R.J.; Nagpal, T.S.; Meah, V.L.; James, M.; Riske, L.; Sobierajski, F.; Kathol, A.J.; Marchand, A.A.; et al. Effectiveness of exercise interventions in the prevention of excessive gestational weight gain and postpartum weight retention: A systematic review and meta-analysis. *Br. J. Sports Med.* **2018**, *52*, 1347–1356. [CrossRef] [PubMed]
24. Galazis, N.; Docheva, N.; Simillis, C.; Nicolaides, K.H. Maternal and neonatal outcomes in women undergoing bariatric surgery: A systematic review and meta-analysis. *Eur. J. Obstet. Gynecol. Reprod. Biol.* **2014**, *181*, 45–53. [CrossRef] [PubMed]
25. Yi, X.Y.; Li, Q.F.; Zhang, J.; Wang, Z.H. A meta-analysis of maternal and fetal outcomes of pregnancy after bariatric surgery. *Int. J. Gynaecol. Obstet.* **2015**, *130*, 3–9. [CrossRef] [PubMed]
26. Kwong, W.; Tomlinson, G.; Feig, D.S. Maternal and neonatal outcomes after bariatric surgery; a systematic review and meta-analysis: Do the benefits outweigh the risks? *Am. J. Obstet. Gynecol.* **2018**, *218*, 573–580. [CrossRef]
27. Al-Nimr, R.I.; Hakeem, R.; Moreschi, J.M.; Gallo, S.; McDermid, J.M.; Pari-Keener, M.; Stahnke, B.; Papoutsakis, C.; Handu, D.; Cheng, F.W. Effects of bariatric surgery on maternal and infant outcomes of pregnancy-an evidence analysis center systematic review. *J. Acad. Nutr. Diet.* **2019**, *119*, 1921–1943. [CrossRef]
28. Brown, J.; Alwan, N.A.; West, J.; Brown, S.; McKinlay, C.J.; Farrar, D.; Crowther, C.A. Lifestyle interventions for the treatment of women with gestational diabetes. *Cochrane Database Syst. Rev.* **2017**, *5*, CD011970. [CrossRef]
29. Garner, P.; Okun, N.; Keely, E.; Wells, G.; Perkins, S.; Sylvain, J.; Belcher, J. A randomized controlled trial of strict glycemic control and tertiary level obstetric care versus routine obstetric care in the management of gestational diabetes: A pilot study. *Am. J. Obstet. Gynecol.* **1997**, *177*, 190–195. [CrossRef]
30. Crowther, C.A.; Hiller, J.E.; Moss, J.R.; McPhee, A.J.; Jeffries, W.S.; Robinson, J.S. Effect of treatment of gestational diabetes mellitus on pregnancy outcomes. *N. Engl. J. Med.* **2005**, *352*, 2477–2486. [CrossRef] [PubMed]
31. Landon, M.B.; Spong, C.Y.; Thom, E.; Carpenter, M.W.; Ramin, S.M.; Casey, B.; Wapner, R.J.; Varner, M.W.; Rouse, D.J.; Thorp, J.M., Jr.; et al. A multicenter, randomized trial of treatment for mild gestational diabetes. *N. Engl. J. Med.* **2009**, *361*, 1339–1348. [CrossRef] [PubMed]
32. Viana, L.V.; Gross, J.L.; Azevedo, M.J. Dietary intervention in patients with gestational diabetes mellitus: A systematic review and meta-analysis of randomized clinical trials on maternal and newborn outcomes. *Diabetes Care* **2014**, *37*, 3345–3355. [CrossRef] [PubMed]
33. Wei, J.; Heng, W.; Gao, J. Effects of low glycemic index diets on gestational diabetes mellitus: A meta-analysis of randomized controlled clinical trials. *Med. Baltim.* **2016**, *95*, e3792. [CrossRef]
34. Han, S.; Middleton, P.; Shepherd, E.; Van Ryswyk, E.; Crowther, C.A. Different types of dietary advice for women with gestational diabetes mellitus. *Cochrane Database Syst. Rev.* **2017**, *2*, CD009275. [CrossRef]
35. Yamamoto, J.M.; Kellett, J.E.; Balsells, M.; Garcia-Patterson, A.; Hadar, E.; Sola, I.; Gich, I.; van der Beek, E.M.; Castaneda-Gutierrez, E.; Heinonen, S.; et al. Gestational diabetes mellitus and diet: A systematic review and meta-analysis of randomized controlled trials examining the impact of modified dietary interventions on maternal glucose control and neonatal birth weight. *Diabetes Care* **2018**, *41*, 1346–1361. [CrossRef]
36. Brown, J.; Ceysens, G.; Boulvain, M. Exercise for pregnant women with gestational diabetes for improving maternal and fetal outcomes. *Cochrane Database Syst. Rev.* **2017**, *6*, CD012202. [CrossRef] [PubMed]

37. Davenport, M.H.; Meah, V.L.; Ruchat, S.M.; Davies, G.A.; Skow, R.J.; Barrowman, N.; Adamo, K.B.; Poitras, V.J.; Gray, C.E.; Jaramillo Garcia, A.; et al. Impact of prenatal exercise on neonatal and childhood outcomes: A systematic review and meta-analysis. *Br. J. Sports Med.* **2018**, *52*, 1386–1396. [CrossRef]
38. Van Poppel, M.N.M.; Simmons, D.; Devlieger, R.; van Assche, F.A.; Jans, G.; Galjaard, S.; Corcoy, R.; Adelantado, J.M.; Dunne, F.; Harreiter, J.; et al. A reduction in sedentary behaviour in obese women during pregnancy reduces neonatal adiposity: The dali randomised controlled trial. *Diabetologia* **2019**, *62*, 915–925. [CrossRef]
39. Catalano, P.M. Trying to understand gestational diabetes. *Diabet. Med.* **2014**, *31*, 273–281. [CrossRef]
40. Catalano, P.M.; Shankar, K. Obesity and pregnancy: Mechanisms of short term and long term adverse consequences for mother and child. *BMJ* **2017**, *356*, j1. [CrossRef]
41. Gallo, L.A.; Barrett, H.L.; Dekker Nitert, M. Review: Placental transport and metabolism of energy substrates in maternal obesity and diabetes. *Placenta* **2017**, *54*, 59–67. [CrossRef] [PubMed]
42. Falcone, V.; Stopp, T.; Feichtinger, M.; Kiss, H.; Eppel, W.; Husslein, P.W.; Prager, G.; Gobl, C.S. Pregnancy after bariatric surgery: A narrative literature review and discussion of impact on pregnancy management and outcome. *BMC Pregnancy Childbirth* **2018**, *18*, 507. [CrossRef] [PubMed]
43. Dabelea, D.; Crume, T. Maternal environment and the transgenerational cycle of obesity and diabetes. *Diabetes* **2011**, *60*, 1849–1855. [CrossRef] [PubMed]
44. Kim, S.Y.; England, J.L.; Sharma, J.A.; Njoroge, T. Gestational diabetes mellitus and risk of childhood overweight and obesity in offspring: A systematic review. *Exp. Diabetes Res.* **2011**, *2011*, 541308. [CrossRef]
45. Philipps, L.H.; Santhakumaran, S.; Gale, C.; Prior, E.; Logan, K.M.; Hyde, M.J.; Modi, N. The diabetic pregnancy and offspring bmi in childhood: A systematic review and meta-analysis. *Diabetologia* **2011**, *54*, 1957–1966. [CrossRef]
46. Lowe, W.L., Jr.; Lowe, L.P.; Kuang, A.; Catalano, P.M.; Nodzenski, M.; Talbot, O.; Tam, W.H.; Sacks, D.A.; McCance, D.; Linder, B.; et al. Maternal glucose levels during pregnancy and childhood adiposity in the hyperglycemia and adverse pregnancy outcome follow-up study. *Diabetologia* **2019**, *62*, 598–610. [CrossRef]
47. Lowe, W.L., Jr.; Scholtens, D.M.; Kuang, A.; Linder, B.; Lawrence, J.M.; Lebenthal, Y.; McCance, D.; Hamilton, J.; Nodzenski, M.; Talbot, O.; et al. Hyperglycemia and adverse pregnancy outcome follow-up study (hapo fus): Maternal gestational diabetes mellitus and childhood glucose metabolism. *Diabetes Care* **2019**, *42*, 372–380. [CrossRef]
48. Yu, Y.; Arah, O.A.; Liew, Z.; Cnattingius, S.; Olsen, J.; Sorensen, H.T.; Qin, G.; Li, J. Maternal diabetes during pregnancy and early onset of cardiovascular disease in offspring: Population based cohort study with 40 years of follow-up. *BMJ* **2019**, *367*, l6398. [CrossRef]
49. Goldstein, R.; Teede, H.; Thangaratinam, S.; Boyle, J. Excess gestational weight gain in pregnancy and the role of lifestyle intervention. *Semin. Reprod. Med.* **2016**, *34*, e14–e21. [CrossRef]

8

Temporal Trends in Maternal Food Intake Frequencies and Associations with Gestational Diabetes: The Cambridge Baby Growth Study

Clive J. Petry [1,*], Ken K. Ong [1,2,3], Ieuan A. Hughes [1], Carlo L. Acerini [1,†] and David B. Dunger [1,3]

1 Department of Paediatrics, University of Cambridge, Cambridge Biomedical Campus, Cambridge CB2 0QQ, UK; Ken.Ong@mrc-epid.cam.ac.uk (K.K.O.); iah1000@cam.ac.uk (I.A.H.); dbd25@cam.ac.uk (D.B.D.)
2 MRC Epidemiology Unit, University of Cambridge, Cambridge Biomedical Campus, Cambridge CB2 0QQ, UK
3 Institute of Metabolic Science, University of Cambridge, Cambridge Biomedical Campus, Cambridge CB2 0QQ, UK
* Correspondence: cjp1002@cam.ac.uk
† Deceased.

Abstract: Previous studies have suggested that in the first decade of this century the incidence of gestational diabetes (GDM) in pregnancy rose worldwide. In the Cambridge Baby Growth Study cohort we observed that this temporal trend was associated with an index of multiple deprivation and reductions in indices of insulin secretion. Deprivation level was not directly associated with GDM, suggesting that the temporal trend may relate more to other factors linked to it, such as dietary composition. In this study we investigated temporal trends in perceived food intake frequencies, derived from a qualitative, short questionnaire, in 865 pregnant Cambridge Baby Growth Study (CBGS) recruits. A number of food frequency ranks showed both temporal trends and associations with GDM, but of note is the frequency of egg consumption (negative temporal trend $p = 0.03$, slope = −6.2 ranks/year; negative association with GDM $p = 3.0 \times 10^{-8}$, slope = −0.002 increased risk/rank) as it was also positively associated with the insulin disposition index ($p = 1.17 \times 10^{-3}$, slope = 0.42 ranks. L/mmoL). These results are consistent with a potential protective effect of factors related to the frequency of egg consumption in pregnancy. Such factors may have contributed to the observed temporal trend in GDM risk but the overall detectable effect appears to have been small.

Keywords: pregnancy; diet; food frequency questionnaire; glucose; insulin secretion

1. Introduction

Prevalence rates of gestational diabetes (GDM), traditionally defined as any form of glucose intolerance first recognised in pregnancy [1], are rising worldwide [2]. The tempo at which this is happening makes this likely to be predominantly environmentally rather than genetically mediated, although this does not exclude potential interactions between genetic variation and the environment, such as is found between dietary factors and obesity-enhancing genetic variants [3]. Environmental factors that could alter the susceptibility to GDM include changes to dietary intakes (both before and during pregnancy) and physical activity. A recent review [4] found that compliance to a Mediterranean-style diet, categorized as one with relatively higher bread, cereal, legume, vegetable, fruit, fish and olive oil intakes and lower or limited animal fat, meat and egg intakes [5], led to a reduction in GDM risk of between 15–38%. Similarly, a trial where the intervention group ate a Mediterranean diet supplemented with olive oil and pistachio nuts led to a relative risk for GDM of 73% of that of a control group fed a standard diet [6] and a similar effect in a follow-up real world (non-trial) situation [7]. Consumption of this diet was also associated with a reduced risk of other adverse effects of pregnancy [8]. In another study adherence to diet with a high alternate healthy eating index [9], a measure of diet quality that assesses conformance to federal dietary guidance, led to a reduction in GDM risk of 19–46% in a different population. In meta-analyses of studies assessing the effect of physical activity in more than 30,000 pregnancies, exercise regimes showed a reduction in GDM odds in women engaging in any type of pre-pregnancy physical activity (odds ratio 0.70 (0.57–0.85), $p = 6 \times 10^{-4}$, $I^2 = 52\%$ (medium heterogeneity)) or in physical activity early in pregnancy (odds ratio 0.79 (0.64–0.97), $p = 0.03$, $I^2 = 26\%$ (low heterogeneity)) [4]. A recent Cochrane systematic review concluded that there were reduced risks of GDM resulting from combined diet and exercise interventions during pregnancy compared with standard care [10]. Although it has been suggested that modifying dietary factors alone in pregnancy rather than prior to it may not be sufficient to alter the GDM risk very much [11], the RADIEL randomized controlled trial found that in high-risk women recruited less than 20 weeks into their pregnancy, lifestyle intervention focusing on dietary counselling, physical activity and weight gain in pregnancy was able to reduce the incidence of GDM by 39% [12]. Diet quality was improved over this time and there was lower pregnancy weight gain, perhaps not surprisingly given that there was a particular extra emphasis put on dietary factors when the ability of a study recruit to exercise was limited, such as if antenatal contractions occurred.

In the United Kingdom, as in many developed countries elsewhere [13], there has been a dietary shift since the 1970s toward diets with lower total fat contents that includes greater consumption of meats with lower fat contents such as poultry rather than pork, beef and lamb, and the drinking of semi-skimmed rather than full fat milk [14]. The reduced energy intake coming from fats induced by this dietary change has, however, not matched the decreased energy expenditure of less manual jobs and more restful leisure pursuits, contributing to a sharp rise in the prevalence of obesity [15]. This is true for pregnancy where diets in the U.K. appear to be very similar to those consumed by women who are not pregnant [16]. With temporal dietary trends and other dietary factors potentially able to alter circulating glucose concentrations, and therefore possibly GDM risk, it is conceivable that dietary factors could, at least partially, underpin changes in the incidence of GDM. Following studies in Canada [17], the United States [18,19], Israel [20] and Germany [21] all of which showed GDM becoming more prevalent in the first decade of this century, our recent analysis of women recruited to the Cambridge Baby Growth Study (CBGS) in this same decade showed a significant increase in the incidence of GDM that was associated more with a temporal reduction in indices of insulin secretion than insulin sensitivity [22]. In risk factor analysis there was a significant, albeit modestly sized, temporal trend in the index of multiple deprivation. This index was not itself directly associated with GDM, however. This led us to suggest that the temporal trend in the deprivation index could relate to GDM indirectly through changes in other factors that are themselves related to both changes in deprivation and glucose tolerance in pregnancy, such as diet [23] and exercise [24]. Therefore the primary outcome of the present study, rather than being hypothesis driven per se, was to try and find one or more food types whose frequency of consumption during pregnancy most closely reflected the temporal trend in GDM prevalence (and other indices of glucose and insulin secretion and sensitivity) that we had previously observed in the CBGS [22]. Both the year of analysis and the development of GDM were therefore our primary analyses. We found a number of statistically significant associations with these variables, generally with rather small effect sizes. These and other associations are therefore consistent with the possibility that factors related to the frequency of consumption of certain foods in pregnancy may have contributed to the observed temporal trend in GDM risk and changes in insulin secretion rates, but that the overall detectable effect was small.

2. Materials and Methods

2.1. *Cambridge Baby Growth Study*

The prospective and longitudinal CBGS was designed as an observational cohort initially including pregnancy, birth and infancy [25]. In its first phase of recruitment, between April 2001 and March 2009,

2229 mothers aged over 16 years of age were enrolled to it when attending early pregnancy ultrasound clinics at the Rosie Maternity Hospital, Cambridge, U.K. Of these, 571 mothers withdrew before the birth of their infant so were not considered further. Most of the clinical characteristics of the study participants were collected either during nurse-led interviews or by questionnaire with the exception of offspring birth weights, gestational ages and dates of birth, which were compiled from hospital notes. In this cohort 95.3% of the offspring were white, 1.7% were Asian, 1.3% were black (African or Caribbean) and 1.7% were other ethnicities (mainly mixed race), reflective of the population served by the Rosie Maternity Hospital [25].

2.2. Ethics

Ethical approval for the CBGS was granted by the Cambridge Local Research Ethics Committee, Addenbrooke's Hospital, Cambridge, United Kingdom (00/325). All procedures followed were in accordance with the institutional guidelines. All the study participants gave written informed consent.

2.3. Pregnancy (Including Food Frequency) Questionnaire

A wide-ranging pregnancy questionnaire (Appendix A), that was adapted from one developed in Denmark where the self-administered form was validated through phone interviews [26], was given out to all participants at recruitment to the CBGS (around week 12 of pregnancy). Participants were requested to fill the questionnaire in as the pregnancy progressed (with assistance from research nurses if required) and the questionnaires were then collected after the birth of their baby. The questions that were asked were wide-ranging but as part of a section about lifestyle there was a short (specific) food frequency questionnaire covering most of the major food and drink types (Appendix A). For drinks, the participants were asked the number of times they drank a particular drink per day or per week (depending upon the likely consumption frequency of that drink). For food the participants were asked, 'How often did you eat the following foods during pregnancy?' and the response involved ticking one of the following options: never, 1–3 times per month, 1–3 times per week, 4–6 times per week or once or more per day. Participants were encouraged to tick the option that most closely resembled their food or drink intakes in pregnancy. The questionnaires were completed by 1239 of the CBGS recruits and were collected shortly after birth.

2.4. Oral Glucose Tests and Gestational Diabetes

At a median (inter-quartile range) of 28.4 (28.1–28.7) weeks gestation 1074 of the CBGS mothers underwent a 75 g oral glucose tolerance test (OGTT) after fasting overnight [27]. Venous blood was collected just before and 60 min after the glucose load was administered for the measurement of plasma glucose and insulin concentrations. 120 min plasma glucose concentrations were only measured from May 2007 onwards so were not used in this analysis to define GDM (only 7% of U.K. women with GDM receive a diagnosis based solely on the 120 min measurement in any case [28]). The International Association of Diabetes in Pregnancy Study Groups (IADPSG)/World Health Organization (WHO) 2013 thresholds for 0 and 60 min OGTT glucose concentrations (i.e., >5.1 and 10.0 mmol/L, respectively [29,30]) were used retrospectively to define the presence of GDM in this analysis. However when the women were recruited to the CBGS the clinical decision to treat women with GDM was broadly based on WHO 1999 guidelines [31], which considered just fasting and 2-h glucose concentrations. Based on available records and information from treating clinicians, GDM was mostly treated with diet and lifestyle modification, with or without insulin supplementation [32]. Around 19% (16 out of 83) of the women whose OGTT glucose concentrations exceeded the IADPSG/WHO (2013) thresholds for GDM [29,30] did not exceed those that were used clinically at the time and therefore did not receive dietary advice as a frontline therapy for GDM, only standard pregnancy care [32].

2.5. Assays

All biochemical kit-based assays were run according to the manufacturer's instructions. Glucose concentrations were measured using a routine glucose oxidase-based method. OGTT plasma insulin concentrations were measured by ELISA (Dako UK Ltd., Ely, Cambs, UK). Intra-assay imprecision (CV) was 4.3% at 82 pmol/L, 3.0% at 402 pmol/L and 5.7% at 907 pmol/L. Equivalent inter-assay imprecision at these concentrations was 4.3, 5.1 and 5.4%, respectively.

2.6. Calculations

Insulin resistance and pancreatic β-cell function were estimated using the homeostasis model assessment (HOMA IR and B, respectively), calculated using the week 28 fasting circulating glucose and insulin concentrations, and the online HOMA calculator [33]. Insulin secretion (corrected for insulin sensitivity) was estimated using the insulin disposition index, calculated as the change in insulin concentrations over the first hour of the OGTT divided by the change in glucose concentrations, all divided by the reciprocal of the fasting insulin concentration. The maternal body mass index (BMI) was calculated as the pre-pregnancy weight divided by the height squared. Pregnancy weight gain was calculated as the mother's pre-pregnancy body weight taken away from the partum body weight. The index of multiple deprivation was derived and imputed from the postcode of the participants' home addresses as described [34].

2.7. Statistical Analysis and Strategy

The present analysis was restricted to those 865 pregnancies where the women underwent OGTTs (thereby excluding women with pre-existing type 1 diabetes) with 0- and 60-min plasma glucose concentrations available to us, who also completed and returned their pregnancy questionnaires. Because of being ordinal rather than continuous in nature, responses to questions about food and drink consumption frequencies were converted into ranks using standard methods before participant selection and analysis. Associations between food frequency ranks and key phenotypic variables (OGTT year, GDM, the index of multiple deprivation, HOMA IR, HOMA B, the insulin disposition index, OGTT 0 and 60 min glucose concentrations) were tested by non-parametric regression performed using the Siegel repeated medians procedure (deploying the R package 'mblm', version 0.12.1). Multiple testing of these non-parametric regression analyses was accounted for using the Benjamini-Hochberg procedure [35], using a false discovery rate of 0.05. Categorical analysis was performed using Fisher's exact test. Data used in other parametric analyses were logarithmically transformed prior to analyses if the distributions of the statistical model residuals were positively skewed and transformed into reciprocals if the distributions of the residuals were negatively skewed. Further analysis was performed by standard logistic (for binary variables) or linear (for continuous variables whose model residuals using untransformed or transformed data were normally distributed) regression. Unless stated all the other statistical analyses were performed using Stata (version 13.1; Stata Corp., from Timberlake Consultants Ltd., Richmond, Surrey, UK). Statistical significance was assumed at $p < 0.05$ or lower depending on the Benjamini-Hochberg adjustment.

To be consistent with our temporal trends in GDM incidence [22] we sought statistically significant associations with both OGTT year and GDM where the slopes of the regression lines in the two models were in the same direction (i.e., either both positive or both negative). When they were, the food frequency ranks were used as confounders in logistic regression models assessing associations between OGTT year and GDM to see if they attenuated such associations. Associations with the remaining key phenotypic variables were then examined in linear regression models to assess whether they were in the same direction as the temporal trends observed in our original study [22].

To group food types that tended to be eaten with similar frequency ranks we analysed perceived food intake ranks by principal component analysis (using R version 3.6.1 (The R Foundation for Statistical Computing, Vienna, Austria), the R function "princomp" and the R packages "ggplot2" (version 3.2.0) and "factoextra" (version 1.0.5)) on a complete dataset where missing data were imputed to the median. All the R packages that we used were downloaded from http://cran.r-project.org/web/packages/mblm/index.html.

3. Results

3.1. Characteristics of Study Participants

Those women included in the present analysis tended to be representative of the CBGS cohort, albeit that on average they gave birth around 2 days later than those not included in the study (which is unlikely to have been clinically significant), were more likely to have been nulliparous and were less likely to have smoked in pregnancy (Table 1).

Table 1. Clinical characteristics of those Cambridge Baby Growth Study participants who were included in the current analysis and those that were not.

Characteristic	Included	Not-Included	*p*-Value
Mother's age at the birth of her baby (years)	33.4 (33.1, 33.7) (n = 787)	33.7 (33.3, 34.0) (n = 548)	0.3
Parity (n, of increasing parity and starting with 0)	415/310/103/24/4/2	302/330/112/37/4/4	2.0×10^{-3}
GDM (n yes/no)	85 yes, 780 no	26 yes, 193 no	0.4
OGTT fasting glucose concentration (mmol/L)	4.3 (4.3, 4.4) (n = 865)	4.4 (4.3, 4.5) (n = 218)	0.1
OGTT fasting insulin concentration (pmol/L)	45 (44, 47) (n = 846)	46 (44, 49) (n = 290)	0.8
Pre-pregnancy BMI (kg/m^2)	23.5 (23.2, 23.7) (n = 776)	23.3 (22.9, 23.6) (n = 411)	0.4
Index of multiple deprivation	8.0 (7.7, 8.3) (n = 597)	8.1 (7.8, 8.5) (n = 401)	0.6
Maternal highest qualification (category GCSE/A levels/degree) (n)	75/123/337	38/62/155	0.8
Sex of baby (n males/females)	443/413	412/386	1.0
Baby's birth weight (kg) *	3.490 (3.459, 3.552) (n = 774)	3.449 (3.406, 3.492) (n = 408)	0.1
Gestational age at birth of baby (weeks)	39.9 (39.8, 40.0) (n = 857)	39.6 (39.5, 39.7) (n = 800)	5.1×10^{-4}
Reported smoking during pregnancy (n yes/no)	31/825	55/744	3.0×10^{-3}

* adjusted for maternal pre-pregnancy BMI, gestational age at birth, sex of baby and parity. Data are either the number of participants or mean (95% confidence interval).

3.2. Associations with Food Intake Frequencies

3.2.1. Year of OGTT (Temporal Trends)

The numbers of women who were recruited to the CBGS whose data contributed to this analysis in the nine calendar years of recruitment were: 2001→46, 2002→130, 2003→81, 2004→75, 2005→158, 2006→144, 2007→130, 2008→91 and 2009→10 (recruitment to this phase of the CBGS having closed in March 2009). Several different food and drinks showed significant temporal trends (associations between their intake frequency ranks and the year in which the pregnancy OGTT was performed (Table 2)). The largest effect size was observed in the negative association with the frequency of drinking spirits, although this is caused by only a small proportion of study participants drinking spirits with a median (and lower and upper quartile) for this population of 0 glasses of spirits drunk per week. Smaller negative temporal trends were also observed for other alcoholic drinks such as beer and wine (both with medians of zero bottles or glasses consumed per week in this population), and non-alcoholic cola (with a median (interquartile range) consumption of 0 (0, 0.5) litres per week) and fresh fruit juice (with a median intake frequency corresponding to drinking it 4–6 times per week). The only drink with a positive temporal trend was tap water. The largest significant positive effect sizes with food frequency ranks were observed with pulses (loose and canned) and tinned fruit. Comparatively much smaller, but the largest negative effect sizes were observed with food frequency ranks for eggs, canned fish and baked beans.

For clarity the temporal trends for the three dietary components with the highest absolute value for the slope (spirits, pulses and tinned fruit) are shown in bar chart form in Figure S1.

Table 2. Statistically significant associations between the food/drink intake frequency ranks and year of oral glucose tolerance test (OGTT) testing in the Cambridge Baby Growth Study (CBGS) presented in descending order of the absolute value of the slope.

Food/Drink Type	Slope (Ranks/Year)	*p*-Value
Spirits	−155.06	2.12×10^{-2}
Pulses	95.90	1.37×10^{-24}
Tinned fruit	69.81	2.33×10^{-5}
Other canned beans/pulses	34.29	3.27×10^{-11}
Organic food	33.40	2.51×10^{-12}
Beer	−32.33	2.75×10^{-3}
Soft cheese	29.99	3.00×10^{-11}
Tinned vegetables	29.92	1.07×10^{-2}
Wine	−26.63	1.40×10^{-6}
Tap water	25.25	2.63×10^{-4}
Dried fruit	23.00	1.36×10^{-8}
Organic fruit and vegetables	22.75	2.19×10^{-13}
Organic dairy	19.67	2.88×10^{-9}
Organic meat	17.98	1.07×10^{-8}
Yogurt	17.04	5.69×10^{-8}
Cola	−15.17	5.75×10^{-3}
Salad	15.00	2.22×10^{-5}
Other fresh vegetables	13.33	1.38×10^{-3}
Bean curd	10.13	2.42×10^{-3}
Fresh fruit	8.98	1.20×10^{-3}
Fresh fish with bread	8.88	1.92×10^{-3}
Hard cheese	8.41	5.54×10^{-3}
Soya	7.05	1.68×10^{-2}
Fresh fish with salad pasta	6.44	9.48×10^{-3}
Eggs	−6.19	3.03×10^{-2}
Organic others	6.13	7.16×10^{-3}
Chocolate	5.25	2.54×10^{-3}
Fresh fruit juice	−3.37	7.46×10^{-3}
Canned fish	−3.28	1.64×10^{-2}
Baked beans	−1.36	1.21×10^{-4}
Shellfish	-1.28×10^{-5}	2.44×10^{-2}

p-values are presented unadjusted for the Benjamini-Hochberg procedure. All food types in the food frequency questionnaire that are not shown did not have a significant association with the year of OGTT testing (Benjamini-Hochberg adjusted $p > 0.05$).

3.2.2. Gestational Diabetes, Including Attenuation of the Association with Year of OGTT

A number of different food and drink intake frequency ranks showed significant (positive or negative) associations with GDM (Table 3). Not surprisingly though, none of the effect sizes of these associations were large enough to attenuate the association between GDM and year of OGTT testing. Food whose intake frequency ranks were significantly positively associated with both OGTT year and GDM (Tables 2 and 3) were salad and fresh fruit. Equivalent significant negative associations were found with baked beans, shellfish and eggs. Drinks whose intake frequency ranks were also significantly negatively associated with both OGTT year and GDM were beer, wine and spirits. The only drink whose intake frequency was significantly positively associated with both OGTT year and GDM (albeit weakly) was tap water. The positive association between the frequency of tap water intake and GDM may seem unexpected but probably reflects the fact that the food frequency questions were designed to reflect the whole of pregnancy, not just the time preceding the development and diagnosis of GDM. Hence women diagnosed with GDM may have drunk more tap water in preference to less healthy beverages such as alcoholic drinks, in the overall context of a positive temporal trend for the frequency of tap water consumption, and negative temporal trends for beer, wine and spirits. An alternative explanation for the positive association between the frequency of tap water consumption and GDM is that polydipsia in women with poorly controlled GDM [36] could have caused them to drink tap water more often.

3.2.3. Indices of Insulin Secretion & Sensitivity, OGTT Glucose Concentrations

The associations between food/drink intake frequency ranks and HOMA IR, HOMA B, the insulin disposition index, OGTT fasting and 60 min glucose concentrations (where the Benjamini-Hochberg modified p-value of at least one of these associations was <0.05) are shown in Table S1. Of the ranks that showed significant temporal trends and associations with GDM (in the same direction) (Tables 2 and 3) the following also showed negative associations with indices of insulin secretion, as we observed in our original study [22]: salad, fresh fruit, tap water, wine and beer. The ranks of the frequency of the consumption of baked beans also showed a significant negative association with the insulin indisposition index, although this rules out the factors related to them having a causal role in contributing towards the temporal trend in GDM and reduced insulin secretion in the CBGS, as their intake was also negatively associated with GDM. Again, rather than reflecting factors related to them contributing towards causality, the other negative associations with the intake ranks of these specific food/drinks may be more likely to reflect dietary modifications in GDM women post-development and diagnosis. Egg intake frequency ranks were negatively associated with both year of testing and GDM, as well as positively significantly associated with the insulin disposition index. These results are consistent with either the consumption of eggs themselves, or factors related to the frequency of eggs being eaten somehow to protect against the development of GDM. Further evidence in support of this concept is gained from the fact that egg intake frequency ranks were negatively associated with both fasting and 60 min OGTT glucose concentrations.

3.2.4. Index of Multiple Deprivation

Increased deprivation (a lowering of the index of multiple deprivation) was significantly associated with eating baked beans and drinking tea more frequently (the only drink whose intake frequency was significantly associated with the index of multiple deprivation), as well as eating hard cheese and white fish more frequently (Table 4). In contrast decreased deprivation was associated with eating bean curd, soya, beans/pulses, salad and organic food more frequently (amongst other foodstuffs).

Table 3. Statistically significant associations between the food/drink intake frequencies and GDM in the CBGS presented in descending order of the absolute value of the slope.

Food/Drink Type	Slope (Ranks/ Diagnosis of GDM)	p-Value	Association between Year of OGTT Testing and GDM in These Women		Association between Year of OGTT Testing and GDM in These Women (Adjusted for Food/Drink Type)	
			OR	p-Value	OR	p-Value
Bean curd	-2.00×10^{-3}	6.42×10^{-13}	1.2 (1.1, 1.3) (n = 890)	1.3×10^{-3}	1.2 (1.1, 1.3) (n = 890)	1.3×10^{-3}
Eggs	-1.86×10^{-3}	3.03×10^{-8}	1.2 (1.1, 1.3) (n = 893)	1.7×10^{-3}	1.2 (1.1, 1.3) (n = 893)	1.6×10^{-3}
White fish	-1.83×10^{-3}	3.88×10^{-6}	1.2 (1.1, 1.3) (n = 888)	1.5×10^{-3}	1.2 (1.1, 1.3) (n = 888)	1.6×10^{-3}
Soya	-1.66×10^{-3}	9.02×10^{-9}	1.2 (1.1, 1.3) (n = 890)	1.9×10^{-3}	1.2 (1.1, 1.3) (n = 888)	2.1×10^{-3}
Meat	1.63×10^{-3}	4.86×10^{-8}	1.2 (1.1, 1.3) (n = 893)	1.5×10^{-3}	1.2 (1.1, 1.3) (n = 893)	1.6×10^{-3}
Spirits	-1.63×10^{-3}	1.20×10^{-17}	1.2 (1.1, 1.3) (n = 857)	3.1×10^{-3}	1.2 (1.1, 1.3) (n = 857)	3.0×10^{-3}
Beer	-1.62×10^{-3}	1.97×10^{-12}	1.2 (1.1, 1.3) (n = 856)	3.3×10^{-3}	1.2 (1.1, 1.3) (n = 856)	4.5×10^{-3}
Liver	-1.57×10^{-3}	1.50×10^{-15}	1.2 (1.1, 1.3) (n = 889)	1.3×10^{-3}	1.2 (1.1, 1.3) (n = 889)	1.2×10^{-3}
Canned meat	-1.57×10^{-3}	4.49×10^{-14}	1.2 (1.1, 1.3) (n = 892)	1.5×10^{-3}	1.2 (1.1, 1.3) (n = 892)	1.1×10^{-3}
Poultry	1.56×10^{-3}	7.14×10^{-5}	1.2 (1.1, 1.3) (n = 892)	1.5×10^{-3}	1.3 (1.1, 1.3) (n = 892)	1.1×10^{-3}
Cocoa	-1.50×10^{-3}	1.46×10^{-6}	1.2 (1.1, 1.3) (n = 856)	2.7×10^{-3}	1.2 (1.1, 1.3) (n = 856)	2.8×10^{-3}
Fresh fish with salad pasta	-5.22×10^{-4}	4.43×10^{-6}	1.2 (1.1, 1.3) (n = 877)	1.5×10^{-3}	1.2 (1.1, 1.3) (n = 877)	1.3×10^{-3}
Salad	3.54×10^{-4}	2.57×10^{-2}	1.2 (1.1, 1.3) (n = 881)	1.1×10^{-3}	1.2 (1.1, 1.3) (n = 881)	1.2×10^{-3}
Fresh fruit	3.01×10^{-4}	8.53×10^{-6}	1.2 (1.1, 1.3) (n = 895)	1.5×10^{-3}	1.2 (1.1, 1.3) (n = 895)	1.7×10^{-3}
Wine	-2.99×10^{-4}	1.74×10^{-4}	1.2 (1.1, 1.3) (n = 867)	2.0×10^{-3}	1.2 (1.1, 1.3) (n = 867)	3.9×10^{-3}
Organic bread	-2.83×10^{-4}	7.89×10^{-3}	1.2 (1.1, 1.4) (n = 603)	4.4×10^{-3}	1.2 (1.1, 1.4) (n = 603)	4.9×10^{-3}
Fresh fish with bread	-2.53×10^{-4}	2.00×10^{-3}	1.2 (1.1, 1.3) (n = 864)	1.2×10^{-3}	1.2 (1.1, 1.3) (n = 864)	1.2×10^{-3}
Hard cheese	-2.31×10^{-4}	1.49×10^{-3}	1.2 (1.1, 1.3) (n = 894)	1.5×10^{-3}	1.2 (1.1, 1.3) (n = 894)	1.5×10^{-3}

Table 3. *Cont.*

Food/Drink Type	Slope (Ranks/ Diagnosis of GDM)	p-Value	Association between Year of OGTT Testing and GDM in These Women		Association between Year of OGTT Testing and GDM in These Women (Adjusted for Food/Drink Type)	
			OR	p-Value	OR	p-Value
Soft cheese	-2.15×10^{-4}	5.32×10^{-4}	1.2 (1.1, 1.3) (n = 877)	3.2×10^{-3}	1.2 (1.1, 1.3) (n = 877)	3.2×10^{-3}
Canned fish	2.13×10^{-4}	8.82×10^{-5}	1.2 (1.1, 1.3) (n = 893)	1.5×10^{-3}	1.2 (1.1, 1.3) (n = 893)	1.6×10^{-3}
Fresh fruit juice	1.66×10^{-4}	2.17×10^{-3}	1.2 (1.1, 1.3) (n = 888)	1.5×10^{-3}	1.2 (1.1, 1.3) (n = 888)	1.5×10^{-3}
Dried fruit	-1.34×10^{-4}	5.76×10^{-4}	1.2 (1.1, 1.3) (n = 892)	1.4×10^{-3}	1.2 (1.1, 1.3) (n = 892)	7.9×10^{-4}
Shellfish	-5.92×10^{-5}	8.47×10^{-3}	1.2 (1.1, 1.3) (n = 886)	1.9×10^{-3}	1.2 (1.1, 1.3) (n = 886)	1.8×10^{-3}
Tea	-5.10×10^{-5}	1.16×10^{-3}	1.2 (1.1, 1.3) (n = 876)	2.2×10^{-3}	1.2 (1.1, 1.3) (n = 876)	2.6×10^{-3}
Fresh fish as main course	-3.19×10^{-5}	3.92×10^{-4}	1.2 (1.1, 1.3) (n = 888)	1.4×10^{-3}	1.2 (1.1, 1.3) (n = 888)	9.5×10^{-3}
Baked beans	-1.55×10^{-5}	6.05×10^{-3}	1.2 (1.1, 1.3) (n = 894)	1.5×10^{-3}	1.2 (1.1, 1.3) (n = 894)	1.1×10^{-3}
Tap water	1.43×10^{-5}	2.06×10^{-3}	1.2 (1.1, 1.3) (n = 894)	1.5×10^{-3}	1.2 (1.1, 1.3) (n = 894)	1.9×10^{-3}

Data are mean (95% confidence interval where shown). OR = odds ratio. p-values are presented unadjusted for the Benjamini-Hochberg procedure. All food/drink types in the food frequency questionnaire that are not shown in this Table did not have a significant association with GDM (Benjamini-Hochberg adjusted $p > 0.05$).

Table 4. Statistically significant associations between the food/drink intake frequency ranks and the index of multiple deprivation in the CBGS presented in descending order of the absolute value of the slope.

Food/Drink Type	Slope (Ranks/Index of Multiple Deprivation Units)	p-Value
Bean curd	38.24	9.82×10^{-4}
Soya	20.07	1.29×10^{-2}
Other canned beans/pulses	18.41	4.21×10^{-3}
Pulses	17.83	5.39×10^{-5}
Organic food	16.36	1.20×10^{-4}
Salad	11.58	7.05×10^{-3}
Dried fruit	10.82	1.07×10^{-2}
Organic dairy	10.23	2.46×10^{-4}
Baked beans	−9.81	1.67×10^{-3}
Tea	−9.77	1.04×10^{-3}
Organic bread	9.47	9.65×10^{-3}
Organic meat	9.47	1.43×10^{-2}
Organic others	8.97	1.42×10^{-4}
Hard cheese	−8.24	4.94×10^{-3}
Fish	7.89	2.48×10^{-3}
Eggs	6.70	1.56×10^{-3}
White fish	−6.58	1.49×10^{-2}

p-values are presented unadjusted for the Benjamini-Hochberg procedure. All food types in the food frequency questionnaire that are not shown did not have a significant association with the index (Benjamini-Hochberg adjusted $p > 0.05$).

3.3. Principal Component Analysis of Food Intake Frequency Ranks

Principal component analysis of maternal food intake frequency ranks in pregnancy produced 32 principal components that explained more than 1% of the variance in food intake frequency ranks. The first two principal components explained a little more than 20% of the total variance in the reported food intake frequency ranks of those food types included in the questionnaire (Figure S2). Plotting the different contributions to the first two principal components (Figure 1) (where positively correlated food intake frequencies point to the same side of the plot, and negatively correlated food intake frequencies point to the opposite side of the plot) shows several food types where the intake frequencies can be grouped (e.g., fish frequency intake in the bottom left quadrant). The frequency of egg consumption (or factors related to it), which appeared to be somewhat protective against the development of GDM in our analyses, was most closely positively related to the intake frequency of fresh fruit, salad, fresh green vegetables, tap water and yogurt. It was most negatively related to the frequency of cola intake.

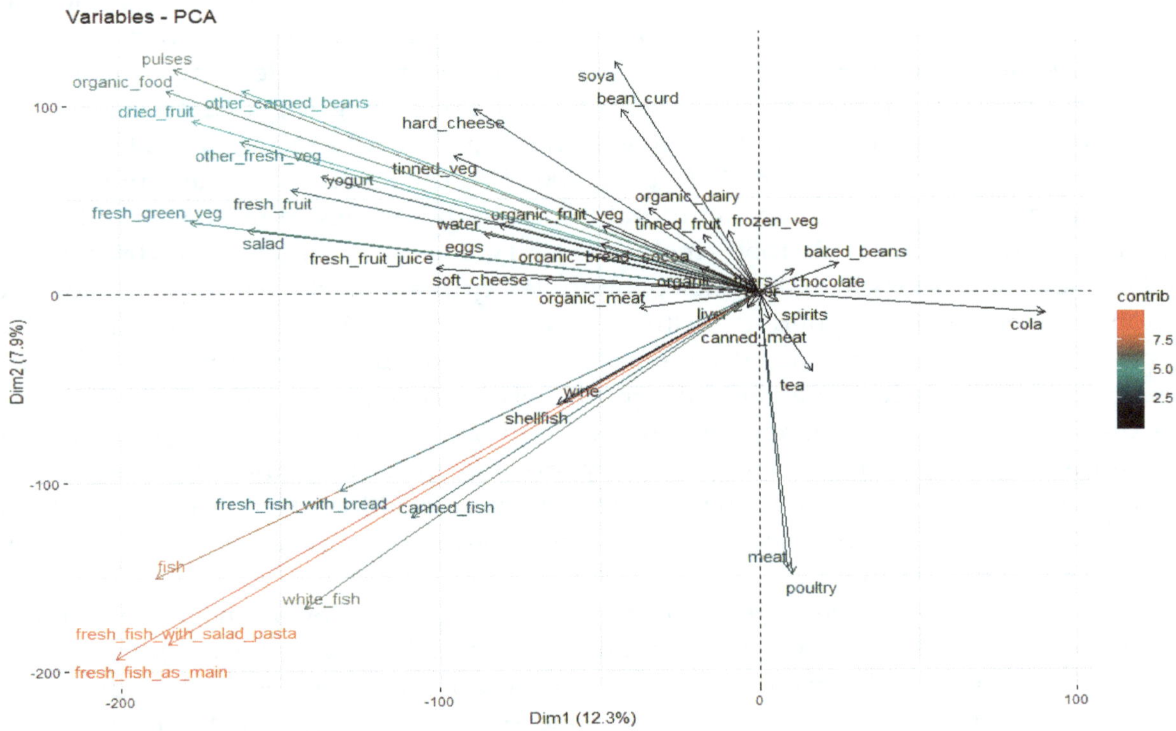

Figure 1. Variables plot of the first two principal components (dimensions) of maternal food intake frequency ranks in pregnancy, showing basic grouping of dietary patterns and their likely contributions to the overall variance.

4. Discussion

In this study we observed a number of significant associations between perceived food intake frequencies and both year of analysis (i.e., temporal trends) and GDM in the CBGS. In this cohort we had previously observed a strong positive temporal trend in the prevalence of GDM [22] and wanted to investigate the possible trends in perceived food/drink intake frequencies over the same period of time which could have contributed to this themselves or been markers of dietary factors that contributed to this. One limitation of using food intake frequencies is that associations cannot infer causality (not that changing the frequency of intake of one particular food or drink would be expected to have a big direct effect on GDM risk in any case). Indeed, of the significant food and drink intake frequencies the positive associations between frequencies of salad and tap water intakes with GDM (which also gave a positive temporal trend) are examples of food and drink types that seem particularly unlikely to have positive causal effects on GDM development. As our questionnaires were designed to be filled in across pregnancy, however, the significant positive association with salad (and tap water) intake frequency could reflect an increased frequency of consumption with GDM post-development in those women who were clinically diagnosed with the condition, in an effort for them to consume a healthier diet. Alternatively, potential confounders of this association, especially since the effect size is small, could include increased consumption of salad dressing that may be high in saturated fat and sugar content which could have slightly alter the risk of GDM [37]. Other food/drink intake frequencies showing associations in the same direction for both the year of analysis and risk of GDM include negative associations with the consumption of spirits, beer, wine, eggs, baked beans and shellfish, and a positive association with the frequency of consumption of fresh fruit. All of these associations were of modest effect sizes, and most may be more attributable to dietary modifications following a clinical diagnosis of GDM.

In the present analysis a number of perceived intake frequencies of specific foods/drinks showed temporal trends but were not associated with GDM or were associated with both but in opposite directions and could not explain the temporal trends in GDM incidence observed in the CBGS [22]. These specific foods and drink included pulses (loose or canned), fruit (dried, tinned and fresh juice), vegetables (tinned and other fresh), organic food (including fruit, vegetables, dairy, meat and others), cheese (soft and hard), fresh fish (with bread and salad pasta), yogurt, soya, bean curd, cola and chocolate. The temporal trends with the intake of these foods could relate, at least partially, to the upsurge in food prices observed in the U.K. from 2007 [38] especially in women living with a high degree of deprivation. More likely the temporal trends in the perceived intakes of pulses (loose or canned), bean curd, soya, organic food (including dairy, meat and others) and dried fruit can be explained by their associations with the index of multiple deprivation, which rose (signifying decreased deprivation) as the recruitment period for the study progressed [22]. Of the remaining food and drink types, the only one with a negative temporal trend was in the consumption of cola, which was presumably in the context of a general trend in certain populations of the U.K. for consuming healthier diets [39,40], and pregnancy diets reflecting those of non-pregnancy [16]. The observed positive temporal trends for the consumption of various forms of fruit and vegetables, and yogurt and fresh fish may also reflect the national trend for eating a healthier diet. In contrast, the positive temporal trends for chocolate and cheese intakes seem to have gone against the national trend [40,41] and may be population-specific.

With the positive temporal trend with incidence of GDM in the CBGS, a negative temporal trend was also previously observed in indices of insulin secretion [22]. There were a number of significant associations between the insulin disposition index and perceived frequencies of particular food/drink intakes in the present study. However the only food type in the pregnancy questionnaire whose frequency of intakes had statistically significant associations in directions consistent with our key phenotypes (positive with year of analysis and GDM, and negative with the insulin disposition index) were eggs, albeit in each case the associations were in the opposite direction to those associated with increased risk with time. This suggests a possible protective effect either of eggs themselves or of factors related to the frequency of egg intakes on GDM development. Consistent with the idea that is eggs themselves, at least one other study [42] has found a negative association between egg intake in pregnancy and GDM risk. However other evidence from a meta-analysis suggests that egg intakes in pregnancy may be positively related to GDM development [43] rather than protective, with the positive effect on GDM development thought to be related to one or more of the nutritive components of eggs, namely cholesterol, ω-polyunsaturated fatty acids and lutein [44]. In the present study, because of the basic (and incomplete in terms of food groups) nature of the food frequency questionnaire that was used, we analysed the food intake frequencies using simple associations with ranks, with no reference to nutritional databases to convert food intake frequencies into nutrient intakes. However we did perform principal component analysis in an attempt to group the egg intake frequencies into a basic dietary pattern. The frequencies of egg intakes appeared to be most closely positively related to intake frequencies of fresh fruit, salad, fresh green vegetables and yogurt (as may be enriched in diets such as the Mediterranean diet, which has been shown to have positive effects on reducing GDM prevalence [5–7]) when plotting the first two principal components of food/drink intake frequency ranks. These two components between them explained just over 20% of their variance. In the analysis by Shin et al. [37] of the National Health and Nutrition Examination Survey from around the same period of time that the CBGS participants were recruited, the biggest absolute weighting by far given for eggs was a negative one for the 'high added sugar and organ meats; low fruits, vegetables and seafood' dietary pattern which was associated with the highest risk for the development of GDM in pregnant women in that study. In another study from Northern Sweden, egg consumption was associated with intakes of fish, fruits, cereals and whole grain products which are noted to reduce the risk of GDM [45]. Our data from the present analysis therefore seems consistent with these two other studies [37,45], perhaps not surprisingly given the similarities in dietary habits between these countries [46]. In each case it would appear that eating more eggs might be associated with eating a 'healthy' diet which leads to a lower risk for the development of GDM. Using findings from the present study, plus those other cited studies [5–7,37,45], consumption of these 'healthy' rather than more standard Westernized diets would therefore appear to have beneficial effects on the development of GDM. However even with the key, highly statistically significant associations in our study, including the one with the index of multiple deprivation, and plausible explanations as to why the frequency of egg intakes in pregnancy may be related to a lower risk of developing GDM, the detectable effect size appears to be very small so will only have explained a modest proportion of the risk in the CBGS.

In the present study we analysed a short, qualitative (in terms of lack of portion size) food frequency questionnaire that was part of a much larger lifestyle questionnaire where the answers were supposed to reflect the whole of pregnancy (so in the context of GDM both pre- and post- a possible clinical diagnosis). The questions related to food and drink intake frequencies were restricted to the items listed in the questionnaire and were not designed to be comprehensive. Indeed they did not include questions related to intake frequencies of high carbohydrate foods such as potatoes and rice. Like all such questionnaires, it was therefore not reliable for assessing the total diet, energy or nutrient intakes. In addition it did not contain questions about the method of cooking of the food that was consumed. It was, however, the only form of dietary record that we had for mothers in this cohort. Another shortcoming of using the questionnaire could have been the requirement for the participants to have good recall, literacy and numerical skills, although CBGS participants tended to be relatively highly qualified [25], so this may have been less of a problem than it might otherwise have been. Participants were encouraged to fill in their questionnaires as their pregnancy progressed to further abrogate this potential shortcoming. Whilst the use of the questionnaire had a number of limitations it also had strengths. First, after the initial withdrawals from the study, 74.7% of the CBGS participants completed and returned their questionnaires so there was a relatively high response rate suggesting that the results from the present analysis were likely to be representative of those of the whole CBGS. Second, by listing specific food items (even in combination) it also made it easy for the participants to complete, which may have contributed to this high response rate. Third, by being qualitative in terms of portion sizes of specific food types eaten (but semi-quantitative in terms of food intake frequencies) the respondents did not have to estimate food intakes which could have helped limit inaccuracies (albeit by doing this they indirectly inferred that portion sizes were average and uniform). Finally, by covering the whole of pregnancy the questionnaire was not confounded by trimester.

5. Conclusions

Within the limitations of the short (specific) food frequency questionnaire that was analysed in this study, the food and drink intake frequency ranks with the associations that most closely resembled those linking year of analysis with GDM and related metabolic indices [22] were those linked to the frequency of egg consumption. All these relevant associations were in the opposite direction to those with the year of analysis in the CBGS, suggesting that either the frequency of egg consumption themselves or factors related to the frequency of egg intake during pregnancy (which our analysis suggests could be related to the intake of a healthier diet in pregnancy) appeared protective against GDM and reductions in insulin secretion. However the detectable effect sizes of all the individual associations were small, and certainly, these associations with GDM were not strong enough to attenuate the observed temporal trend in GDM incidence (although realistically the consumption frequencies of the single food or drink types would not be expected to do this). We conclude that in the CBGS there was a potential protective effect of dietary factors related to the frequency of egg consumption in pregnancy, a reduction in which over time could have contributed modestly to the observed temporal trend in GDM risk.

Author Contributions: Conceptualization, C.J.P. and D.B.D.; methodology, C.J.P. and K.K.O.; formal analysis and investigation, C.J.P.; resources, K.K.O., I.A.H., C.L.A. and D.B.D.; data curation, C.J.P. and C.L.A.; writing—original draft preparation, C.J.P.; writing—review and editing, K.K.O., I.A.H. and D.B.D.; project administration, K.K.O., I.A.H., C.L.A. and D.B.D.; funding acquisition, K.K.O., I.A.H., C.L.A. and D.B.D.

Acknowledgments: The authors would like to thank all the families that took part in the Cambridge Baby Growth Study, and acknowledge the crucial role played by the research nurses especially Suzanne Smith, Ann-Marie Wardell and Karen Forbes, staff at the Addenbrooke's Wellcome Trust Clinical Research Facility, and midwives at the Rosie Maternity Hospital in collecting data for this study. We would also like to thank Angie Watts, Karen Whitehead and Dianne Wingate for excellent laboratory assistance.

Appendix A

The prenatal questionnaire (which included the food/drink intake frequency questions) that were given out to all pregnant women recruited to the CBGS.

References

1. American Diabetes Association. Diagnosis and classification of diabetes mellitus. *Diabetes Care* **2010**, *33*, S62–S69. [CrossRef] [PubMed]
2. International Diabetes Federation. *IDF Diabetes Atlas*, 8th ed.; International Diabetes Federation: Brussels, Belgium, 2017.
3. Heianza, Y.; Qi, L. Gene-diet interaction and precision nutrition in obesity. *Int. J. Mol. Sci.* **2017**, *18*, 787. [CrossRef] [PubMed]
4. Mijatovic-Vukas, J.; Capling, L.; Cheng, S.; Stamatakis, E.; Louie, J.; Cheung, N.W.; Markovic, T.; Ross, G.; Senior, A.; Brand-Miller, J.C.; et al. Associations of diet and physical activity with risk for Gestational Diabetes Mellitus: A Systematic Review and Meta-Analysis. *Nutrients* **2018**, *10*, 698. [CrossRef] [PubMed]
5. Radd-Vagenas, S.; Kouris-Blazos, A.; Singh, M.F.; Flood, V.M. Evolution of Mediterranean diets and cuisine: Concepts and definitions. *Asia Pac. J. Clin. Nutr.* **2017**, *26*, 749–763. [PubMed]
6. Assaf-Balut, C.; García de la Torre, N.; Durán, A.; Fuentes, M.; Bordiú, E.; Del Valle, L.; Familiar, C.; Ortolá, A.; Jiménez, I.; Herraiz, M.A.; et al. A Mediterranean diet with additional extra virgin olive oil and pistachios reduces the incidence of gestational diabetes mellitus (GDM): A randomized controlled trial: The St. Carlos GDM prevention study. *PLoS ONE* **2017**, *12*, e0185873. [CrossRef] [PubMed]
7. De la Torre, N.G.; Assaf-Balut, C.; Jiménez Varas, I.; Del Valle, L.; Durán, A.; Fuentes, M.; Del Prado, N.; Bordiú, E.; Valerio, J.J.; Herraiz, M.A.; et al. Effectiveness of following Mediterranean diet recommendations in the real world in the incidence of Gestational Diabetes Mellitus (GDM) and adverse maternal-foetal outcomes: A prospective, universal, interventional study with a single group. The St Carlos Study. *Nutrients* **2019**, *11*, 1210.
8. Assaf-Balut, C.; García de la Torre, N.; Duran, A.; Fuentes, M.; Bordiú, E.; Del Valle, L.; Familiar, C.; Valerio, J.; Jiménez, I.; Herraiz, M.A.; et al. A Mediterranean diet with an enhanced consumption of extra virgin olive oil and pistachios improves pregnancy outcomes in women without Gestational Diabetes Mellitus: A Sub-analysis of the St. Carlos Gestational Diabetes Mellitus Prevention Study. *Ann. Nutr. Metab.* **2019**, *74*, 69–79. [CrossRef]
9. McCullough, M.L.; Feskanich, D.; Stampfer, M.J.; Giovannucci, E.L.; Rimm, E.B.; Hu, F.B.; Spiegelman, D.; Hunter, D.J.; Colditz, G.A.; Willett, W.C. Diet quality and major chronic disease risk in men and women: Moving toward improved dietary guidance. *Am. J. Clin. Nutr.* **2002**, *76*, 1261–1271. [CrossRef]
10. Shepherd, E.; Gomersall, J.C.; Tieu, J.; Han, S.; Crowther, C.A.; Middleton, P. Combined diet and exercise interventions for preventing gestational diabetes mellitus. *Cochrane Database Syst. Rev.* **2017**. [CrossRef]

11. Donazar-Ezcurra, M.; López-Del Burgo, C.; Bes-Rastrollo, M. Primary prevention of gestational diabetes mellitus through nutritional factors: A systematic review. *BMC Pregnancy Childbirth* **2017**, *17*, 30. [CrossRef]
12. Koivusalo, S.B.; Rönö, K.; Klemetti, M.M.; Roine, R.P.; Lindström, J.; Erkkola, M.; Kaaja, R.J.; Pöyhönen-Alho, M.; Tiitinen, A.; Huvinen, E.; et al. Gestational Diabetes Mellitus can be prevented by lifestyle intervention: The Finnish Gestational Diabetes Prevention Study (RADIEL): A randomized controlled trial. *Diabetes Care* **2016**, *39*, 24–30. [CrossRef] [PubMed]
13. Drewnowski, A.; Popkin, B.M. The nutrition transition: New trends in the global diet. *Nutr. Rev.* **1997**, *55*, 31–43. [CrossRef] [PubMed]
14. Foster, R.; Lunn, J. 40th Anniversary Briefing Paper: Food availability and our changing diet. *Nutr. Bull.* **2007**, *32*, 187–249. [CrossRef]
15. Ferro-Luzzi, A.; Martino, L. Obesity and physical activity. *Ciba Found. Symp.* **1996**, *201*, 207–221.
16. Crozier, S.R.; Robinson, S.M.; Godfrey, K.M.; Cooper, C.; Inskip, H.M. Women's dietary patterns change little from before to during pregnancy. *J. Nutr.* **2009**, *139*, 1956–1963. [CrossRef]
17. Feig, D.S.; Hwee, J.; Shah, B.R.; Booth, G.L.; Bierman, A.S.; Lipscombe, L.L. Trends in incidence of diabetes in pregnancy and serious perinatal outcomes: A large, population-based study in Ontario, Canada, 1996–2010. *Diabetes Care* **2014**, *37*, 1590–1596. [CrossRef]
18. Khalifeh, A.; Breathnach, F.; Coulter-Smith, S.; Robson, M.; Fitzpatrick, C.; Malone, F. Changing trends in diabetes mellitus in pregnancy. *J. Obstet. Gynaecol.* **2014**, *34*, 135–137. [CrossRef]
19. Wang, Y.; Chen, L.; Xiao, K.; Horswell, R.; Besse, J.; Johnson, J.; Ryan, D.H.; Hu, G. Increasing incidence of gestational diabetes mellitus in Louisiana, 1997–2009. *J. Women's Health* **2012**, *21*, 319–325. [CrossRef]
20. Sella, T.; Shalev, V.; Elchalal, U.; Chovel-Sella, A.; Chodick, G. Screening for gestational diabetes in the 21st century: A population-based cohort study in Israel. *J. Matern. Fetal Neonatal Med.* **2013**, *26*, 412–416. [CrossRef]
21. Huy, C.; Loerbroks, A.; Hornemann, A.; Röhrig, S.; Schneider, S. Prevalence, Trend and determining factors of Gestational Diabetes in Germany. *Geburtshilfe Frauenheilkd* **2012**, *72*, 311–315. [CrossRef]
22. Petry, C.J.; Fisher, B.G.; Ong, K.K.; Hughes, I.A.; Acerini, C.L.; Dunger, D.B. Temporal trends without seasonal effects on gestational diabetes incidence relate to reductions in indices of insulin secretion: The Cambridge Baby Growth Study. *Acta Diabetol.* **2019**, *56*, 1133–1140. [CrossRef] [PubMed]
23. Haggarty, P.; Campbell, D.M.; Duthie, S.; Andrews, K.; Hoad, G.; Piyathilake, C.; McNeill, G. Diet and deprivation in pregnancy. *Br. J. Nutr.* **2009**, *102*, 1487–1497. [CrossRef] [PubMed]
24. Laraia, B.; Messer, L.; Evenson, K.; Kaufman, J.S. Neighborhood factors associated with physical activity and adequacy of weight gain during pregnancy. *J. Urban Health* **2007**, *84*, 793–806. [CrossRef] [PubMed]
25. Prentice, P.; Acerini, C.L.; Eleftheriou, A.; Hughes, I.A.; Ong, K.K.; Dunger, D.B. Cohort Profile: The Cambridge Baby Growth Study (CBGS). *Int. J. Epidemiol.* **2016**. [CrossRef] [PubMed]
26. Damgaard, I.N.; Jensen, T.K.; Petersen, J.H.; Skakkebaek, N.E.; Toppari, J.; Main, K.M. Cryptorchidism and maternal alcohol consumption during pregnancy. *Environ. Health Perspect.* **2007**, *115*, 272–277. [CrossRef] [PubMed]
27. Petry, C.J.; Seear, R.V.; Wingate, D.L.; Manico, L.; Acerini, C.L.; Ong, K.K.; Hughes, I.A.; Dunger, D.B. Associations between paternally transmitted fetal *IGF2* variants and maternal circulating glucose concentrations in pregnancy. *Diabetes* **2011**, *60*, 3090–3096. [CrossRef]
28. National Collaborating Centre for Women's and Children's Health. *Diabetes in Pregnancy: Management of Diabetes and Its Complications from Preconception to the Postnatal Period*; RCOG Press: London, UK, 2015.
29. Metzger, B.E.; Gabbe, S.G.; Persson, B.; Buchanan, T.A.; Catalano, P.A.; Damm, P.; Dyer, A.R.; Leiva, A.D.; Hod, M.; International Association of Diabetes and Pregnancy Study Groups Consensus Panel; et al. International Association of Diabetes and Pregnancy Study Groups recommendations on the diagnosis and classification of hyperglycemia in pregnancy. *Diabetes Care* **2010**, *33*, 676–682. [CrossRef]
30. World Health Organization. Diagnostic Criteria and Classification of Hyperglycaemia First Detected in Pregnancy: A World Health Organization Guideline. 2013. Available online: http://apps.who.int/iris/bitstream/10665/85975/1/WHO_NMH_MND_13.2_eng.pdf (accessed on 3 June 2019).
31. World Health Organization Department of Noncommunicable Disease Surveillance Geneva. *Definition, Diagnosis and Classification of Diabetes Mellitus and Its Complications*; WHO: Geneva, Switzerland, 1999.

32. Prentice, P.M.; Olga, L.; Petry, C.J.; Simmons, D.; Murphy, H.; Hughes, I.A.; Acerini, C.L.; Ong, K.K.; Dunger, D.B. Reduced size at birth and persisting reductions in adiposity in recent compared with earlier cohorts of infants born to mothers with gestational diabetes mellitus. *Diabetologia* **2019**, *62*, 1977–1987. [CrossRef]
33. Levy, J.C.; Matthews, D.R.; Hermans, M.P. Correct homeostasis model assessment (HOMA) evaluation uses the computer program. *Diabetes Care* **1998**, *21*, 2191–2192. [CrossRef]
34. De Lauzon-Guillain, B.; Wijndaele, K.; Clark, M.; Acerini, C.L.; Hughes, I.A.; Dunger, D.B.; Wells, J.C.; Ong, K.K. Breastfeeding and infant temperament at age three months. *PLoS ONE* **2012**, *7*, e29326. [CrossRef]
35. Benjamini, Y.; Hochberg, Y. Controlling the false discovery rate: A practical and powerful approach to multiple testing. *J. R. Stat. Soc.* **1995**, *57*, 289–300. [CrossRef]
36. Tieu, J.; Crowther, C.A.; Middleton, P. Dietary advice in pregnancy for preventing gestational diabetes mellitus. *Cochrane Database Syst. Rev.* **2008**. [CrossRef]
37. Shin, D.; Lee, K.W.; Song, W.O. Dietary patterns during pregnancy are associated with risk of gestational diabetes mellitus. *Nutrients* **2015**, *7*, 9369–9382. [CrossRef] [PubMed]
38. Lang, T.; Dibb, S.; Reddy, S. *Looking Back, Looking forward: Sustainability and UK Food Policy 2000–2011*; Sustainable Development Commission: London, UK, 2011; pp. 1–54. Available online: http://www.sd-commission.org.uk/data/files/publications/FoodPolicy10_Report_final_w.pdf (accessed on 3 June 2019).
39. Vartanian, L.R.; Schwartz, M.B.; Brownell, K.D. Effects of soft drink consumption on nutrition and health: A systematic review and meta-analysis. *Am. J. Public Health* **2007**, *97*, 667–675. [CrossRef] [PubMed]
40. Pot, G.K.; Prynne, C.J.; Almoosawi, S.; Kuh, D.; Stephen, A.M.; NSHD Scientific and Data Collection Teams. Trends in food consumption over 30 years: Evidence from a British birth cohort. *Eur. J. Clin. Nutr.* **2015**, *69*, 817–823. [CrossRef]
41. Whitton, C.; Nicholson, S.K.; Roberts, C.; Prynne, C.J.; Pot, G.K.; Olson, A.; Fitt, E.; Cole, D.; Teucher, B.; Bates, B.; et al. National Diet and Nutrition Survey: UK food consumption and nutrient intakes from the first year of the rolling programme and comparisons with previous surveys. *Br. J. Nutr.* **2011**, *106*, 1899–1914. [CrossRef]
42. Qiu, C.; Frederick, I.O.; Zhang, C.; Sorensen, T.K.; Enquobahrie, D.A.; Williams, M.A. Risk of gestational diabetes mellitus in relation to maternal egg and cholesterol intake. *Am. J. Epidemiol.* **2011**, *173*, 649–658. [CrossRef]
43. Schoenaker, D.A.; Mishra, G.D.; Callaway, L.K.; Soedamah-Muthu, S.S. The role of energy, nutrients, foods, and dietary patterns in the development of gestational diabetes mellitus: A systematic review of observational studies. *Diabetes Care* **2016**, *39*, 16–23. [CrossRef]
44. Milajerdi, A.; Tehrani, H.; Haghighatdoost, F.; Larijani, B.; Surkan, P.J.; Azadbakht, L. Associations between higher egg consumption during pregnancy with lowered risks of high blood pressure and gestational diabetes mellitus. *Int. J. Vitam. Nutr. Res.* **2018**, *88*, 166–175. [CrossRef]
45. Stråvik, M.; Jonsson, K.; Hartvigsson, O.; Sandin, A.; Wold, A.E.; Sandberg, A.S.; Barman, M. Food and nutrient intake during pregnancy in relation to maternal characteristics: Results from the NICE Birth Cohort in Northern Sweden. *Nutrients* **2019**, *11*, 1680. [CrossRef]
46. Blumfield, M.L.; Hure, A.J.; Macdonald-Wicks, L.; Smith, R.; Collins, C.E. Systematic review and meta-analysis of energy and macronutrient intakes during pregnancy in developed countries. *Nutr. Rev.* **2012**, *70*, 322–336. [CrossRef] [PubMed]

9

Effect of High Versus Low Carbohydrate Intake in the Morning on Glycemic Variability and Glycemic Control Measured by Continuous Blood Glucose Monitoring in Women with Gestational Diabetes Mellitus

Louise Rasmussen [1,†], Maria Lund Christensen [1,†], Charlotte Wolff Poulsen [2], Charlotte Rud [3], Alexander Sidelmann Christensen [4,5], Jens Rikardt Andersen [1], Ulla Kampmann [6,*] and Per Glud Ovesen [2]

1 Department of Nutrition, Exercise and Sports, University of Copenhagen, Rolighedsvej 26, 1958 Frederiksberg C, Copenhagen, Denmark; louiseras90@gmail.com (L.R.); mclund89@gmail.com (M.L.C.); jra@nexs.ku.dk (J.R.A.)
2 Department of Obstetrics and Gynecology, Aarhus University Hospital, Palle Juul-Jensens Boulevard 99, 8200 Aarhus N, Denmark; charpoul@rm.dk (C.W.P.); per.ovesen@clin.au.dk (P.G.O.)
3 Department of Hepatology and Gastroenterology, Aarhus University Hospital, Palle Juul-Jensens Boulevard 99, 8200 Aarhus N, Denmark; charru@rm.dk
4 Steno Diabetes Center Copenhagen, Niels Steensens Vej 2-4, 2820 Gentofte, Denmark; alexander.sidelmann.christensen@regionh.dk
5 Clinic for Clinical Metabolic Research, Herlev and Gentofte Hospital, University of Copenhagen, Gentofte Hospitalsvej 7, 3. Sal, 2800 Hellerup, Denmark
6 Steno Diabetes Center Aarhus, Aarhus University Hospital, Hedeager 3, 8200 Aarhus N, Denmark
* Correspondence: ulla@opstrup.dk
† Shares first author ship.

Abstract: Carbohydrate is the macronutrient that has the greatest impact on blood glucose response. Limited data are available on how carbohydrate distribution throughout the day affects blood glucose in women with gestational diabetes mellitus (GDM). We aimed to assess how a high-carbohydrate morning-intake (HCM) versus a low-carbohydrate-morning-intake (LCM), affect glycemic variability and glucose control. In this randomized crossover study continuous glucose monitoring (CGM) was performed in 12 women with diet treated GDM (75 g, 2-h OGTT $\geq$ 8.5 mmol/L), who went through 2 $\times$ 3 days of HCM and LCM. A within-subject-analysis showed a significantly higher mean amplitude of glucose excursions (MAGE) (0.7 mmol/L, $p = 0.004$) and coefficient of variation (CV) (5.1%, $p = 0.01$) when comparing HCM with LCM, whereas a significantly lower mean glucose (MG) (-0.3 mmol/L, $p = 0.002$) and fasting blood glucose (FBG) were found (-0.4 mmol/L, $p = 0.01$) on the HCM diet compared to the LCM diet. In addition, insulin resistance, expressed as Homeostatic Model Assessment for Insulin Resistance (HOMA-IR), decreased significantly during HCM. Results indicate that a carbohydrate distribution of 50% in the morning favors lower blood glucose and improvement in insulin sensitivity in women with GDM, but in contrary gives a higher glycemic variability.

Keywords: glycemic variability; carbohydrate distribution; gestational diabetes mellitus; mean amplitude of glucose; breakfast diet

1. Introduction

Pregnant women develop decreased insulin sensitivity with increasing gestational age. The adapted insulin sensitivity in the mother ensures sufficient nutrients supply for the growing fetus [1]. In women with Gestational diabetes mellitus (GDM) insulin sensitivity is reduced even further and GDM is defined as decreased glucose tolerance developed during pregnancy [2,3]. The prevalence of GDM varies worldwide, ranging from 1% to over 30% in some countries and the number of women diagnosed with GDM is increasing [4,5].

With repeated episodes of hyperglycemia, the fetus receives too much glucose [4,6] and several studies on GDM patients have shown a correlation between increasing blood glucose levels and birth complications [7–9]. According to studies including pregnant women with type 1 diabetes and type 2 diabetes, large variations in blood glucose levels cause more complications than constantly elevated blood glucose levels [10,11]. Twenty-four hours continuous glucose measurements (CGM) detect a more detailed glycemic profile than self-monitored blood glucose (SMGB) by better measuring the duration and magnitude of fluctuation, especially for fasting and postprandial measurements [12,13].

Carbohydrate is the macronutrient with the greatest impact on postprandial blood glucose response. Treatment of GDM involves dietary guidance on the amount, type and distribution of carbohydrate [14–16]. However, there is currently no evidence on how carbohydrate intake should be distributed during the day. Distributing carbohydrate intake throughout the day into multiple meals and snacks may be beneficial for controlling postprandial blood glucose levels [14]. It is customary in Denmark to recommend 5–6 daily meals for patients with GDM and a maximum of 30 g of carbohydrates at breakfast [17]. However, only few intervention studies have been conducted focusing on meal pattern [14], including the optimal timing of carbohydrate intake during the day. Patients with type 2 diabetes who consume breakfast with a high energy and carbohydrate content and a low energy and carbohydrate intake in the evening showed a beneficial effect on the postprandial blood glucose response and led to an increase in Glucagon-like-peptide-1 (GLP-1), insulin response and C-peptide excretion compared to an energy and carbohydrate-reduced breakfast [18]. These findings contradict the recommendation that GDM patients should consume only a few carbohydrates for breakfast. This recommendation is given because of the usually marked postprandial rise in blood glucose during mornings, with insulin resistance being most pronounced at this time of day [19]. High carbohydrate breakfast and carbohydrate-reduced dinner could also be beneficial for blood glucose response in GDM patients. As far as the authors are aware, it has not yet been studied whether a high carbohydrate intake in the morning is beneficial in patients with GDM.

The aim of the present study was to investigate the effects of a High-carbohydrate-morning-intake (HCM) compared to a low-carbohydrate-morning-intake (LCM), both diets isocaloric for each participant and with the same total carbohydrate content, on glycemic variability in GDM patients measured by mean amplitude of glucose excursions (MAGE) and coefficient of variation (CV), using CGM. Secondarily we investigated the effect of HCM compared with LCM on parameters of glycemic control; mean glucose (MG) and fasting blood glucose (FBG). In addition, we assessed the effect of the two diets on insulin resistance expressed as Homeostatic Model Assessment for Insulin Resistance (HOMA-IR).

2. Materials and Methods

2.1. Study Design and Population

We conducted a randomized crossover clinical trial to investigate the effect of the carbohydrate distribution on different blood glucose measurements. The study participants included women of at least 18 years of age with diet treated GDM and gestational age of at least 30 weeks. Participants were randomized through the web-based application Research Electronic Data Capture (RedCap) [20]. An independent administrative employee created a randomization-key, balanced 1:1, blinding the investigators of the allocation sequence of participants until assignment.

Fifteen participants with GDM according to WHO diagnostic criteria (75 g, 2-h OGTT ≥ 8.5 mmol/L) [21] were enrolled. We did not include women on any type of diabetes medication, and if a participant was prescribed insulin treatment during the intervention period, the woman was excluded as well. The primary outcome was to assess the overall effect on glycemic variability in both meal plans (HCM vs. LCM) expressed by MAGE. Secondarily to investigate the effect on CV%, MG, FBG and HOMA-IR.

All clinical data were entered in RedCap. The Danish National Committee on Health Research Ethics approved the study. All participants gave their informed consent. The study was registered at ClinicalTrials.gov (NCT03835208).

2.2. *Intervention*

All participants received two different dietary-treatments in two independent but continuous periods of 4 days each with four to five days of wash-out period in between. The dietary treatments consisted of two different meal timing schedules with either "breakfast diet" with a high **carbohydrate** and energy content in the morning and a low carbohydrate and energy content in the evening (HCM) or a "dinner diet" with a low carbohydrate and energy content in the morning and a high carbohydrate and energy content at dinner (LCM). The total macronutrient content and composition was identical in the two periods but the meal distribution differed.

The participants visited the clinic four times during the two intervention periods; at the start and end of each intervention. Meal plans with different carbohydrate distribution was handed out followed by careful instructions from the investigators at the beginning of each intervention period. The meal plans were followed in home settings. The participants were provided with a grocery list and pictures of specific food items for shopping and the meal plans contained pictures of each meal in order to control the dietary intake as much as possible without handing out any food.

In general, the meal plans followed the standard care of the Department of Obstetrics and Gynecology Aarhus University Hospital, apart from the carbohydrate distribution during the day. All meal plans were according to the recommendations in Table 1. All meals contained only whole grain products. The participants were asked not to ingest or drink anything besides the food components of the meal plan. All participants received a kitchen scale and were asked to weigh all foods.

Table 1. Meal plans recommendations.

Nutrient	
Carbohydrates	45–60 E%
Fibers	>28 g
Sugar (added)	10 E%
Protein	10–20 E%
Fat	25–40 E%
SFA	<10 E%
PUFA	5–10 E%
MUFA	10–20 E%

SFA, saturated fatty acid; PUFA, polyunsaturated fatty acid; MUFA, monounsaturated fatty acid.

Calorie content of both the HCM and LCM meal plans were either 1800, 2000, 2200 or 2400 kcal according to the individual needs. Calorie-needs were calculated by the use of equations calculating for resting energy expenditure (REE) by Henry [22] based on pre-pregnancy weight and height multiplied by a factor of physical activity level (PAL). All participants were in their third trimester and an additional 537 kcal were added. The estimated calorie-needs were reduced by 30% if the patient was overweight (based on pre-gestational BMI >25) or already had reached the optimal weight gain, according to the recommendation of IOM [23] at the time for study inclusion. After calculating each participant's individual energy-needs, the nearest 200-calorie step was used for guidance purposes. The two meal plans representing the two intervention periods (HCM and LCM) were kept isocaloric

+/−2,5% for each participant. Both meal plans provided a total of five meals a day and had the same overall macronutrients distribution; 46 E% carbohydrates, 34 E% fat and 20 E% protein. All values +/−2 E%.

The distribution of energy and carbohydrate content during the day for the meal plans in both intervention periods (HCM and LCM) are shown in Table 2. During both intervention-periods two 24-h diet recalls were obtained by one of the investigators to check for compliance and the participants were also asked to take pictures of the main meals and of the plate if any leftovers.

Table 2. Meal plan structure and diet compositions of HCM and LCM.

	HCM	LCM
Energy distribution Calories as a percentage of total calorie content during the day	Breakfast: 25%–30% morning-snack: 15%–20% Lunch: 25%–30% Afternoon-snack: 10%–15% Dinner: 15%–20%	Breakfast: 15%–20% Lunch: 25%–30% Afternoon-snack: 10%–15% Dinner: 30%–35% Late-night-snack: 15%–20%
Carbohydrate distribution Carbohydrate as a percentage of total carbohydrate content during the day	morning: 50% • Breakfast: 30%–35% • morning-snack: 15%–20% Lunch: 40% • Lunch: 25%–30% • Afternoon-snack: 10%–15% Dinner: 10%	morning: 10% Lunch: 40% • Lunch: 25%–30% • Afternoon-snack: 10%–15% Dinner: 50% • Dinner: 30%–35% • Late-night-snack: 15%–20%

HCM, high carbohydrate and energy content in the morning; LCM, low carbohydrate and energy content in the morning.

2.3. CGM-Measurements and -Parameter Calculation

Glucose levels were monitored continuously in all participants by CGMs (Medtronic, Ipro 2 (Medtronic MiniMed, Northridge, CA, USA)) for 72 h in each intervention period. On day 1 of each of the intervention periods, the sensor was attached to the triceps of the participant by one of the investigators immediately before serving breakfast. The sensor was affixed with an adhesive bandage and removed at the end of each intervention period by an investigator. The women were instructed to do pre-prandial SMBG four times a day (before breakfast, lunch, dinner and before bedtime) with a glucometer (Accu-Chek Mobile, Roche Diagnostics GmbH, Mannheim, Germany) for calibrating the CGMs. Accuracy of the glucometer was tested in comparison with the fasting blood glucose tested in the laboratory and a 15% deviation was accepted.

Calibrated glucose profiles recorded for each patient over a period of 48 h of each intervention period (day 2 and day 3) was used for statistical analysis and quantification of glycemic variability. Parameters of glycemic variability included the standard deviation of blood glucose (SD), MAGE and the CV%. MG was also calculated from the CGM data as a measurement of glycemic control.

2.4. Blood Samples

Fasting blood samples were drawn at all four visits. C-peptide, fasting blood glucose, lipid-profile (triglycerides, HDL, LDL and total cholesterol), 3-hydroxy-butyrat and C-reactive protein (CRP) were measured. All blood samples were drawn at the same time of the day at all four visits and analyzed by a certified medical laboratory technician immediately after sampling.

HOMA-IR was calculated based on fasting C-peptide and fasting blood glucose at baseline and at the end of each intervention period using the HOMA Calculator v2.2.3 [24].

2.5. Sample Size and Power Analysis

Power calculation on the primary outcome MAGE was based on a study by Dalfrá et al. [25]. A sample size of 12 participants was required to ensure adequate power of 80%, to detect a 5% difference between interventions. With an estimated dropout range of 20%, it was necessary to include a total of 15 participants.

2.6. Statistical Analysis

Data of baseline characteristics are presented by descriptive statistics for all included participants ($n = 12$). The efficacy of the two interventions was assessed based on the within-subject difference between the two meal schedules regarding the outcome variable. Outcome from CGM data are calculated by the use of the excel-based workbook software called "EasyGV" [26].

To ensure that treatment effects were distinguished from carry-over effects, test of carry-over effect was done by performing a pre-test for unpaired samples. An unpaired two sample t-test was used.

Comparison of treatment effects of HCM and LCM was conducted using paired sample t-tests on the difference between periods. Assumptions of equal mean and SD was tested using Bland-Altman plots. Whether or not outcome differences were normally distributed were assessed with QQ-plots. A p-value ≤ 0.05 was considered statistically significant. Statistical analysis was performed using R-statistics software.

All data are represented as mean ± standard deviation (SD).

3. Results

3.1. Participants

A total of 12 out of 15 participants completed the study. Two of the excluded participants were randomized to sequence LCM|HCM and one to sequence HCM|LCM, leaving a total of six participants in each sequence-group for the final analysis. A flow chart of all study participants is shown in Figure 1.

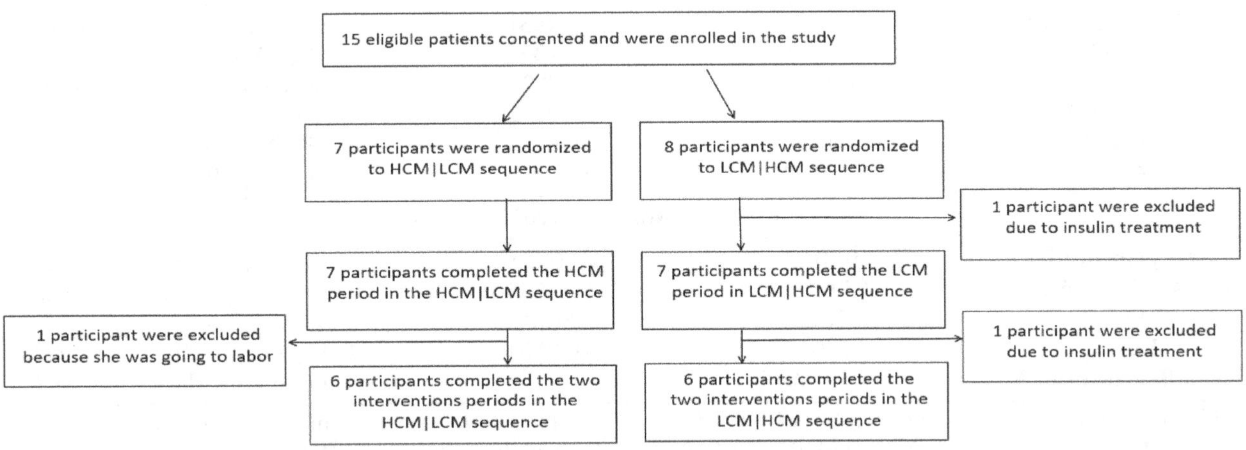

Figure 1. Flow chart of the study. HCM, high carbohydrate and energy content in the morning; LCM, low carbohydrate and energy content in the morning.

Baseline characteristics of the study population are shown in Table 3. Study population had a mean gestational age (GA) of 33.5 ± 2.3 weeks at the beginning of the intervention, a mean age of 33.6 ± 6.7 years and a mean BMI of 25.2 ± 4.0 kg/m^2.

Table 3. Baseline characteristics of the participants (n = 12) included in the final analysis.

	All Study Participants (n = 12)
Age at Debut (year)	33.6 (6.7)
Pregestational weight (kg)	68.6 (11.3)
GA (weeks)	33.5 (2.3)
Parity (n (%))	
0	6 (50)
1	2 (17)
2	4 (33)
BMI (kg/m^2)	25.2 (4.0)
GWG (kg)	12.8 (7.7)
OGTT (mmol/L)	9.7 (0.7)
HbA1C	5.3 (2.5)
(%) (mmol/mol)	(34.4 (4.2))
Average BS (mmol/mol)	5.8 (0.6)
Systolic BP (mmHg)	115.1 (9.4)
Diastolic BP (mmHg)	75.4 (6.3)

Results are mean (SD) except parity which is n (%). GA, gestational age; GWG, gestational weight gain.

3.2. *Comparison between HCM and LCM-Diet on Parameters of Glycemic Variability and Glycemic Control*

Table 4 shows the mean values of MAGE, CV, SD, TIR, TBR, TAR and MG of both HCM and LCM and the difference in C-peptide and FBG of the two attendance days in each period (day 4 minus day 1). Statistically significant estimates of the treatment effect from within-subject differences (HCM minus LCM) were observed for measurements of glycemic variability (MAGE and CV) and glycemic control (MG and FBG).

Table 4. Results of treatment effect.

	HCM (n = 12) Mean (SD)	LCM (n = 12) Mean (SD)	Difference (95% CI)	p-Value
	Glycemic Variability			
MAGE (mmol/L)	2.5 (1.8)	1.9 (0.5)	0.7 (0.3;1.2)	0.004
CV (%)	20.1 (5.9)	14.9 (3.6)	5.1 (1.5;8.8)	0.01
SD	1.0 (0.3	0.8 (0.2)	0.2 (0.0;0.4)	0.02
TIR (%)	93.46(8.7)	97.96(3.2)	−4.5(−9.7;0.7)	0.08
TBR (%)	6.42(8.5)	2.04(3.2)	4.38(-0.7-9.5)	0.09
TAR (%)	1.64(2.6)	1.06(2.5)	0.58(-0.78;1.93)	0.37
	Glycemic Control			
MG (mmol/L)	4.9 (0.3)	5.2 (0.5)	−0.3 (−0.6; −0.1)	0.02
ΔC-peptide (pmol/L)	−82.3 (109.1)	71.9 (363.9)	−154.2 (−381.4;73.0)	0.16
FBG_{start}	4.85(0.5)	4.88(0.6)	−0.025(−0.2;0.1)	0.75
FBG_{end}	4.62(0.4)	5.07(0.5)	−0.45(−0.7; −02)	0.0007
ΔFBG (mmol/L)	−0.2 (0.2)	0.2 (0.5)	−0.4 (−0.7; −0.1)	0.01

All variables are given as mean (SD). HCM, high carbohydrate and energy content in the morning; LCM, low carbohydrate and energy content in the morning; MAGE, mean amplitude of glucose excursions; CV, coefficient of variation; TIR, time in range; TBR, time below range; TAR, time above; MG, mean glucose; FBG, fasting blood glucose. All FBG values are taking in the morning. FBG_{start} is day 1 in each period. FBG_{end} is day 4 in each period. Values of MAGE, CV and MG are all based on calculation of the calibrated glucose profiles recorded for each patient over a period of 48 h of each intervention period (day 2 and day 3). Δ: Delta values are based on day 4 minus day 1 in both HCM and LCM intervention period.

Both measurements of glycemic variability indicated a significantly higher variability in the HCM-diet compared to the LCM diet. MAGE was significantly higher on the HCM-diet (2.5 ± 1.8 mmol/L) compared to the LCM-diet (1.9 ± 0.5 mmol/L) with a mean difference of 0.7 mmol/L

(0.3; 1.2) ($p = 0.004$) (Table 4 and Figure 2). A higher CV was found with a mean difference of 5.1% (1.5; 8.8) ($p = 0.01$) on the HCM-diet compared to the LCM-diet.

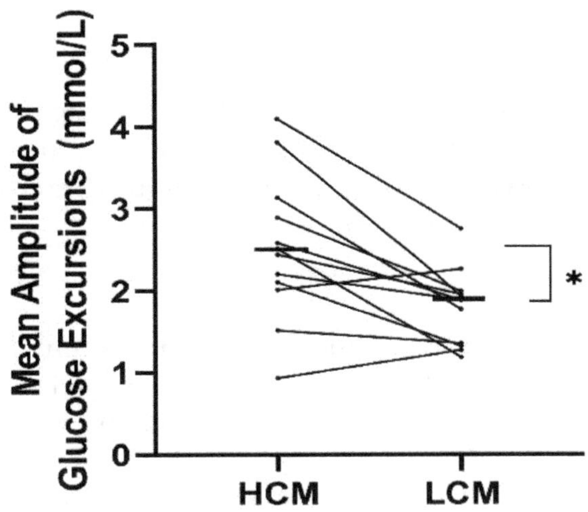

Figure 2. Treatment effect on mean amplitude of glucose excursions (MAGE) for each participant following a diet with two days of high carbohydrate load (HCM) and two days of low carbohydrate load (LCM) in the morning. Mean values of the treatment effect of each period are marked with black lines. HCM, high carbohydrate and energy content in the morning; LCM, low carbohydrate and energy content in the morning; MAGE, mean amplitude of glucose excursions.

Both measurements of glycemic control were significantly higher for LCM- compared with HCM-diet. A treatment effect with a mean difference of −0.3 mmol/L (−0.6; 0.1) ($p = 0.02$) in MG was observed when comparing HCM-diet to LCM-diet (Table 4 and Figure 3). A decrease in FBG was observed for the HCM-diet with a mean FBG at baseline of 4.9 mmol/L and 4.6 mmol/L at the end (mean difference of −0.2 mmol/L), while an increase was found for the LCM-diet with a mean FBG at baseline of 4.9 mmol/L and 5.1 mmol/L at the end (mean difference of 0.2 mmol/L). There was a significant difference of FBG between the two diets of −0.4 mmol/L (−0.7; −0.1) ($p = 0.01$) when comparing the mean difference (day 4 minus day 1) of HCM- to LCM-diet. C-peptide did also tend to decrease during HCM-diet with −82.3 pmol/L, while increasing during LCM-diet with 71.9 pmol/L between end of each period and baseline.

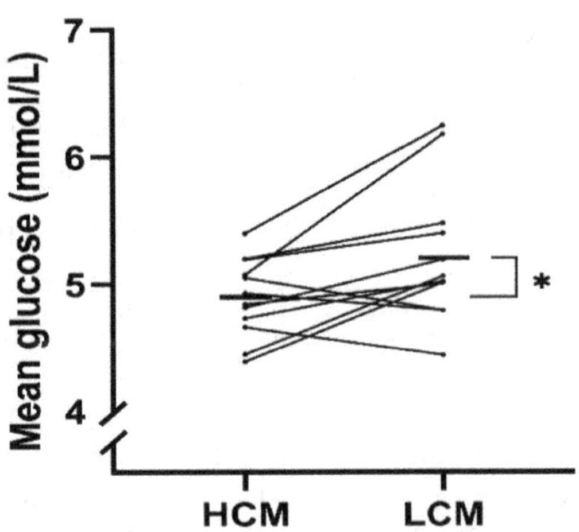

Figure 3. Treatment effect on mean glucose (MG) for each participant following a diet with high carbohydrate load (HCM) and a diet with low carbohydrate load (LCM) in the morning. Mean values of the treatment effect of each period are marked with black lines. HCM, high carbohydrate and energy content in the morning; LCM, low carbohydrate and energy content in the morning; MG, mean glucose.

In summary, the HCM-diet seemed to give a higher glycemic variability but a better glycemic control when comparing with the LCM-diet.

3.3. HOMA-IR

To assess insulin resistance HOMA-IR was calculated based on fasting C-peptide and FBG at baseline and at the end of each intervention. HOMA-IR decreased significantly during the HCM-period with a mean difference of −0.214 ($p = 0.02$) and tended to increase during the LCM-period with a mean difference of −0.107 ($p = 0.68$). However, there was not a significant difference when comparing the HCM- with the LCM-period with a mean difference of −0.321.

3.4. Tertiary Outcomes

Table 5 shows the mean values of the differences (day 4 minus day 1) between the two interventions, regarding the lipid-profile, 3-hydroxy-butyrat and C-reactive protein. Comparisons between the two diets by a paired t-test did not reveal any significant within-subject differences ($p > 0.05$ for all).

Table 5. Effect on tertiary outcomes.

	HCM (n = 12) Mean (SD)	LCM (n = 12) Mean (SD)	Difference (95% CI)	p-Value
Δp-total cholesterol (mmol/L)	0.0 (0.250)	0.1 (0.2)	−0.0 (−0.2; 0.2)	0.87
Δp-LDL cholesterol (mmol/L)	−0.2 (0.408)	0.2 (0.4)	−0.4 (−0.9; 0.0)	0.07
Δp-HDL cholesterol (mmol/L)	0.0 (0.1)	0.1 (0.1)	−0.0 (−0.1; 0.1)	0.83
Δp-triglycerides (mmol/L)	−0.0 (0.3)	−0.2 (0.5)	0.3 (−0.1; 0.6)	0.15
ΔCRP (mg/L)	−0.8 (2.1)	1.4 (4.5)	−2.2 (−6.3; 1.9)	0.27
Δ3-hydroxy-byturat (mmol/L)	−0.2 (0.8)	−0.5 (1.0)	0.2 (−0.7; 1.1)	0.57

HCM, high carbohydrate and energy content in the morning; LCM, low carbohydrate and energy content in the morning. p-values and 95% CI are based on paired t-tests with an assumption of equal variance (all except CRP) and approximately normally distributed data. Δ: Delta values are based on day 4 minus day 1 in both HCM and LCM intervention period.

3.5. Food Intake

Table 6 shows the comparison of food intake in the two diets based on the mean of the two 24-h recalls.

Table 6. Intra-individual comparison of food intake between HCM and LCM.

	HCM Mean (SD)	LCM Mean (SD)	Difference (95% CI)	p-Value
Energy, kcal	2012 (263)	2055 (2740)	−43.33 (−126.6; 40.0)	$p = 0.28$
Carbohydrates, g	222 (28)	215 (36)	6.2 g (−2.9; 15.4)	$p = 0.16$
Dietary fiber, g	38.79 (5.8)	39.50 (8.0)	−0.71(4.3; 2.9)	$p = 0.68$
Fat, g	73 (10)	82 (10)	−9.9 g (−16.5; −3.2)	$p = 0.007$
Protein, g	98 (15)	94 (14)	4.2 g (−0.6; 8.9)	$p = 0.08$

HCM, high carbohydrate and energy content in the morning; LCM, low carbohydrate and energy content in the morning. Mean difference, 95% CI and p-values are based on a paired t-test between HCM and LCM based on raw data.

Some intake of the participants deviated by more than the acceptable (2.5% from intended energy content (approximately +/−50 kcal) and +/−2 E% for macronutrient). Even though there were no significant difference within-subject in intake of energy, carbohydrate and protein when comparing the two intervention periods (HCM vs. LCM) (Table 6), there was a significant difference in the intake of fat between the two periods with a mean difference of 9.9 g.

The difference in fat intake between the two intervention diets might have been due to misunderstandings. One participant thought that she was supposed to put butter on every piece of bread in the LCM intervention and some participants used recipes for wok (also in the LCM intervention) in which they did not use light coconut milk as prescribed, but used regular coconut milk instead.

4. Discussion

4.1. Glycemic Variability and Glycemic Control

This study showed that a HCM diet (with a high carbohydrate intake in the morning) gave a higher MAGE and CV%, indicating a higher glycemic variability, when comparing with a LCM diet (with a low carbohydrate intake in the morning and a higher carbohydrate intake in the evening). On the other hand, the HCM diet seemed to lower mean glycemia compared to LCM-diet; MG was significantly lower in the HCM-diet and likewise was FBG. Similar findings have to our knowledge not been shown before. However, Jakubowicz et al. reported that morning carbohydrate intake compared to low carbohydrate intake lowered postprandial hyperglycemia in non-pregnant type 2 diabetic patients [18]. Though, comparison of results between the two studies are complicated, because our study evaluated treatment effect over a period, whereas Jakubowicz evaluated a single meal response, our results of glycemic control expressed as MG and FBG, seem to be in accordance with the results of Jakubowicz; a high carbohydrate intake in the morning seems beneficial. The results of glycemic variability are on the other hand not in accordance with the study by Jakubowicz as these parameters seem to be in favor of the LCM-diet in our study.

Large variations in blood glucose levels may cause more complications than constantly elevated glucose levels in patients with type 1 diabetes and type 2 diabetes [10]. Limited evidence are available for the consequence of high glycemic variability in pregnancies complicated by gestational diabetes [25]. It is evident that hyperglycemia, one characteristic of higher variability, is a strong predictor of adverse pregnancy outcomes, especially LGA [7]. However, in a new study from 2018 in GDM patients, glycemic variability in the third trimester was not a predictor of fetal birthweight and had no significant association to adverse pregnancy outcomes [27]. In the present study all participants had a stable glucose values defined as CV <36% [28], why one could argue that the difference in glycemic variability between the diets only have a small impact. We also found a mean difference of 0.7 mmol/L for MAGE, and it is debatable if this has any clinical relevance. In addition, TIR was highest on the LCM diet compared to HCM diet, primarily due to a decrease in TBR supporting the LCM diet as most favorable. In an ATTD consensus report from 2019 on clinical CGM targets of the metrics TIR, TBR and TAR, consensus was reached on glycemic cut point: Target range 3.5–7.8 mmol/L in pregnancy along with a target for time pr. day of 70% in late gestation (>34 weeks). No significant differences were observed in TIR between groups and despite diet the average TIR was above the recommended 70%. Whether glycemic control or variability is the best measurement to predict complications in diabetic pregnancies is also debatable, but ongoing studies will contribute to a clarification.

4.2. Carbohydrate Content of the Two Diets

In this crossover study, it can be argued that the LCM-diet is comparable to standard care at Department of Obstetrics and Gynecology at Aarhus University Hospital, as the carbohydrate content of the LCM-diet was approximate similar to the 30 g of carbohydrate usually recommended in standard care. In this way, the study contributes with new knowledge that contradicts the recommendations used in practice.

The study has a number of strengths and limitations. First, the crossover design made it possible to use within subject analyzes thus reducing the risk of potential confounders. The calorie-needs were individually calculated which can be seen as a strength as long as within-subject analyzes are used.

It is important that the total carbohydrate intake is the same during the two periods and this was the case in our study. According to the 24-h recall the total carbohydrate content did not differ significantly between the two interventions (Table 6). There was however a significant difference in the total intake of fat between the two groups. The higher intake of fat might have interfered with some of the outcomes, but because carbohydrate is the macronutrient with the highest impact on the blood glucose, we do not expect that this has affected the results noticeably.

Two be able to compare the two diets the breakfast meal of the HCM diet had the same carbohydrate content +/−2 E% as the dinner meal of the LCM diet. The dinner usually contains a higher carbohydrate load than breakfast. In the matter of transferring the results to clinical practice, this therefore needs to be taken into account. However, the participants in our study all reported satiety after dinner and some even had trouble finishing the whole meal even though most of the participants were energy reduced due to either BMI ≥25 or large weight gain at enrollment.

Clinical guidelines recommend a daily meal frequency of 3 main meals and 2–3 snack meals in between. This is advised in order to avoid high energy intake at main meals and distribute the carbohydrate intake over the day, and thereby decreasing the risk of postprandial hyperglycemia. Both diets in our study had a meal frequency of 5 meals pr. day. The HCM diet had a snack meal between breakfast and lunch, but no late evening snack and the LCM diet had no snack between breakfast and lunch, but a late evening snack.

4.3. CGM Data

Verification of CGM data was necessary to make sure that data on glycemic patterns was reliable and representative. No standard is currently available for CGM validation and performance, but the ATTD consensus recommendations are used as the best alternative [28].

The CGM system was calibrated based on measurements of SMBG with a personal glucometer (Accu-chek mobile). According to our analyzes the accuracy of the glucometer was within a range of +/−15% as advised by the ISO standard and ADA. Furthermore, the CGM IPro has been validated and used in pregnant women before [29,30].

Instructions were given to do pre-prandial SMBG four times a day. Not all participants managed to do all instructed measurements which weakens the calibration of the CGM system and implies a weakness in data reliability when dependent on compliance. The ATTD consensus report also recommends a minimum of 2 weeks to secure a sufficient data collection period. Our results were only based on data of 2 full days (2 × 24 h) of each intervention period. However, we did find significant differences on the parameters MAGE, CV%, FBG and MG between the two diets. The differences might have been even greater if we had a larger data set.

Another limitation of this study is the small sample size. However, the power was fulfilled, and it would be unethical to include more patients, and despite a small dataset, we were able to detect significant differences on several parameters between the two diets.

5. Conclusions

In conclusion, a diet with a high carbohydrate intake in the morning seem to result in a higher glycemic variability, but a lower MG and FBG, when comparing with a diet with a low carbohydrate intake in the morning and a higher carbohydrate intake in the evening. In addition, insulin resistance expressed as HOMA-IR decreased significantly during the HCM diet, indicating that a carbohydrate distribution of 50% in the morning favors lower blood glucose and improvement in insulin sensitivity in women with GDM.

Further research may clarify the impact of carbohydrate distribution on the complex matter of blood sugar regulation, and the use of CGM data to quantify glycemic variability, glucose control and their interactions.

Author Contributions: C.W.P., L.R., M.L.C., P.G.O., J.R.A and U.K. conceived and designed the experiments; L.R. and M.L.C. performed the experiments; L.R. and M.L.C analyzed the data in collaboration with a biostatistician as well as A.S.C. and C.R.; L.R. and M.L.C. wrote the paper. All authors read and approved the final manuscript.

Acknowledgments: We would like to thank all participants of the study, who were willing to give their time and effort to the intervention. We are also very grateful to the staff at Department of Obstetrics and Gynecology, Aarhus University Hospital for their support in field facilitation and data collection. Finally, we would like to thank University of Copenhagen for education of the investigators.

References

1. Sonagra, A.D.; Biradar, S.M.; Dattatreya, K.; Murthy, D.S.J. Normal pregnancy- a state of insulin resistance. *J. Clin. Diagn. Res.* **2014**, *8*, C01–C03. [CrossRef]
2. Wendland, E.M.; Torloni, M.R.; Falavigna, M.; Trujillo, J.; Dode, M.A.; Campos, M.A.; Duncan, B.B.; Schmidt, M.I. Gestational diabetes and pregnancy outcomes–a systematic review of the World Health Organization (WHO) and the International Association of Diabetes in Pregnancy Study Groups (IADPSG) diagnostic criteria. *BMC Pregnancy Childbirth* **2012**, *12*, 23. [CrossRef]
3. Ulla Kampmann, S.K.; Jens, F.; Per, O. Determinants of Maternal Insulin Resistance during Pregnancy: An Updated Overview. *J. Diabetes Res.* **2019**, *2019*, 9. [CrossRef] [PubMed]
4. Ovesen, P.G.; Fuglsang, J.; Andersen, M.B.; Wolff, C.; Petersen, O.B.; David McIntyre, H. Temporal trends in gestational diabetes prevalence, treatment, and outcomes at Aarhus university hospital, skejby, between 2004 and 2016. *J. Diabetes Res.* **2018**, *2018*, 5937059. [CrossRef] [PubMed]
5. McIntyre, H.D.; Catalano, P.; Zhang, C.; Desoye, G.; Mathiesen, E.R.; Damm, P. Gestational diabetes mellitus. *Nat. Rev. Dis. Primers* **2019**, *5*, 47. [CrossRef] [PubMed]
6. Mathiesen, E.R.; Vaz, J.A. Insulin treatment in diabetic pregnancy. *Diabetes/Metab. Res. Rev.* **2008**, *24*, S3–S20. [CrossRef]
7. Dalfra, M.G.; Sartore, G.; Di Cianni, G.; Mello, G.; Lencioni, C.; Ottanelli, S.; Sposato, J.; Valgimigli, F.; Scuffi, C.; Scalese, M.; et al. Glucose variability in diabetic pregnancy. *Diabetes Technol. Ther.* **2011**, *13*, 853–859. [CrossRef] [PubMed]
8. Zawiejska, A.; Wender-Ozegowska, E.; Radzicka, S.; Brazert, J. Maternal hyperglycemia according to IADPSG criteria as a predictor of perinatal complications in women with gestational diabetes: A retrospective observational study. *J. Matern. Fetal. Neonatal Med.* **2014**, *27*, 1526–1530. [CrossRef]
9. Kampmann, U.; Madsen, L.R.; Skajaa, G.O.; Iversen, D.S.; Moeller, N.; Ovesen, P. Gestational diabetes: A clinical update. *World J. Diabetes* **2015**, *6*, 1065–1072. [CrossRef]
10. Ceriello, A.; Ihnat, M.A. 'Glycaemic variability': A new therapeutic challenge in diabetes and the critical care setting. *Diabet. Med. J. Br. Diabet. Assoc.* **2010**, *27*, 862–867. [CrossRef]
11. Herranz, L.; Pallardo, L.F.; Hillman, N.; Martin-Vaquero, P.; Villarroel, A.; Fernandez, A. Maternal third trimester hyperglycaemic excursions predict large-for-gestational-age infants in type 1 diabetic pregnancy. *Diabetes Res. Clin. Pract.* **2007**, *75*, 42–46. [CrossRef] [PubMed]
12. Kestila, K.K.; Ekblad, U.U.; Ronnemaa, T. Continuous glucose monitoring versus self-monitoring of blood glucose in the treatment of gestational diabetes mellitus. *Diabetes Res. Clin. Pract.* **2007**, *77*, 174–179. [CrossRef]
13. Su, J.B.; Wang, X.Q.; Chen, J.F.; Wu, G.; Jin, Y.; Xu, F.; Wang, X.H.; Liu, Y.T. Glycemic variability in gestational diabetes mellitus and its association with beta cell function. *Endocrine* **2013**, *43*, 370–375. [CrossRef] [PubMed]
14. Moreno-Castilla, C.; Mauricio, D.; Hernandez, M. Role of Medical Nutrition Therapy in the Management of Gestational Diabetes Mellitus. *Curr. Diabetes Rep.* **2016**, *16*, 22. [CrossRef] [PubMed]
15. Peterson, C.M.; Jovanovic-Peterson, L. Percentage of carbohydrate and glycemic response to breakfast, lunch, and dinner in women with gestational diabetes. *Diabetes* **1991**, *40*, 172–174. [CrossRef] [PubMed]
16. Gunderson, E.P. Gestational diabetes and nutritional recommendations. *Curr. Diabetes Rep.* **2004**, *4*, 377–386. [CrossRef]
17. Ovesen, P.; Damm, P.; Renault, K.; Holm, A.M.; Wolff, C.; Knold, B.; Jensen, B.P.; Møller, M.; Svare, J.; Bødker, B.; et al. *Sandbjerg 2007–GUIDELINE*; Behandling af gestationel diabetes mellitus; DSOG (Danish Society of Obstetrics and Gynecology): Middelfart, Denmark, 2007.
18. Jakubowicz, D.; Wainstein, J.; Ahren, B.; Bar-Dayan, Y.; Landau, Z.; Rabinovitz, H.R.; Froy, O. High-energy breakfast with low-energy dinner decreases overall daily hyperglycaemia in type 2 diabetic patients: A randomised clinical trial. *Diabetologia* **2015**, *58*, 912–919. [CrossRef]

19. 1Tamas, G.; Kerenyi, Z. Gestational diabetes: Current aspects on pathogenesis and treatment. *Exp. Clin. Endocrinol. Diabetes* **2001**, *109*, S400–S411. [CrossRef]
20. Read, K.; LaPolla, F.W.Z. A new hat for librarians: providing REDCap support to establish the library as a central data hub. *J. Med. Libr. Assoc.* **2018**, *106*, 120–126. [CrossRef]
21. WHO. Diagnostic criteria and classification of hyperglycaemia first detected in pregnancy: A World Health Organization Guideline. *Diabetes Res. Clin. Pract.* **2014**, *103*, 341–363. [CrossRef]
22. Henry, C.J. Basal metabolic rate studies in humans: Measurement and development of new equations. *Public Health Nutr.* **2005**, *8*, 1133–1152. [CrossRef]
23. Ann, L.Y.; Kathleen, M.; Rasmussen; National Research Council; Institute of Medicine; Board on Children; Youth, F.; Committee to Reexamine IOM Pregnancy Weight Guidelines. *Weight Gain During Pregnancy: Reexamining the Guidelines (2009)*; Rasmussen, K.M., Yaktine, A.L., Eds.; The National Academies Press: Washington, DC, USA, 2009.
24. Oxford, U.o. HOMA2 CALCULATOR. Available online: https://www.dtu.ox.ac.uk/homacalculator/download.php (accessed on 18 August 2019).
25. Dalfra, M.G.; Chilelli, N.C.; Di Cianni, G.; Mello, G.; Lencioni, C.; Biagioni, S.; Scalese, M.; Sartore, G.; Lapolla, A. Glucose Fluctuations during Gestation: An Additional Tool for Monitoring Pregnancy Complicated by Diabetes. *Int. J. Endocrinol.* **2013**, *2013*, 279021. [CrossRef]
26. Yu, X.; Lin, L.; Shen, J.; Chen, Z.; Jian, J.; Li, B.; Xin, S.X. Calculating the Mean Amplitude of Glycemic Excursions from Continuous Glucose Data Using an Open-Code Programmable Algorithm Based on the Integer Nonlinear Method. *Comput. Math. Methods Med.* **2018**, *2018*, 6286893. [CrossRef] [PubMed]
27. Panyakat, W.S.; Phatihattakorn, C.; Sriwijitkamol, A.; Sunsaneevithayakul, P.; Phaophan, A.; Phichitkanka, A. Correlation Between Third Trimester Glycemic Variability in Non-Insulin-Dependent Gestational Diabetes Mellitus and Adverse Pregnancy and Fetal Outcomes. *J. Diabetes Sci. Technol.* **2018**, *12*, 622–629. [CrossRef] [PubMed]
28. Danne, T.; Nimri, R.; Battelino, T.; Bergenstal, R.M.; Close, K.L.; DeVries, J.H.; Garg, S.; Heinemann, L.; Hirsch, I.; Amiel, S.A.; et al. International Consensus on Use of Continuous Glucose Monitoring. *Diabetes Care* **2017**, *40*, 1631–1640. [CrossRef] [PubMed]
29. Kerssen, A.; de Valk, H.W.; Visser, G.H. The Continuous Glucose Monitoring System during pregnancy of women with type 1 diabetes mellitus: Accuracy assessment. *Diabetes Technol. Ther.* **2004**, *6*, 645–651. [CrossRef] [PubMed]
30. Kerssen, A.; De Valk, H.W.; Visser, G.H. Validation of the Continuous Glucose Monitoring System (CGMS) by the use of two CGMS simultaneously in pregnant women with type 1 diabetes mellitus. *Diabetes Technol. Ther.* **2005**, *7*, 699–706. [CrossRef] [PubMed]

10

Bisphenol A and Phthalates in Diet: An Emerging Link with Pregnancy Complications

Tiziana Filardi, Francesca Panimolle, Andrea Lenzi and Susanna Morano *

Department of Experimental Medicine, "Sapienza" University, Viale del Policlinico 155, 00161 Rome, Italy; tiziana.filardi@uniroma1.it (T.F.); francesca.panimolle@uniroma1.it (F.P.); andrea.lenzi@uniroma1.it (A.L.)
* Correspondence: susanna.morano@uniroma1.it

Abstract: Endocrine-disrupting chemicals (EDCs) are exogenous substances that are able to interfere with hormone action, likely contributing to the development of several endocrine and metabolic diseases. Among them, Bisphenol A (BPA) and phthalates contaminate food and water and have been largely studied as obesogenic agents. They might contribute to weight gain, insulin resistance and pancreatic β-cell dysfunction in pregnancy, potentially playing a role in the development of pregnancy complications, such as gestational diabetes mellitus (GDM), and adverse outcomes. Pregnancy and childhood are sensitive windows of susceptibility, and, although with not univocal results, preclinical and clinical studies have suggested that exposure to BPA and phthalates at these stages of life might have an impact on the development of metabolic diseases even many years later. The molecular mechanisms underlying this association are largely unknown, but adipocyte and pancreatic β-cell dysfunction are suspected to be involved. Remarkably, transgenerational damage has been observed, which might be explained by epigenetic changes. Further research is needed to address knowledge gaps and to provide preventive measure to limit health risks connected with exposure to EDCs.

Keywords: gestational diabetes; diet; endocrine disruptors; endocrine-disrupting chemicals; pregnancy; bisphenol A; BPA; phthalates; pregnancy outcomes

1. Introduction

The prevalence of obesity and metabolic diseases has been increasing over the last decades, and a complex interaction between multiple environmental and genetic factors might explain this trend [1]. Remarkably, there is mounting evidence that several metabolic adult-onset conditions, such as metabolic syndrome, type 2 diabetes (T2D) and cardiovascular diseases (CVD), might take roots in a hostile intrauterine environment related to an unfavourable maternal diet or lifestyle [2].

Diabetes occurring in the second or third trimester of pregnancy is known as gestational diabetes mellitus (GDM) [3]. Over the last decades, the prevalence of this condition has dramatically grown, along with the epidemic spread of obesity [4]. Overall, the prevalence of GDM is largely influenced by ethnicity, ranging between 12.9% and 5.8%, and by the diagnostic criteria applied [5]. High body mass index (BMI) has a considerable impact on the risk of developing GDM, as well as first degree family history of T2D and advanced maternal age [6,7]. GDM contributes to adverse gestational outcomes, such as the increased rates of preterm delivery and caesarean section [8]. The most common neonatal complications include dystocia, neonatal hypoglycaemia, jaundice and acute respiratory distress syndrome [8,9]. Besides the recognized short-term consequences, there is rising concern about the negative consequences observed several years later, such as the high risk of T2D occurrence [10,11]. It is estimated that, in European countries, the cumulative incidence of T2D in mothers previously affected by GDM ranges from 2.1% to 35.7% in a follow-up time of 5.5 months–15 years [5]. There is consistent evidence in longitudinal studies that previous GDM is linked with an increased risk of obesity, metabolic syndrome and T2D, not only in mothers but also in offspring [12–14]. Furthermore, children of mothers previously affected by GDM exhibit increased rates of CVD in adulthood, even of early onset [15,16].

Interestingly, a suboptimal milieu in utero, especially in the context of a particular window of susceptibility, might contribute to the development of pathological conditions, even with a long latency. For instance, in pregnancy complicated by GDM, foetal hyperglycaemia and hyperinsulinemia might influence vascular gene expression, resulting in endothelial dysfunction and contributing to the increased CVD risk in offspring [17]. In addition to the possible role played by endogenous factors, in recent years, increasing attention has been focused on the suspected contribution of environmental chemicals exposure in the development of metabolic and endocrine conditions, specifically during pregnancy [2]. According to the World Health Organization (WHO) definition, an endocrine disruptor (ED) is "an exogenous substance or mixture that alters function(s) of the endocrine system and consequently causes adverse health effects in an intact organism, or its progeny, or (sub) populations" [18]. Humans and animals come constantly into contact with endocrine-disrupting chemicals (EDCs), which are thought to interfere with hormone action at different stages. To date, plenty of substances are suspected to have a negative impact on human health, although only a few have been extensively evaluated in proper studies. Over the last decades, an association between EDCs and the development of metabolic diseases has emerged, and there is rising concern about the risk of adverse health outcomes, which might be largely underestimated.

2. Endocrine Disruptors in Diet

EDCs are ubiquitous and extensively pollute food and water. Industrial processes of food production allow them to unintentionally enter the food chain and to accumulate in wildlife and in humans. Almost 800 chemicals are suspected to interfere with endocrine functions and, among them, bisphenol A (BPA) and phthalates have been broadly studied as "obesogenic" factors [18].

BPA is a chemical compound obtained from a reaction of condensation between phenol and acetone. It is considered the first synthetic estrogen, although without a steroid structure, as it does not include the phenanthrene nucleus [19]. Due to its property of acting as a linker between chemicals, BPA is adopted by the chemical industry to produce plastic polymers.

Phthalates are diesters of phthalic acid classified into high and low molecular weight phthalates. The first category includes several compounds that are largely adopted to make plastic more flexible and durable. Among them, the most commonly employed additive is di(2-ethylhexyl) phthalate (DEHP). Low molecular weight phthalates are mainly used in personal care products and cosmetics, but they are also widespread in insecticides and in food packaging plastic [20]. In particular, diethyl phthalate (DEP) is one of the major phthalates in commerce [20]. BPA and phthalates are therefore widely diffused, due to the considerable volume of plastic production [21]. Basically, plastic materials for food storage, such as bottles and containers, are the main source of these chemicals. Although released even at room temperature, cooling and heating considerably facilitate the leaching of chemicals from containers, resulting in the contamination of food and beverages [22,23]. Another major source of BPA is the inner layer of cans (made of epoxy resins). As a result, products stored in cans and plastic casings have the highest concentrations of BPA independently of the specific nutrient category. Fish, vegetables and dairy products which are not packed in plastic containers or cans have therefore low concentrations of BPA and phthalates [24–26]. Conversely, ready-to-eat food stored in plastic bags is a major exposure source [27]. After ingestion, BPA is partially metabolized by the intestinal microbiota and largely absorbed in the intestinal tract [28]. BPA is transformed in the liver mainly by glucuronidation and, to a lesser extent, by sulfation, being eventually eliminated by the kidney [29]. Thus, BPA-glucuronide is the main metabolite of BPA in humans. As for phthalates, exposure to DEHP is reflected by the presence of its metabolites in urine, such as mono(2-ethylhexyl) phthalate (MEHP), mono(2-ethyl-5-hydroxyhexyl) phthalate, mono(2-ethyl-5-carboxypentyl) phthalate and mono(2-ethyl-5-oxohexyl) phthalate. Whereas the main urinary metabolite of DEP is mono-ethyl phthalate (MEP). Remarkably, the bioactivity of phthalate metabolites is superior to that of the original substance [29].

Since BPA does not accumulate in fat, a reduction in the intake of food stored in plastic materials and the adoption of BPA-free plastic containers considerably limit exposure [30,31]. In contrast, high molecular weight phthalates are more lipophilic and accumulate in fat food. Indeed, high concentrations of DEHP and BPA in dairy, meat and fast food products, such as hamburgers, have been reported [32,33]. Valvi et al. observed an inverse association between consumption of organic food and phthalate urinary levels in pregnant women [34]. Although evidence from clinical studies is still limited, a short course diet excluding food in plastic or cans was able to produce a significant drop in the urinary levels of BPA and DEHP [35].

BPA and phthalate concentrations have been evaluated in different biologic fluids at various stages of life. In the general population, urinary levels of BPA are reported to be on average 1.63 ng/mL in men and 1.12 ng/mL in women, whereas in serum BPA concentrations range between 0.3–4.4 ng/mL [36]. As regards phthalates, levels in urine vary among different countries, ranging from 1 to 100 μg/L [20]. Differences between ethnic groups might be explained by genetic polymorphisms in enzymes involved in biotransformation processes [37]. Overall, phthalate metabolites, mainly DEHP and DEP, have considerably lower concentrations in serum than in urine [38].

Pregnancy and childhood are particularly sensitive windows of susceptibility to chemicals, and exposure is potentially more harmful. Given the reduced ability to metabolize and eliminate BPA compared to adults, foetuses and children have considerably high levels of BPA in blood and urine [39,40]. A widespread exposure to EDCs has been consistently reported in pregnancy. Phthalate metabolites have been found in urine of about 98–100% of pregnant women [41,42]. In a sample of 378 pregnant women, at least 93% exhibited detectable concentrations of eight phthalate metabolites in urine between 18 and 22 weeks [43]. A positive association between phthalate concentrations and BMI in pregnancy has been reported in several studies [34,44–48], and higher phthalate levels in urine were observed in African American pregnant women compared to Caucasian [43,49,50]. In pregnant women, MEP is the predominant phthalate metabolite in urine, reaching a median concentration of 30 μg/L in most studies. Interestingly, maternal education and income were inversely related with phthalates levels, suggesting that sociocultural and lifestyle patterns might significantly influence exposure [34,43]. Data on urinary concentrations of phthalates in newborns are controversial. While some authors reported similar levels to those in the mothers [51], others observed two- or three times lower concentrations in offspring [52]. As for children, higher levels of urinary phthalates compared to adults have been found [53].

Many EDCs, such as high molecular weight phthalates and, to a lesser extent, low molecular weight phthalates, are quite lipophilic and are stored in adipose tissue [54]. Remarkably, almost all EDCs are able to cross the placenta, reaching the cord blood and the amniotic fluid [55,56]. They are also transferred from mother to child with lactation [57]. BPA in foetal circulation and amniotic fluid is almost 1–3 ng/mL, although in the latter, changes have been observed throughout pregnancy, averaging 8.3 ng/mL in the second trimester and then dropping to almost 1.1 ng/mL at the end of gestation [40]. In breastmilk, an average BPA concentration of 0.61 ng/mL has been reported [58]. As regards phthalates, amniotic fluid and breastmilk showed similar concentrations, generally far lower than those observed in urine and in serum [59].

3. General Aspects of EDCs

Endocrine functions are disrupted by EDCs through several complex mechanisms which are still not completely understood. Nuclear receptors (NR) are targeted by most of these substances, as well as steroid synthesis and metabolism [60,61]. NRs are located in the cytoplasm or nucleus in a monomeric state. The interaction with endogenous or exogenous ligands induces the translocation in the nucleus, the dimerization and the activation of gene transcription [62].

Several EDCs, including BPA and phthalate metabolites, are able to bind to estrogen receptors α (ERα) and β (ERβ). These receptors regulate the growth and the differentiation of many tissues, such as the female reproductive tract and the mammary gland [63].

Androgens intervene in the differentiation of male foetuses. EDCs, mainly pesticides but also bisphenols, have displayed anti-androgenic activities, interfering with the function of the androgen receptor (AR) [64].

Notably, the "obesogenic" effect attributed to EDCs has been linked to the activity of peroxisome proliferator-activated receptors (PPARs), which are crucially involved in lipid and glucose metabolism and energy homeostasis. Specifically, PPARγ are highly expressed in adipose tissue, and MEHP-induced activation of these receptors stimulates adipogenesis in vitro and in vivo [65,66]. The PPARα is principally expressed in the liver and in brown adipose tissue, and it is a target of MEHP as well [67].

EDCs disrupt thyroid hormone signalling, mainly acting as antagonists of thyroid receptors α (TRα) and β (TRβ), resulting in hypothyroidism and alterations of brain development [68].

The biotransformation of exogenous substances in the liver is regulated by the pregnane X receptor (PXR) and the constitutive androstane receptor (CAR). PXR induces the transcription of genes coding for cytochrome P450 and other enzymes involved in the clearance of xenobiotic substances. Notably, CAR regulates also lipid metabolism by eliminating cholesterol in the small intestine [69]. The activation of PXR and CAR pathways therefore protects the endocrine systems against EDCs. However, several substances, including bisphenols, are able to disrupt their activity, causing adverse effects [64]. Similarly, the aryl hydrocarbon receptor (AhR) exerts protective functions by sensing the presence of xenobiotic compounds and leading to the activation of cytochrome P450 enzymes. Interestingly, AhR can influence adipogenesis by altering PPARγ expression, and some "obesogenic" EDCs act specifically by disrupting this pathway [70].

Retinoid X receptors (RXR) are targeted by EDCs as well. These receptors are able to heterodimerize with other partners, such as PPARs, PXR, CAR, RARs and TRs. Thus, a multitude of adverse responses can be triggered by the exogenous ligand of RXRs, affecting human health [71].

Generally, the interaction between hormones and their receptors is not linear but sigmoidal [72,73]. When receptors are downregulated by high concentration of ligands, a U-shaped dose-response curve, implying high responses at low and high concentrations, or an inverted U-shaped curve, showing a stronger effect at medium doses, are frequently observed as well [72]. Despite their agonist and antagonist actions, EDCs are potentially able to modulate almost every aspect of hormone metabolism. Notably, the effects of EDCs exerted at low doses can be quite different from those induced by high doses, and it is fairly difficult to define a clear cut-off above which damage occurs. As EDCs can act at extremely low concentrations, their negative effects in real settings is often caused by a chronic low-dose exposure [74,75]. The U.S. Environmental Protection Agency (EPA) established for BPA a reference dose, or safe dose (i.e., the highest acceptable oral dose of a toxic substance), of 50 μg/kg/day, based on a "lowest observed adverse effect level" (LOAEL) of 50 mg/kg/day, whereas a "no observed adverse effect level" (NOAEL) has not emerged from toxicological studies [76]. As regards DEHP, the reference dose is 20 μg/kg/day, based on a LOAEL of 29 mg/kg/day, whereas the NOAEL is 5.8 mg/kg/day [20]. The estimated range exposure in humans is 0.4–5.0 μg/kg/day for BPA and 0.5–25.0 μg/kg/day for DEHP [76].

Another critical aspect of EDCs' actions is that their impact on health might not be immediately evident. In light of this, early contact with a substance might lead to long-term damage. Accordingly, most adult diseases that are suspected of being related to EDCs might be a result of intrauterine life exposure. EDCs are able to modulate gene expression and directly modify the epigenome by DNA methylation [77,78]. Notably, epigenetic modifications can be transmitted throughout generations, and the transgenerational effects might become manifest only several years later [79,80].

Although it is broadly accepted that chemicals interfering with hormone pathways are therefore able to cause adverse outcomes, in the evaluation of the risks connected to exposure, other factors should be considered, such as dose and duration of exposure [73]. Additionally, the specific period of the life cycle in which exposure occurs is crucial for the prediction of adverse outcomes. An extremely sensitive window is the time between conception and birth, when critical cellular processes (such as replication and differentiation) and organ development take place [81].

Interestingly, gender differences have consistently emerged in several studies, suggesting that similar conditions of exposure to an EDC may lead to different clinical manifestations which might be explained by several factors, such as the different expression of receptors or enzymes in EDCs target tissues and organs between male and female sexes [82].

4. Effects of Gestational Exposure to BPA and Phthalates

Exposure to BPA and phthalates during sensitive windows such as pregnancy can lead to metabolic dysfunction in the mother and interfere with foetal development. The disrupting effect might result in long-term consequences, both in the mother and in the offspring (Figure 1).

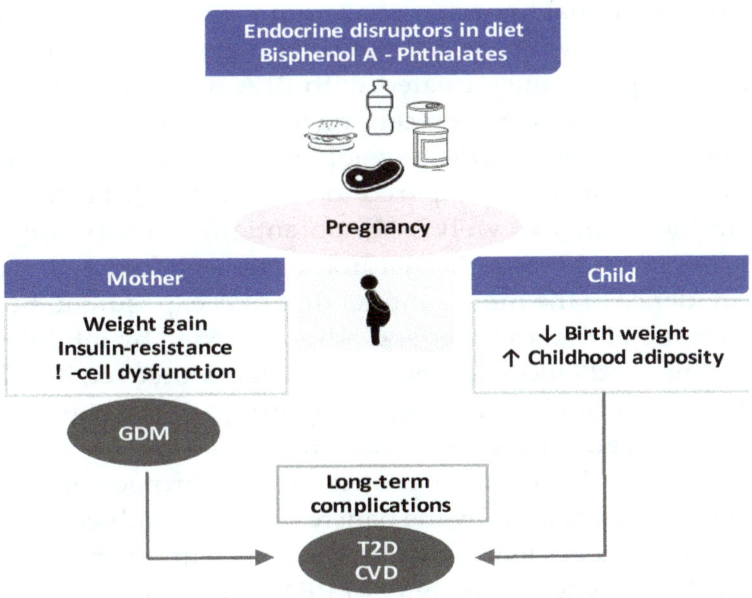

Figure 1. Endocrine disruptors in diet and pregnancy outcomes. GDM: gestational diabetes mellitus, T2D: type 2 diabetes and CVD: cardiovascular disease.

4.1. Impact on the Mother and Risk of GDM

It is well-known that both adipose tissue and gestational tissues (such as the placenta) release a wide number of molecules that promote insulin resistance [83]. As a result, a progressive fall in insulin sensitivity is observed until the second trimester, even in healthy pregnancies. Nevertheless, the increase in insulin secretion by pancreatic β-cell prevents the development of GDM. GDM therefore occurs when the compensatory effect of the pancreatic β-cell is insufficient [84]. Furthermore, a low-grade pro-inflammatory state [85–87] has been described even in physiological pregnancy, and it was found to be enhanced in GDM, possibly contributing to the development of insulin resistance and adverse pregnancy outcomes [88–90].

BPA and phthalates seem to target several pathophysiological features of GDM, potentially playing a role in the pathogenesis of GDM. Indeed, they have been linked to weight gain, insulin resistance and pancreatic β-cell dysfunction.

Gestational weight gain is a well-known risk factor for GDM [5]. In the Lifecodes cohort study, which enrolled 350 pregnant women, mean levels of maternal urinary MEP throughout pregnancy were positively associated with weight gain. Accordingly, the risk of impaired glucose tolerance (IGT) increased with high levels of this phthalate metabolite at the second trimester [91,92].

More recently, Shaffer et al. found that high mean levels (average concentration between first and third trimesters) of maternal urinary MEP significantly increased the odds of IGT and GDM [93]. Similarly, BPA urinary levels at the second trimester of pregnancy were positively associated with post-load glycaemia levels [94]. However, other cohort studies did not confirm the association between EDCs exposure and IGT, showing contrasting results for both BPA [95–99] and phthalates [97]. A possible reason for these controversial outcomes lies in the confounding effect of adiposity. Indeed, in a further analysis of the Lifecodes cohort study, Bellavia et al. investigated the association between first and second trimester BPA urinary levels and post-load glycaemia both in the overall sample and stratifying by BMI categories. Remarkably, although not any significant relationship emerged when considering the full sample, in the overweight/obese subgroup, higher concentrations of BPA at both trimesters were significantly associated with high post-load glycaemia [100].

Besides hyperglycaemia, in a prospective study, phthalate exposure in a low-risk cohort of pregnant women has been linked to increased diastolic blood pressure within 20 weeks of gestation and to the development of gestational hypertension and pre-eclampsia in late pregnancy [101].

Long-term adverse outcomes have been observed in mothers with BPA-associated insulin resistance in pregnancy. Specifically, pregnant mice treated with BPA had significantly higher body weights four months after delivery than control mice receiving vehicle [102]. Furthermore, the same authors reported that pregnant mice exposed to BPA developed insulin resistance and glucose intolerance later, along with significant weight gain, compared to controls [103]. Phthalates have been linked to long-term weight gain in the mother as well [104], potentially contributing to the development of metabolic diseases, such as T2D and metabolic syndrome, the well-known long-term complications of GDM [12,105]. There is evidence in the mouse model that BPA exposure in pregnancy targets insulin signalling pathways in peripheral tissues (liver and adipose tissue) by inhibiting the phosphorylation of Akt, therefore inducing impaired glucose homeostasis [102]. Moreover, BPA has a 17-β estradiol-like (E2) effect, as it is able to bind both ERα and ERβ, activating several signalling pathways. Notably, estrogen receptors are widespread throughout different tissues and are known to play a role in the regulation of glucose homeostasis [106]. In the mouse model, chronic administration of both E2 and BPA increased insulin synthesis and release by the pancreatic β-cell, inducing chronic hyperinsulinemia. Chronic hyperinsulinemia eventually led to insulin resistance in this model [107,108]. There is also evidence indicating that BPA increases the activity of PPARγ in adipocytes [109,110].

EDCs target the pancreatic β-cell as well [111]. Given that GDM occurs when the compensative effect of the pancreatic β-cell fails, the interference of EDCs might contribute to the development of hyperglycaemia. Furthermore, inflammation and oxidative stress are thought to be involved in the pathogenesis of insulin resistance in pregnancy. A positive correlation between BPA, inflammation and oxidative stress markers (IL-6, 8-isoprostane and 8-hydroxydeoxyguanosine) was also observed in pregnant women in early pregnancy [112].

4.2. Impact on Offspring: Short-Term and Long-Term Outcomes

Low birth weight is a well-known risk factor for obesity and T2D [113]. Interestingly, EDCs are reported to affect foetal growth and the length of pregnancy in cohort studies. In a study involving 482 pregnancies, levels of maternal urinary DEHP metabolites were inversely associated with foetal growth parameters (femur length, head circumference and weight) [114]. Other authors found that phthalate exposure at the third trimester of gestation was positively linked to the risk of preterm birth as well [115]. Several studies have investigated the relationship between BPA exposure and pregnancy outcomes, with controversial results. Indeed, in the prospective Upstate KIDS study, BPA levels in the blood of 6171 infants after delivery were negatively associated with the length of pregnancy, birth weight and head circumference [116]. Veiga-Lopez et al. observed similar results only regarding birth weight, although gender differences emerged. Indeed, the negative correlation between maternal urinary BPA at the first trimester and birth weight was stronger in pregnancies with a female foetus. Conversely, a significant increase in the lengths of the pregnancies was observed, although more marked when the foetus was a female [117]. In another cohort study, increased BPA concentrations in maternal and cord blood were predictive of a higher risk of low birth weights in male foetuses [118]. However, in a recent meta-analysis of eight studies, no significant correlation emerged between BPA exposure and birth weight [119].

Overall, in a large meta-analysis of 13 European cohort studies enrolling 133,957 pregnancies, exposure to EDCs was associated with a significant increase in the risk of low birth weight [120].

The molecular mechanisms underlying the possible association between exposure to EDCs during pregnancy and reduced foetal growth are not completely uncovered. The disrupting effect of phthalates is suspected to target placental TR. In mice exposed to the phthalate metabolite DEHP, placental levels of TR mRNA were found to be reduced in small for gestational age progeny [121]. Similarly, the expression of several factors involved in the regulation of placental angiogenesis, such as vascular endothelial growth factor, placental growth factor, insulin-like growth factor-1 and insulin-like growth factor-2, was reduced. In parallel, a lower number of micro-vessels emerged histologically in placentas [121]. Other mechanisms, such as the alteration of patterns of placental micro-RNA expression, DNA methylation and gene imprinting in the placenta, might be involved [82]. Interestingly, it has been observed that phthalates interfere with the expression of multiple genes, including epidermal growth factor, in the placenta at the first trimester by altering DNA methylation [78].

Besides short-term pregnancy outcomes, several cohort studies have focused on the effects of prenatal and early life exposure to EDCs on childhood adiposity. As regards BPA, the main findings are controversial. The Maternal-Infant Research on Environmental Chemicals (MIREC) study enrolled 719 mother-child pairs, and urinary levels of BPA were determined in mothers at 12 weeks of gestation. Anthropometric parameters were obtained at 3.5 years in children, and a positive association between BPA concentration and waist-to-hip ratio was observed [122]. In the RHEA cohort study, relevant sex differences emerged, since maternal BPA in urine was inversely related to BMI in females and positively in males at 4 years of age, whereas increasing postnatal levels of urinary BPA in progeny were significantly predictive of higher BMI, waist circumference and skinfold thickness (an indicator of central adiposity) in both genders [123]. Harley et al. observed that BPA concentration in maternal urine associated inversely with fat mass and BMI only in girls of 9 years of age, whilst urinary BPA measured at 9 years of age correlated positively with BMI, waist circumference and fat mass at the same determination time both in females and in males [124]. The specific time of exposure might therefore explain the different effects of a substance in the same population. However, in other cohort studies, no association between both prenatal and early life levels of BPA and childhood adiposity emerged [122,125]. In the Eden Mother-Child Cohort study, 520 mothers and children (of male sex only) were recruited and followed up for 5 years. Phthalate metabolites during pregnancy were positively linked to BMI at 5 years and to weight increase from 2 to 5 years of age in children [126].

The effect of multiple substances has been evaluated as well in a Spanish cohort study of 470 mother-child pairs with a 7-year follow-up, and phthalate exposure during pregnancy was a negative predictor of overweightness at 7 years of age [127].

Overall, although the results from cohort studies are not univocal, exposure to EDCs during pregnancy or early in life might have obesogenic properties, possibly playing a role in the development of metabolic diseases many years later. It is recognized that adipocyte dysfunction and inflammation contribute to the development of T2D and GDM [128,129]. Preclinical studies have investigated the action of EDCs on adipocytes. Indeed, adipocyte hypertrophy occurred in the progeny of rats that received BPA during pregnancy, along with a rise in the expression of pro-adipogenic factors. Proliferation of pre-adipocyte induced by BPA has been described in vitro as well [109,110,130]. In cultures of 3T3-L1 pre-adipocytes, the expression of PPARγ was enhanced by BPA, and lipid content in mature cells increased. In parallel, reduced insulin sensitivity and the enhanced expression of both leptin and the pro-inflammatory cytokine IL-6 were observed [110]. In a cohort study,

250 mother-offspring pairs were followed up until 8–14 years. A positive association was found between urinary phthalate metabolites measured in mothers during pregnancy and circulating leptin levels in females and an inverse association with insulin secretion in males at puberty [131]. In the MIREC study, high BPA urinary levels measured at the first trimester of pregnancy were predictive of low adiponectin in cord blood at birth, although only in male foetuses. Furthermore, a significant association between the metabolite of DEHP mono-(3-carboxypropyl)-phthalate and increased circulating leptin levels were observed in males [132].

Studies in animal models have reported that BPA exposure during pregnancy leads to the same metabolic alterations induced by high fat diets in offspring later in life, such as hyperglycaemia, IGT and high levels of non-esterified fatty acids [133,134]. This effect might be explained not only by the disruption of adipocyte function but also by the induction of β-cell dysfunction. Indeed, in male offspring of pregnant mice, β-cell inflammation, mitochondrial dysfunction and β-cell death were observed after exposure to BPA, and the damage persisted even in the next generation. Interestingly, gene expression in the β-cell was modified by altering DNA methylation [135].

5. Conclusions

It is well-established that an unfavourable maternal diet can lead to poor pregnancy outcomes. EDCs are broadly diffused in food, and the risks connected with exposure are suspected to be largely uncovered. Overall, there is evidence that BPA and phthalates are able to affect pregnancy and early life, influencing foetal growth and childhood adiposity. Their disrupting effect is likely to have long-term and transgenerational consequences in the field of metabolic diseases occurrences. Further research is mandatory to clarify the real impact of these substances on the risk of developing GDM and, importantly, to assess whether the limitation of exposure through the adoption of appropriate preventive measures might effectively reduce the incidence of this condition.

The synergistic effect deriving from exposure to multiple substances at the same time is a key aspect as well. Providing that EDCs are ubiquitous, the interactions between different EDCs and the overall effect should also be considered in real settings, rather than focusing on the actions of a single substance.

Remarkably, several studies have reported sex-specific findings, and more research should also clarify the mechanisms behind gender differences in pregnancy outcomes.

Finally, long-term follow-up studies are needed to further investigate the association between pregnancy exposure to EDCs and the risk of metabolic dysfunctions in adulthood.

Author Contributions: Conceptualization, S.M.; PubMed search, T.F. and F.P.; writing—draft preparation, T.F.; writing—review and editing, S.M.; and supervision and critical revision, A.L. All authors have read and agreed to the published version of the manuscript.

References

1. Gruss, S.M.; Nhim, K.; Gregg, E.; Bell, M.; Luman, E.; Albright, A. Public Health Approaches to Type 2 Diabetes Prevention: The US National Diabetes Prevention Program and Beyond. *Curr. Diabetes Rep.* **2019**, *19*, 78. [CrossRef] [PubMed]
2. Fernandez-Twinn, D.S.; Hjort, L.; Novakovic, B.; Ozanne, S.E.; Saffery, R. Intrauterine programming of obesity and type 2 diabetes. *Diabetologia* **2019**, *62*, 1789–1801. [CrossRef] [PubMed]
3. American Diabetes Association. 2. Classification and Diagnosis of Diabetes: Standards of Medical Care in Diabetes-2019. *Diabetes Care* **2019**, *42*, S13–S28. [CrossRef] [PubMed]
4. Casagrande, S.S.; Linder, B.; Cowie, C.C. Prevalence of gestational diabetes and subsequent Type 2 diabetes among U.S. women. *Diabetes Res. Clin. Pract.* **2018**, *141*, 200–208. [CrossRef] [PubMed]
5. Zhu, Y.; Zhang, C. Prevalence of Gestational Diabetes and Risk of Progression to Type 2 Diabetes: A Global Perspective. *Curr. Diabetes Rep.* **2016**, *16*, 7. [CrossRef] [PubMed]

6. Filardi, T.; Tavaglione, F.; Di Stasio, M.; Fazio, V.; Lenzi, A.; Morano, S. Impact of risk factors for gestational diabetes (GDM) on pregnancy outcomes in women with GDM. *J. Endocrinol. Investig.* **2018**, *41*, 671–676. [CrossRef] [PubMed]
7. Hedderson, M.; Ehrlich, S.; Sridhar, S.; Darbinian, J.; Moore, S.; Ferrara, A. Racial/ethnic disparities in the prevalence of gestational diabetes mellitus by BMI. *Diabetes Care* **2012**, *35*, 1492–1498. [CrossRef]
8. HAPO Study Cooperative Research Group; Metzger, B.E.; Lowe, L.P.; Dyer, A.R.; Trimble, E.R.; Chaovarindr, U.; Coustan, D.R.; Hadden, D.R.; McCance, D.R.; Hod, M.; et al. Hyperglycemia and adverse pregnancy outcomes. *N. Engl. J. Med.* **2008**, *358*, 1991–2002. [CrossRef]
9. Pintaudi, B.; Fresa, R.; Dalfra, M.; Dodesini, A.R.; Vitacolonna, E.; Tumminia, A.; Sciacca, L.; Lencioni, C.; Marcone, T.; Lucisano, G.; et al. The risk stratification of adverse neonatal outcomes in women with gestational diabetes (STRONG) study. *Acta Diabetol.* **2018**, *55*, 1261–1273. [CrossRef]
10. Damm, P.; Houshmand-Oeregaard, A.; Kelstrup, L.; Lauenborg, J.; Mathiesen, E.R.; Clausen, T.D. Gestational diabetes mellitus and long-term consequences for mother and offspring: A view from Denmark. *Diabetologia* **2016**, *59*, 1396–1399. [CrossRef]
11. Rayanagoudar, G.; Hashi, A.A.; Zamora, J.; Khan, K.S.; Hitman, G.A.; Thangaratinam, S. Quantification of the type 2 diabetes risk in women with gestational diabetes: A systematic review and meta-analysis of 95,750 women. *Diabetologia* **2016**, *59*, 1403–1411. [CrossRef]
12. Bellamy, L.; Casas, J.P.; Hingorani, A.D.; Williams, D. Type 2 diabetes mellitus after gestational diabetes: A systematic review and meta-analysis. *Lancet* **2009**, *373*, 1773–1779. [CrossRef]
13. Clausen, T.D.; Mathiesen, E.R.; Hansen, T.; Pedersen, O.; Jensen, D.M.; Lauenborg, J.; Damm, P. High prevalence of type 2 diabetes and pre-diabetes in adult offspring of women with gestational diabetes mellitus or type 1 diabetes: The role of intrauterine hyperglycemia. *Diabetes Care* **2008**, *31*, 340–346. [CrossRef] [PubMed]
14. Clausen, T.D.; Mathiesen, E.R.; Hansen, T.; Pedersen, O.; Jensen, D.M.; Lauenborg, J.; Schmidt, L.; Damm, P. Overweight and the metabolic syndrome in adult offspring of women with diet-treated gestational diabetes mellitus or type 1 diabetes. *J. Clin. Endocrinol. Metab.* **2009**, *94*, 2464–2470. [CrossRef] [PubMed]
15. Yu, Y.; Arah, O.A.; Liew, Z.; Cnattingius, S.; Olsen, J.; Sorensen, H.T.; Qin, G.; Li, J. Maternal diabetes during pregnancy and early onset of cardiovascular disease in offspring: Population based cohort study with 40 years of follow-up. *BMJ* **2019**, *367*, l6398. [CrossRef] [PubMed]
16. Marco, L.J.; McCloskey, K.; Vuillermin, P.J.; Burgner, D.; Said, J.; Ponsonby, A.L. Cardiovascular disease risk in the offspring of diabetic women: The impact of the intrauterine environment. *Exp. Diabetes Res.* **2012**, *2012*, 565160. [CrossRef] [PubMed]
17. Sallam, N.A.; Palmgren, V.A.C.; Singh, R.D.; John, C.M.; Thompson, J.A. Programming of Vascular Dysfunction in the Intrauterine Milieu of Diabetic Pregnancies. *Int. J. Mol. Sci.* **2018**, *19*, 3665. [CrossRef]
18. World Health Organization. Global Assessment of the State-of-the-Science of Endocrine Disruptors. Available online: https://www.who.int/ipcs/publications/new_issues/endocrine_disruptors/en/ (accessed on 20 January 2020).
19. Gramec Skledar, D.; Peterlin Masic, L. Bisphenol A and its analogs: Do their metabolites have endocrine activity? *Environ. Toxicol. Pharmacol.* **2016**, *47*, 182–199. [CrossRef]
20. Wang, Y.; Zhu, H.; Kannan, K. A Review of Biomonitoring of Phthalate Exposures. *Toxics* **2019**, *7*, 21. [CrossRef]
21. Frederiksen, H.; Jensen, T.K.; Jorgensen, N.; Kyhl, H.B.; Husby, S.; Skakkebaek, N.E.; Main, K.M.; Juul, A.; Andersson, A.M. Human urinary excretion of non-persistent environmental chemicals: An overview of Danish data collected between 2006 and 2012. *Reproduction* **2014**, *147*, 555–565. [CrossRef]
22. Li, C.; Xu, J.; Chen, D.; Xiao, Y. Detection of phthalates migration from disposable tablewares to drinking water using hexafluoroisopropanol-induced catanionic surfactant coacervate extraction. *J. Pharm. Anal.* **2016**, *6*, 292–299. [CrossRef]
23. Cooper, J.E.; Kendig, E.L.; Belcher, S.M. Assessment of bisphenol A released from reusable plastic, aluminium and stainless steel water bottles. *Chemosphere* **2011**, *85*, 943–947. [CrossRef] [PubMed]
24. Bradley, E.L.; Burden, R.A.; Bentayeb, K.; Driffield, M.; Harmer, N.; Mortimer, D.N.; Speck, D.R.; Ticha, J.; Castle, L. Exposure to phthalic acid, phthalate diesters and phthalate monoesters from foodstuffs: UK total diet study results. *Food Addit. Contam. Part A Chem. Anal. Control Expo. Risk Assess* **2013**, *30*, 735–742. [CrossRef] [PubMed]

25. Fierens, T.; Van Holderbeke, M.; Willems, H.; De Henauw, S.; Sioen, I. Transfer of eight phthalates through the milk chain—A case study. *Environ. Int.* **2013**, *51*, 1–7. [CrossRef] [PubMed]
26. Liao, C.; Kannan, K. Concentrations and profiles of bisphenol A and other bisphenol analogues in foodstuffs from the United States and their implications for human exposure. *J. Agric. Food Chem.* **2013**, *61*, 4655–4662. [CrossRef] [PubMed]
27. Pacyga, D.C.; Sathyanarayana, S.; Strakovsky, R.S. Dietary Predictors of Phthalate and Bisphenol Exposures in Pregnant Women. *Adv. Nutr.* **2019**, *10*, 803–815. [CrossRef]
28. Michalowicz, J. Bisphenol A—Sources, toxicity and biotransformation. *Environ. Toxicol. Pharmacol.* **2014**, *37*, 738–758. [CrossRef]
29. Zwierello, W.; Maruszewska, A.; Skorka-Majewicz, M.; Goschorska, M.; Baranowska-Bosiacka, I.; Dec, K.; Styburski, D.; Nowakowska, A.; Gutowska, I. The influence of polyphenols on metabolic disorders caused by compounds released from plastics—Review. *Chemosphere* **2020**, *240*, 124901. [CrossRef]
30. Martina, C.A.; Weiss, B.; Swan, S.H. Lifestyle behaviors associated with exposures to endocrine disruptors. *Neurotoxicology* **2012**, *33*, 1427–1433. [CrossRef]
31. Carwile, J.L.; Luu, H.T.; Bassett, L.S.; Driscoll, D.A.; Yuan, C.; Chang, J.Y.; Ye, X.; Calafat, A.M.; Michels, K.B. Polycarbonate bottle use and urinary bisphenol A concentrations. *Environ. Health Perspect.* **2009**, *117*, 1368–1372. [CrossRef]
32. Mercogliano, R.; Santonicola, S. Investigation on bisphenol A levels in human milk and dairy supply chain: A review. *Food Chem. Toxicol.* **2018**, *114*, 98–107. [CrossRef] [PubMed]
33. Zota, A.R.; Phillips, C.A.; Mitro, S.D. Recent Fast Food Consumption and Bisphenol A and Phthalates Exposures among the U.S. Population in NHANES, 2003–2010. *Environ. Health Perspect.* **2016**, *124*, 1521–1528. [CrossRef] [PubMed]
34. Valvi, D.; Monfort, N.; Ventura, R.; Casas, M.; Casas, L.; Sunyer, J.; Vrijheid, M. Variability and predictors of urinary phthalate metabolites in Spanish pregnant women. *Int. J. Hyg. Environ. Health* **2015**, *218*, 220–231. [CrossRef] [PubMed]
35. Rudel, R.A.; Gray, J.M.; Engel, C.L.; Rawsthorne, T.W.; Dodson, R.E.; Ackerman, J.M.; Rizzo, J.; Nudelman, J.L.; Brody, J.G. Food packaging and bisphenol A and bis(2-ethyhexyl) phthalate exposure: Findings from a dietary intervention. *Environ. Health Perspect.* **2011**, *119*, 914–920. [CrossRef]
36. Vandenberg, L.N.; Hauser, R.; Marcus, M.; Olea, N.; Welshons, W.V. Human exposure to bisphenol A (BPA). *Reprod. Toxicol.* **2007**, *24*, 139–177. [CrossRef]
37. McGraw, J.; Waller, D. Cytochrome P450 variations in different ethnic populations. *Expert Opin. Drug Metab. Toxicol.* **2012**, *8*, 371–382. [CrossRef]
38. Silva, M.J.; Barr, D.B.; Reidy, J.A.; Kato, K.; Malek, N.A.; Hodge, C.C.; Hurtz, D., 3rd; Calafat, A.M.; Needham, L.L.; Brock, J.W. Glucuronidation patterns of common urinary and serum monoester phthalate metabolites. *Arch. Toxicol.* **2003**, *77*, 561–567. [CrossRef]
39. Calafat, A.M.; Ye, X.; Wong, L.Y.; Reidy, J.A.; Needham, L.L. Exposure of the U.S. population to bisphenol A and 4-tertiary-octylphenol: 2003–2004. *Environ. Health Perspect.* **2008**, *116*, 39–44. [CrossRef]
40. Ikezuki, Y.; Tsutsumi, O.; Takai, Y.; Kamei, Y.; Taketani, Y. Determination of bisphenol A concentrations in human biological fluids reveals significant early prenatal exposure. *Hum. Reprod.* **2002**, *17*, 2839–2841. [CrossRef]
41. Cantonwine, D.E.; Meeker, J.D.; Ferguson, K.K.; Mukherjee, B.; Hauser, R.; McElrath, T.F. Urinary Concentrations of Bisphenol A and Phthalate Metabolites Measured during Pregnancy and Risk of Preeclampsia. *Environ. Health Perspect.* **2016**, *124*, 1651–1655. [CrossRef]
42. Woodruff, T.J.; Zota, A.R.; Schwartz, J.M. Environmental chemicals in pregnant women in the United States: NHANES 2003–2004. *Environ. Health Perspect.* **2011**, *119*, 878–885. [CrossRef] [PubMed]
43. Wenzel, A.G.; Brock, J.W.; Cruze, L.; Newman, R.B.; Unal, E.R.; Wolf, B.J.; Somerville, S.E.; Kucklick, J.R. Prevalence and predictors of phthalate exposure in pregnant women in Charleston, SC. *Chemosphere* **2018**, *193*, 394–402. [CrossRef] [PubMed]
44. Buser, M.C.; Murray, H.E.; Scinicariello, F. Age and sex differences in childhood and adulthood obesity association with phthalates: Analyses of NHANES 2007–2010. *Int. J. Hyg. Environ. Health* **2014**, *217*, 687–694. [CrossRef] [PubMed]

45. Peck, J.D.; Sweeney, A.M.; Symanski, E.; Gardiner, J.; Silva, M.J.; Calafat, A.M.; Schantz, S.L. Intra- and inter-individual variability of urinary phthalate metabolite concentrations in Hmong women of reproductive age. *J. Expo. Sci. Environ. Epidemiol.* **2010**, *20*, 90–100. [CrossRef] [PubMed]
46. Stahlhut, R.W.; van Wijngaarden, E.; Dye, T.D.; Cook, S.; Swan, S.H. Concentrations of urinary phthalate metabolites are associated with increased waist circumference and insulin resistance in adult U.S. males. *Environ. Health Perspect.* **2007**, *115*, 876–882. [CrossRef] [PubMed]
47. Yaghjyan, L.; Sites, S.; Ruan, Y.; Chang, S.H. Associations of urinary phthalates with body mass index, waist circumference and serum lipids among females: National Health and Nutrition Examination Survey 1999–2004. *Int. J. Obes.* **2015**, *39*, 994–1000. [CrossRef] [PubMed]
48. American Diabetes Association. Introduction: Standards of Medical Care in Diabetes-2019. *Diabetes Care* **2019**, *42*, S4–S6. [CrossRef]
49. Huang, T.; Saxena, A.R.; Isganaitis, E.; James-Todd, T. Gender and racial/ethnic differences in the associations of urinary phthalate metabolites with markers of diabetes risk: National Health and Nutrition Examination Survey 2001–2008. *Environ. Health* **2014**, *13*, 6. [CrossRef]
50. Kobrosly, R.W.; Parlett, L.E.; Stahlhut, R.W.; Barrett, E.S.; Swan, S.H. Socioeconomic factors and phthalate metabolite concentrations among United States women of reproductive age. *Environ. Res.* **2012**, *115*, 11–17. [CrossRef]
51. Cullen, E.; Evans, D.; Griffin, C.; Burke, P.; Mannion, R.; Burns, D.; Flanagan, A.; Kellegher, A.; Schoeters, G.; Govarts, E.; et al. Urinary Phthalate Concentrations in Mothers and Their Children in Ireland: Results of the DEMOCOPHES Human Biomonitoring Study. *Int. J. Environ. Res. Public Health* **2017**, *14*, 1456. [CrossRef]
52. Kim, J.H.; Park, H.; Lee, J.; Cho, G.; Choi, S.; Choi, G.; Kim, S.Y.; Eun, S.H.; Suh, E.; Kim, S.K.; et al. Association of diethylhexyl phthalate with obesity-related markers and body mass change from birth to 3 months of age. *J. Epidemiol. Community Health* **2016**, *70*, 466–472. [CrossRef] [PubMed]
53. CDC. NHANES. Fourth National Report on Human Exposure to Environmental Chemicals. Available online: https://www.cdc.gov/exposurereport/pdf/fourthreport.pdf (accessed on 14 February 2020).
54. Baldi, F.; Mantovani, A. A new database for food safety: EDID (Endocrine disrupting chemicals—Diet Interaction Database). *Annali dell'Istituto Superiore di Sanità* **2008**, *44*, 57–63. [CrossRef] [PubMed]
55. Chen, M.; Edlow, A.G.; Lin, T.; Smith, N.A.; McElrath, T.F.; Lu, C. Determination of bisphenol-A levels in human amniotic fluid samples by liquid chromatography coupled with mass spectrometry. *J. Sep. Sci.* **2011**, *34*, 1648–1655. [CrossRef] [PubMed]
56. Zbucka-Kretowska, M.; Lazarek, U.; Miltyk, W.; Sidorkiewicz, I.; Pierzynski, P.; Milewski, R.; Wolczynski, S.; Czerniecki, J. Simultaneous analysis of bisphenol A fractions in maternal and fetal compartments in early second trimester of pregnancy. *J. Perinat. Med.* **2019**, *47*, 765–770. [CrossRef]
57. Stefanidou, M.; Maravelias, C.; Spiliopoulou, C. Human exposure to endocrine disruptors and breast milk. *Endocr. Metab. Immune Disord. Drug Targets* **2009**, *9*, 269–276. [CrossRef]
58. Sun, Y.; Irie, M.; Kishikawa, N.; Wada, M.; Kuroda, N.; Nakashima, K. Determination of bisphenol A in human breast milk by HPLC with column-switching and fluorescence detection. *Biomed. Chromatogr.* **2004**, *18*, 501–507. [CrossRef]
59. Silva, M.J.; Reidy, J.A.; Herbert, A.R.; Preau, J.L., Jr.; Needham, L.L.; Calafat, A.M. Detection of phthalate metabolites in human amniotic fluid. *Bull. Environ. Contam. Toxicol.* **2004**, *72*, 1226–1231. [CrossRef]
60. Balaguer, P.; Delfosse, V.; Grimaldi, M.; Bourguet, W. Structural and functional evidences for the interactions between nuclear hormone receptors and endocrine disruptors at low doses. *C. R. Biol.* **2017**, *340*, 414–420. [CrossRef]
61. Rouiller-Fabre, V.; Guerquin, M.J.; N'Tumba-Byn, T.; Muczynski, V.; Moison, D.; Tourpin, S.; Messiaen, S.; Habert, R.; Livera, G. Nuclear receptors and endocrine disruptors in fetal and neonatal testes: A gapped landscape. *Front. Endocrinol.* **2015**, *6*, 58. [CrossRef]
62. Dahlman-Wright, K.; Cavailles, V.; Fuqua, S.A.; Jordan, V.C.; Katzenellenbogen, J.A.; Korach, K.S.; Maggi, A.; Muramatsu, M.; Parker, M.G.; Gustafsson, J.A. International Union of Pharmacology. LXIV. Estrogen receptors. *Pharmacol. Rev.* **2006**, *58*, 773–781. [CrossRef]
63. Couse, J.F.; Korach, K.S. Estrogen receptor null mice: What have we learned and where will they lead us? *Endocr. Rev.* **1999**, *20*, 358–417. [CrossRef] [PubMed]
64. Toporova, L.; Balaguer, P. Nuclear receptors are the major targets of endocrine disrupting chemicals. *Mol. Cell. Endocrinol.* **2019**, *502*, 110665. [CrossRef] [PubMed]

65. Chappell, V.A.; Janesick, A.; Blumberg, B.; Fenton, S.E. Tetrabromobisphenol-A Promotes Early Adipogenesis and Lipogenesis in 3T3-L1 Cells. *Toxicol. Sci.* **2018**, *166*, 332–344. [CrossRef] [PubMed]
66. Watt, J.; Schlezinger, J.J. Structurally-diverse, PPARgamma-activating environmental toxicants induce adipogenesis and suppress osteogenesis in bone marrow mesenchymal stromal cells. *Toxicology* **2015**, *331*, 66–77. [CrossRef] [PubMed]
67. Lapinskas, P.J.; Brown, S.; Leesnitzer, L.M.; Blanchard, S.; Swanson, C.; Cattley, R.C.; Corton, J.C. Role of PPARalpha in mediating the effects of phthalates and metabolites in the liver. *Toxicology* **2005**, *207*, 149–163. [CrossRef] [PubMed]
68. Fini, J.B.; Le Mevel, S.; Palmier, K.; Darras, V.M.; Punzon, I.; Richardson, S.J.; Clerget-Froidevaux, M.S.; Demeneix, B.A. Thyroid hormone signaling in the Xenopus laevis embryo is functional and susceptible to endocrine disruption. *Endocrinology* **2012**, *153*, 5068–5081. [CrossRef]
69. Kobayashi, K.; Hashimoto, M.; Honkakoski, P.; Negishi, M. Regulation of gene expression by CAR: An update. *Arch. Toxicol.* **2015**, *89*, 1045–1055. [CrossRef]
70. Darbre, P.D. Endocrine Disruptors and Obesity. *Curr. Obes. Rep.* **2017**, *6*, 18–27. [CrossRef]
71. le Maire, A.; Teyssier, C.; Balaguer, P.; Bourguet, W.; Germain, P. Regulation of RXR-RAR Heterodimers by RXR- and RAR-Specific Ligands and Their Combinations. *Cells* **2019**, *8*, 1392. [CrossRef]
72. Hill, C.E.; Myers, J.P.; Vandenberg, L.N. Nonmonotonic Dose-Response Curves Occur in Dose Ranges That Are Relevant to Regulatory Decision-Making. *Dose Response* **2018**, *16*, 1559325818798282. [CrossRef]
73. Zoeller, R.T.; Brown, T.R.; Doan, L.L.; Gore, A.C.; Skakkebaek, N.E.; Soto, A.M.; Woodruff, T.J.; Vom Saal, F.S. Endocrine-disrupting chemicals and public health protection: A statement of principles from The Endocrine Society. *Endocrinology* **2012**, *153*, 4097–4110. [CrossRef] [PubMed]
74. Barouki, R. Endocrine disruptors: Revisiting concepts and dogma in toxicology. *C. R. Biol.* **2017**, *340*, 410–413. [CrossRef] [PubMed]
75. Vandenberg, L.N.; Hunt, P.A.; Gore, A.C. Endocrine disruptors and the future of toxicology testing—Lessons from CLARITY-BPA. *Nat. Rev. Endocrinol.* **2019**, *15*, 366–374. [CrossRef] [PubMed]
76. Vandenberg, L.N.; Colborn, T.; Hayes, T.B.; Heindel, J.J.; Jacobs, D.R., Jr.; Lee, D.H.; Shioda, T.; Soto, A.M.; vom Saal, F.S.; Welshons, W.V.; et al. Hormones and endocrine-disrupting chemicals: Low-dose effects and nonmonotonic dose responses. *Endocr. Rev.* **2012**, *33*, 378–455. [CrossRef] [PubMed]
77. Marampon, F.; Megiorni, F.; Camero, S.; Crescioli, C.; McDowell, H.P.; Sferra, R.; Vetuschi, A.; Pompili, S.; Ventura, L.; De Felice, F.; et al. HDAC4 and HDAC6 sustain DNA double strand break repair and stem-like phenotype by promoting radioresistance in glioblastoma cells. *Cancer Lett.* **2017**, *397*, 1–11. [CrossRef] [PubMed]
78. Grindler, N.M.; Vanderlinden, L.; Karthikraj, R.; Kannan, K.; Teal, S.; Polotsky, A.J.; Powell, T.L.; Yang, I.V.; Jansson, T. Exposure to Phthalate, an Endocrine Disrupting Chemical, Alters the First Trimester Placental Methylome and Transcriptome in Women. *Sci. Rep.* **2018**, *8*, 6086. [CrossRef]
79. Franzago, M.; Fraticelli, F.; Stuppia, L.; Vitacolonna, E. Nutrigenetics, epigenetics and gestational diabetes: Consequences in mother and child. *Epigenetics* **2019**, *14*, 215–235. [CrossRef]
80. Hjort, L.; Novakovic, B.; Grunnet, L.G.; Maple-Brown, L.; Damm, P.; Desoye, G.; Saffery, R. Diabetes in pregnancy and epigenetic mechanisms-how the first 9 months from conception might affect the child's epigenome and later risk of disease. *Lancet Diabetes Endocrinol.* **2019**, *7*, 796–806. [CrossRef]
81. Nesan, D.; Sewell, L.C.; Kurrasch, D.M. Opening the black box of endocrine disruption of brain development: Lessons from the characterization of Bisphenol A. *Horm. Behav.* **2018**, *101*, 50–58. [CrossRef]
82. Strakovsky, R.S.; Schantz, S.L. Impacts of bisphenol A (BPA) and phthalate exposures on epigenetic outcomes in the human placenta. *Environ. Epigenet.* **2018**, *4*, dvy022. [CrossRef]
83. Baz, B.; Riveline, J.P.; Gautier, J.F. ENDOCRINOLOGY OF PREGNANCY: Gestational diabetes mellitus: Definition, aetiological and clinical aspects. *Eur. J. Endocrinol.* **2016**, *174*, R43–R51. [CrossRef] [PubMed]
84. Catalano, P.M.; Tyzbir, E.D.; Wolfe, R.R.; Calles, J.; Roman, N.M.; Amini, S.B.; Sims, E.A. Carbohydrate metabolism during pregnancy in control subjects and women with gestational diabetes. *Am. J. Physiol.* **1993**, *264*, E60–E67. [CrossRef] [PubMed]
85. Mor, G.; Cardenas, I.; Abrahams, V.; Guller, S. Inflammation and pregnancy: The role of the immune system at the implantation site. *Ann. N. Y. Acad. Sci.* **2011**, *1221*, 80–87. [CrossRef] [PubMed]

86. Lappas, M.; Permezel, M.; Rice, G.E. Leptin and adiponectin stimulate the release of proinflammatory cytokines and prostaglandins from human placenta and maternal adipose tissue via nuclear factor-kappaB, peroxisomal proliferator-activated receptor-gamma and extracellularly regulated kinase 1/2. *Endocrinology* **2005**, *146*, 3334–3342. [CrossRef] [PubMed]
87. Hauguel-de Mouzon, S.; Guerre-Millo, M. The placenta cytokine network and inflammatory signals. *Placenta* **2006**, *27*, 794–798. [CrossRef] [PubMed]
88. Santangelo, C.; Zicari, A.; Mandosi, E.; Scazzocchio, B.; Mari, E.; Morano, S.; Masella, R. Could gestational diabetes mellitus be managed through dietary bioactive compounds? Current knowledge and future perspectives. *Br. J. Nutr.* **2016**, *115*, 1129–1144. [CrossRef] [PubMed]
89. Lowe, L.P.; Metzger, B.E.; Lowe, W.L., Jr.; Dyer, A.R.; McDade, T.W.; McIntyre, H.D.; Group, H.S.C.R. Inflammatory mediators and glucose in pregnancy: Results from a subset of the Hyperglycemia and Adverse Pregnancy Outcome (HAPO) Study. *J. Clin. Endocrinol. Metab.* **2010**, *95*, 5427–5434. [CrossRef]
90. Lekva, T.; Norwitz, E.R.; Aukrust, P.; Ueland, T. Impact of Systemic Inflammation on the Progression of Gestational Diabetes Mellitus. *Curr. Diabetes Rep.* **2016**, *16*, 26. [CrossRef]
91. Bellavia, A.; Hauser, R.; Seely, E.W.; Meeker, J.D.; Ferguson, K.K.; McElrath, T.F.; James-Todd, T. Urinary phthalate metabolite concentrations and maternal weight during early pregnancy. *Int. J. Hyg. Environ. Health* **2017**, *220*, 1347–1355. [CrossRef]
92. James-Todd, T.M.; Meeker, J.D.; Huang, T.; Hauser, R.; Ferguson, K.K.; Rich-Edwards, J.W.; McElrath, T.F.; Seely, E.W. Pregnancy urinary phthalate metabolite concentrations and gestational diabetes risk factors. *Environ. Int.* **2016**, *96*, 118–126. [CrossRef]
93. Shaffer, R.M.; Ferguson, K.K.; Sheppard, L.; James-Todd, T.; Butts, S.; Chandrasekaran, S.; Swan, S.H.; Barrett, E.S.; Nguyen, R.; Bush, N.; et al. Maternal urinary phthalate metabolites in relation to gestational diabetes and glucose intolerance during pregnancy. *Environ. Int.* **2019**, *123*, 588–596. [CrossRef] [PubMed]
94. Chiu, Y.H.; Minguez-Alarcon, L.; Ford, J.B.; Keller, M.; Seely, E.W.; Messerlian, C.; Petrozza, J.; Williams, P.L.; Ye, X.; Calafat, A.M.; et al. Trimester-Specific Urinary Bisphenol A Concentrations and Blood Glucose Levels Among Pregnant Women From a Fertility Clinic. *J. Clin. Endocrinol. Metab.* **2017**, *102*, 1350–1357. [CrossRef] [PubMed]
95. Fisher, B.G.; Frederiksen, H.; Andersson, A.M.; Juul, A.; Thankamony, A.; Ong, K.K.; Dunger, D.B.; Hughes, I.A.; Acerini, C.L. Serum Phthalate and Triclosan Levels Have Opposing Associations With Risk Factors for Gestational Diabetes Mellitus. *Front. Endocrinol.* **2018**, *9*, 99. [CrossRef] [PubMed]
96. Robledo, C.; Peck, J.D.; Stoner, J.A.; Carabin, H.; Cowan, L.; Koch, H.M.; Goodman, J.R. Is Bisphenol-A exposure during pregnancy associated with blood glucose levels or diagnosis of gestational diabetes? *J. Toxicol. Environ. Health A* **2013**, *76*, 865–873. [CrossRef]
97. Shapiro, G.D.; Dodds, L.; Arbuckle, T.E.; Ashley-Martin, J.; Fraser, W.; Fisher, M.; Taback, S.; Keely, E.; Bouchard, M.F.; Monnier, P.; et al. Exposure to phthalates, bisphenol A and metals in pregnancy and the association with impaired glucose tolerance and gestational diabetes mellitus: The MIREC study. *Environ. Int.* **2015**, *83*, 63–71. [CrossRef]
98. Wang, X.; Wang, X.; Chen, Q.; Luo, Z.C.; Zhao, S.; Wang, W.; Zhang, H.J.; Zhang, J.; Ouyang, F. Urinary Bisphenol A Concentration and Gestational Diabetes Mellitus in Chinese Women. *Epidemiology* **2017**, *28* (Suppl. S1), S41–S47. [CrossRef]
99. Zhang, W.; Xia, W.; Liu, W.; Li, X.; Hu, J.; Zhang, B.; Xu, S.; Zhou, Y.; Li, J.; Cai, Z.; et al. Exposure to Bisphenol a Substitutes and Gestational Diabetes Mellitus: A Prospective Cohort Study in China. *Front. Endocrinol.* **2019**, *10*, 262. [CrossRef]
100. Bellavia, A.; Cantonwine, D.E.; Meeker, J.D.; Hauser, R.; Seely, E.W.; McElrath, T.F.; James-Todd, T. Pregnancy urinary bisphenol-A concentrations and glucose levels across BMI categories. *Environ. Int.* **2018**, *113*, 35–41. [CrossRef]
101. Werner, E.F.; Braun, J.M.; Yolton, K.; Khoury, J.C.; Lanphear, B.P. The association between maternal urinary phthalate concentrations and blood pressure in pregnancy: The HOME Study. *Environ. Health* **2015**, *14*, 75. [CrossRef]
102. Alonso-Magdalena, P.; Vieira, E.; Soriano, S.; Menes, L.; Burks, D.; Quesada, I.; Nadal, A. Bisphenol A exposure during pregnancy disrupts glucose homeostasis in mothers and adult male offspring. *Environ. Health Perspect.* **2010**, *118*, 1243–1250. [CrossRef]

103. Alonso-Magdalena, P.; Garcia-Arevalo, M.; Quesada, I.; Nadal, A. Bisphenol-A treatment during pregnancy in mice: A new window of susceptibility for the development of diabetes in mothers later in life. *Endocrinology* **2015**, *156*, 1659–1670. [CrossRef] [PubMed]
104. Rodriguez-Carmona, Y.; Cantoral, A.; Trejo-Valdivia, B.; Tellez-Rojo, M.M.; Svensson, K.; Peterson, K.E.; Meeker, J.D.; Schnaas, L.; Solano, M.; Watkins, D.J. Phthalate exposure during pregnancy and long-term weight gain in women. *Environ. Res.* **2019**, *169*, 26–32. [CrossRef] [PubMed]
105. Kelstrup, L.; Damm, P.; Mathiesen, E.R.; Hansen, T.; Vaag, A.A.; Pedersen, O.; Clausen, T.D. Insulin resistance and impaired pancreatic beta-cell function in adult offspring of women with diabetes in pregnancy. *J. Clin. Endocrinol. Metab.* **2013**, *98*, 3793–3801. [CrossRef] [PubMed]
106. Rettberg, J.R.; Yao, J.; Brinton, R.D. Estrogen: A master regulator of bioenergetic systems in the brain and body. *Front. Neuroendocrinol.* **2014**, *35*, 8–30. [CrossRef]
107. Alonso-Magdalena, P.; Ropero, A.B.; Carrera, M.P.; Cederroth, C.R.; Baquie, M.; Gauthier, B.R.; Nef, S.; Stefani, E.; Nadal, A. Pancreatic insulin content regulation by the estrogen receptor ER alpha. *PLoS ONE* **2008**, *3*, e2069. [CrossRef]
108. Alonso-Magdalena, P.; Morimoto, S.; Ripoll, C.; Fuentes, E.; Nadal, A. The estrogenic effect of bisphenol A disrupts pancreatic beta-cell function in vivo and induces insulin resistance. *Environ. Health Perspect.* **2006**, *114*, 106–112. [CrossRef]
109. Li, L.; Wang, Q.; Zhang, Y.; Niu, Y.; Yao, X.; Liu, H. The molecular mechanism of bisphenol A (BPA) as an endocrine disruptor by interacting with nuclear receptors: Insights from molecular dynamics (MD) simulations. *PLoS ONE* **2015**, *10*, e0120330. [CrossRef]
110. Ariemma, F.; D'Esposito, V.; Liguoro, D.; Oriente, F.; Cabaro, S.; Liotti, A.; Cimmino, I.; Longo, M.; Beguinot, F.; Formisano, P.; et al. Low-Dose Bisphenol-A Impairs Adipogenesis and Generates Dysfunctional 3T3-L1 Adipocytes. *PLoS ONE* **2016**, *11*, e0150762. [CrossRef]
111. Whitehead, R.; Guan, H.; Arany, E.; Cernea, M.; Yang, K. Prenatal exposure to bisphenol A alters mouse fetal pancreatic morphology and islet composition. *Horm. Mol. Biol. Clin. Investig.* **2016**, *25*, 171–179. [CrossRef]
112. Ferguson, K.K.; Cantonwine, D.E.; McElrath, T.F.; Mukherjee, B.; Meeker, J.D. Repeated measures analysis of associations between urinary bisphenol-A concentrations and biomarkers of inflammation and oxidative stress in pregnancy. *Reprod. Toxicol.* **2016**, *66*, 93–98. [CrossRef]
113. Zanetti, D.; Tikkanen, E.; Gustafsson, S.; Priest, J.R.; Burgess, S.; Ingelsson, E. Birthweight, Type 2 Diabetes Mellitus, and Cardiovascular Disease: Addressing the Barker Hypothesis with Mendelian Randomization. *Circ. Genom. Precis. Med.* **2018**, *11*, e002054. [CrossRef] [PubMed]
114. Ferguson, K.K.; Meeker, J.D.; Cantonwine, D.E.; Mukherjee, B.; Pace, G.G.; Weller, D.; McElrath, T.F. Environmental phenol associations with ultrasound and delivery measures of fetal growth. *Environ. Int.* **2018**, *112*, 243–250. [CrossRef] [PubMed]
115. Broe, A.; Pottegard, A.; Hallas, J.; Ahern, T.P.; Lamont, R.F.; Damkier, P. Phthalate exposure from drugs during pregnancy and possible risk of preterm birth and small for gestational age. *Eur. J. Obstet. Gynecol. Reprod. Biol.* **2019**, *240*, 293–299. [CrossRef] [PubMed]
116. Bell, E.M.; Yeung, E.H.; Ma, W.; Kannan, K.; Sundaram, R.; Smarr, M.M.; Buck Louis, G.M. Concentrations of endocrine disrupting chemicals in newborn blood spots and infant outcomes in the upstate KIDS study. *Environ. Int.* **2018**, *121*, 232–239. [CrossRef]
117. Veiga-Lopez, A.; Kannan, K.; Liao, C.; Ye, W.; Domino, S.E.; Padmanabhan, V. Gender-Specific Effects on Gestational Length and Birth Weight by Early Pregnancy BPA Exposure. *J. Clin. Endocrinol. Metab.* **2015**, *100*, E1394–E1403. [CrossRef]
118. Chou, W.C.; Chen, J.L.; Lin, C.F.; Chen, Y.C.; Shih, F.C.; Chuang, C.Y. Biomonitoring of bisphenol A concentrations in maternal and umbilical cord blood in regard to birth outcomes and adipokine expression: A birth cohort study in Taiwan. *Environ. Health* **2011**, *10*, 94. [CrossRef]
119. Hu, C.Y.; Li, F.L.; Hua, X.G.; Jiang, W.; Mao, C.; Zhang, X.J. The association between prenatal bisphenol A exposure and birth weight: A meta-analysis. *Reprod. Toxicol.* **2018**, *79*, 21–31. [CrossRef]
120. Birks, L.; Casas, M.; Garcia, A.M.; Alexander, J.; Barros, H.; Bergstrom, A.; Bonde, J.P.; Burdorf, A.; Costet, N.; Danileviciute, A.; et al. Occupational Exposure to Endocrine-Disrupting Chemicals and Birth Weight and Length of Gestation: A European Meta-Analysis. *Environ. Health Perspect.* **2016**, *124*, 1785–1793. [CrossRef]

121. Yu, Z.; Han, Y.; Shen, R.; Huang, K.; Xu, Y.Y.; Wang, Q.N.; Zhou, S.S.; Xu, D.X.; Tao, F.B. Gestational di-(2-ethylhexyl) phthalate exposure causes fetal intrauterine growth restriction through disturbing placental thyroid hormone receptor signaling. *Toxicol. Lett.* **2018**, *294*, 1–10. [CrossRef]
122. Braun, J.M.; Lanphear, B.P.; Calafat, A.M.; Deria, S.; Khoury, J.; Howe, C.J.; Venners, S.A. Early-life bisphenol a exposure and child body mass index: A prospective cohort study. *Environ. Health Perspect.* **2014**, *122*, 1239–1245. [CrossRef]
123. Vafeiadi, M.; Georgiou, V.; Chalkiadaki, G.; Rantakokko, P.; Kiviranta, H.; Karachaliou, M.; Fthenou, E.; Venihaki, M.; Sarri, K.; Vassilaki, M.; et al. Association of Prenatal Exposure to Persistent Organic Pollutants with Obesity and Cardiometabolic Traits in Early Childhood: The Rhea Mother-Child Cohort (Crete, Greece). *Environ. Health Perspect.* **2015**, *123*, 1015–1021. [CrossRef] [PubMed]
124. Harley, K.G.; Aguilar Schall, R.; Chevrier, J.; Tyler, K.; Aguirre, H.; Bradman, A.; Holland, N.T.; Lustig, R.H.; Calafat, A.M.; Eskenazi, B. Prenatal and postnatal bisphenol A exposure and body mass index in childhood in the CHAMACOS cohort. *Environ. Health Perspect.* **2013**, *121*, 514–520. [CrossRef] [PubMed]
125. Buckley, J.P.; Herring, A.H.; Wolff, M.S.; Calafat, A.M.; Engel, S.M. Prenatal exposure to environmental phenols and childhood fat mass in the Mount Sinai Children's Environmental Health Study. *Environ. Int.* **2016**, *91*, 350–356. [CrossRef] [PubMed]
126. Botton, J.; Philippat, C.; Calafat, A.M.; Carles, S.; Charles, M.A.; Slama, R.; The Eden Mother-Child Cohort Study Group. Phthalate pregnancy exposure and male offspring growth from the intra-uterine period to five years of age. *Environ. Res.* **2016**, *151*, 601–609. [CrossRef]
127. Agay-Shay, K.; Martinez, D.; Valvi, D.; Garcia-Esteban, R.; Basagana, X.; Robinson, O.; Casas, M.; Sunyer, J.; Vrijheid, M. Exposure to Endocrine-Disrupting Chemicals during Pregnancy and Weight at 7 Years of Age: A Multi-pollutant Approach. *Environ. Health Perspect.* **2015**, *123*, 1030–1037. [CrossRef]
128. Pantham, P.; Aye, I.L.; Powell, T.L. Inflammation in maternal obesity and gestational diabetes mellitus. *Placenta* **2015**, *36*, 709–715. [CrossRef]
129. Esser, N.; Legrand-Poels, S.; Piette, J.; Scheen, A.J.; Paquot, N. Inflammation as a link between obesity, metabolic syndrome and type 2 diabetes. *Diabetes Res. Clin. Pract.* **2014**, *105*, 141–150. [CrossRef]
130. Desai, M.; Ferrini, M.G.; Jellyman, J.K.; Han, G.; Ross, M.G. In vivo and in vitro bisphenol A exposure effects on adiposity. *J. Dev. Orig. Health Dis.* **2018**, *9*, 678–687. [CrossRef]
131. Watkins, D.J.; Peterson, K.E.; Ferguson, K.K.; Mercado-Garcia, A.; Tamayo y Ortiz, M.; Cantoral, A.; Meeker, J.D.; Tellez-Rojo, M.M. Relating Phthalate and BPA Exposure to Metabolism in Peripubescence: The Role of Exposure Timing, Sex, and Puberty. *J. Clin. Endocrinol. Metab.* **2016**, *101*, 79–88. [CrossRef]
132. Ashley-Martin, J.; Dodds, L.; Arbuckle, T.E.; Ettinger, A.S.; Shapiro, G.D.; Fisher, M.; Morisset, A.S.; Taback, S.; Bouchard, M.F.; Monnier, P.; et al. A birth cohort study to investigate the association between prenatal phthalate and bisphenol A exposures and fetal markers of metabolic dysfunction. *Environ. Health* **2014**, *13*, 84. [CrossRef]
133. Garcia-Arevalo, M.; Alonso-Magdalena, P.; Rebelo Dos Santos, J.; Quesada, I.; Carneiro, E.M.; Nadal, A. Exposure to bisphenol-A during pregnancy partially mimics the effects of a high-fat diet altering glucose homeostasis and gene expression in adult male mice. *PLoS ONE* **2014**, *9*, e100214. [CrossRef] [PubMed]
134. Wei, J.; Lin, Y.; Li, Y.; Ying, C.; Chen, J.; Song, L.; Zhou, Z.; Lv, Z.; Xia, W.; Chen, X.; et al. Perinatal exposure to bisphenol A at reference dose predisposes offspring to metabolic syndrome in adult rats on a high-fat diet. *Endocrinology* **2011**, *152*, 3049–3061. [CrossRef] [PubMed]
135. Bansal, A.; Rashid, C.; Xin, F.; Li, C.; Polyak, E.; Duemler, A.; van der Meer, T.; Stefaniak, M.; Wajid, S.; Doliba, N.; et al. Sex- and Dose-Specific Effects of Maternal Bisphenol A Exposure on Pancreatic Islets of First- and Second-Generation Adult Mice Offspring. *Environ. Health Perspect.* **2017**, *125*, 097022. [CrossRef] [PubMed]

11

Influence of GDM Diagnosis and Treatment on Weight Gain, Dietary Intake and Physical Activity in Pregnant Women with Obesity: Secondary Analysis of the UPBEAT Study

La'Shay Atakora [1], Lucilla Poston [2], Louise Hayes [3], Angela C. Flynn [2,†] and Sara L. White [2,4,†,*]

1 London School of Hygiene and Tropical Medicine, London WC1E 7HT, UK; lashay.yeboa-atakora1@alumni.lshtm.ac.uk
2 Department of Women and Children's Health, King's College London, London SE1 7EH, UK; lucilla.poston@kcl.ac.uk (L.P.); angela.flynn@kcl.ac.uk (A.C.F.)
3 Population Health Sciences Institute, Newcastle University, Newcastle upon Tyne NE2 4AX, UK; louise.hayes@newcastle.ac.uk
4 Guy's and St Thomas' NHS Foundation Trust, London SE1 7EH, UK
* Correspondence: sara.white@kcl.ac.uk
† These authors contributed equally to this work.

Abstract: Obesity during pregnancy is associated with the development of gestational diabetes (GDM). This study aimed to assess if the result of an oral glucose tolerance test (OGTT) for GDM influences health (diet and physical activity) behaviours of pregnant women with obesity. In total, 1031 women who participated in the UK Pregnancies Better Eating and Activity Trial (UPBEAT) of a lifestyle intervention from early pregnancy were included. Changes in weight gain, dietary intake and physical activity following an OGTT undertaken between 27^{+0} and 28^{+6} weeks' and 34 and 36 weeks' gestation were examined using linear regression with appropriate adjustment for confounders. Obese women without GDM (IADPSG criteria) gained 1.9 kg (95% CI −2.2, −1.5, $p < 0.001$) more weight than women with GDM. Women with GDM demonstrated greater reductions in energy (−142kcal, 95%CI −242.2, −41.9, $p = 0.006$), carbohydrate intake (−1.5%E 95%CI −2.8, −0.3, $p = 0.016$) and glycaemic load (−15.2, 95%CI −23.6, −6.7, $p < 0.001$) and a greater increase in protein intake (2%E, 95%CI 1.3, 2.7, $p < 0.001$), compared to women without GDM. Trial intervention allocation did not influence any associations observed. The findings emphasise the need for strategies to optimise the health behaviours of pregnant women with obesity, following a negative OGTT for GDM.

Keywords: obesity; pregnancy; gestational diabetes; diet; physical activity; gestational weight gain

1. Introduction

The recent increase in obesity in the UK population [1] is mirrored amongst women in antenatal care, with estimates suggesting that 23% have a BMI ≥ 30 kg/m^2 [2]. Obesity in pregnancy increases the risk of complications [3], most notably, gestational diabetes (GDM), defined by new-onset hyperglycaemia in pregnancy, which now affects up to 30% of pregnancies worldwide [4]. Obesity in pregnancy is related to a 4–9-fold greater risk of GDM compared to pregnant women with a normal weight [5]. The long-term morbidities associated with GDM include progression to type 2 diabetes in approximately 25% of affected mothers [6].

The UK national guidelines for the management of GDM following diagnosis include the provision of advice on diet and physical activity. For women who do not gain adequate glycaemic control through changes in these behaviours, pharmacotherapy with metformin or insulin is prescribed [7].

Whilst differences in diet and weight gain between women with and without a diagnosis of GDM have been reported [8–14], there is a paucity of longitudinal data that explores behaviour change and gestational weight gain following a negative or positive oral glucose tolerance test (OGTT) for the diagnosis and associated treatment of GDM. In a recent longitudinal study of 702 women living in Norway, minimal differences in dietary intake between those with and without GDM were observed, and the women with GDM gained more weight compared to those without GDM [15]. To our knowledge, no previous study has investigated these associations in pregnant women with obesity. Understanding the behavioural patterns of obese women with and without a diagnosis of GDM following testing might help identify suboptimal health behaviours and inform future strategies to improve the health of pregnant women with obesity and their offspring.

The aim of this study was to assess how a negative or positive OGTT for the diagnosis and subsequent treatment of GDM influences the dietary intake, physical activity levels and gestational weight gain of pregnant women with obesity who were participants in UPBEAT, a randomised controlled trial of a lifestyle (diet and physical activity) intervention. We also determined if allocation to the intervention or control arm influenced the association between GDM status and behaviour change. We wished to explore, for example, whether an individual who was randomised to the active arm who subsequently did not develop GDM may show continued adherence to a lifestyle intervention.

2. Materials and Methods

2.1. Study Design and Population

This study is a secondary analysis of data collected from women who participated in the UK Pregnancies Better Eating and Activity Trial (UPBEAT). UPBEAT was a multicentre randomised controlled trial which took place in the UK. UPBEAT assessed whether a behavioural intervention of diet and physical activity advice reduced the incidence of GDM and the delivery of large-for-gestational-age (LGA) infants in pregnant women with obesity [16]. The protocol and main findings of UPBEAT have been previously published [16,17]. In brief, women were eligible to take part if they were aged 16 years or above, had a singleton pregnancy between 15^{+0} and 18^{+6} weeks' gestation and had a body mass index (BMI) of 30 kg/m^2 or above. Women were excluded if they did not give informed consent, were prescribed metformin, or if they had any pre-existing medical conditions. For the purposes of this investigation, only women who had an OGTT were included. Ethical approval was granted by the NHS Research Ethics Committee (UK Integrated Research Application System, reference 09/H0802/5).

The UPBEAT intervention aimed to improve glucose tolerance through dietary and physical activity behaviour change. The participants randomised to the intervention group received eight weekly individual or group-based sessions, in addition to their standard antenatal care appointments. The dietary component of the intervention aimed to encourage a healthier eating pattern through a reduction in glycaemic load and saturated fat intake. To reduce glycaemic load, the participants were encouraged to swap high glycaemic index food and beverages for low glycaemic index alternatives and reduce the consumption of sugar-sweetened beverages including fruit juice. To reduce saturated fat intake, the participants were encouraged to use low fat dairy products and exchange fatty meats and meat products with leaner meat and fish. The physical activity component was tailored to participant preferences and focused on incremental increases in moderate intensity walking and being more active in daily life. Barriers to change were explored and specific, measurable, achievable, relevant, time-specific (SMART) goals were set for the women in the intervention arm. The participants randomised to the control arm were provided with antenatal care in line with local NHS guidelines [16]. We have previously reported that the intervention was not effective in reducing the prevalence of GDM or LGA infants, although several secondary outcomes including diet, weight gain and adiposity demonstrated evidence of improvement [17].

2.2. Data Collection

The maternal social and demographic data obtained at enrolment included age (years), BMI (kg/m^2), ethnicity (Black, White, Asian, other), parity (nulliparous, multiparous), smoking status (smoker, ex-smoker, non-smoker), living in a deprived area (Index of Multiple Deprivation (IMD); scores were calculated for the region of residence) and highest educational attainment. The data were obtained pre-intervention (15^{+0}–18^{+6} weeks' gestation), post-intervention (27^{+0}–28^{+6} weeks' gestation) and in late pregnancy (34–36 weeks' gestation) for diet and physical activity (questionnaires), weight and anthropometric measures.

A semi-quantitative food frequency questionnaire (FFQ) adapted from one used in the UK arm of the European Prospective Investigation into Cancer Study (EPIC) was used to assess the diet of the participants for the preceding month. Glycaemic load was estimated based on the glycaemic index and carbohydrate content of each food, as reported previously [18]. Physical activity was assessed using the International Physical Activity Questionnaire (IPAQ) [16].

The trial protocol required OGTTs to be carried out at 27^{+0}–28^{+6} weeks' gestation. However, a more pragmatic approach was adopted to reflect clinical practice, and women who had OGTTs at 23–30 weeks' gestation were included for the purposes of this analysis. GDM was diagnosed using International Association of Diabetes and Pregnancy Study Groups (IADPSG) criteria: fasting glucose of 5.1 mmol/L or higher, 1 h glucose of 10.0 mmol/L or higher, 2 h glucose of 8.5 mmol/L or higher, or a combination of these (venous blood; post 75 g glucose challenge) [19]. Women diagnosed with GDM were referred to the local antenatal diabetes service and managed according to local practice, with lifestyle dietary management, metformin or insulin treatment as appropriate.

2.3. Outcome Measures

Dietary outcomes included changes in total energy intake (kcal/day), glycaemic index, glycaemic load, carbohydrate (%E), protein (%E), total fat (%E), and saturated fat (%E) intake, from OGTT (27^{+0}—-28^{+6} weeks' gestation) to late pregnancy (34–36 weeks' gestation). Physical activity outcomes included change in moderate or vigorous activity (min/week) and walking (min/week), from OGTT (27^{+0}–28^{+6} weeks' gestation) to late pregnancy (34–36 weeks' gestation). Anthropometric outcomes included change in weight (kg) from OGTT (27^{+0}–28^{+6} weeks' gestation) to late pregnancy (34–36 weeks' gestation).

2.4. Statistical Analysis

The normality of the data was assessed using Shapiro–Wilk tests and visual representations including distributional diagnostic plots and histograms. Summary statistics were calculated for descriptive characteristics. Continuous variables were described as mean (standard deviation) or median (interquartile range). Categorical variables were described as number (percentage). Differences between characteristics at study entry were examined using chi-squared tests for categorical data, and independent sample t-tests for continuous data. The proportion of women who gained weight above or below the National Academy of Medicine (NAM) guidelines for pregnant women with obesity was determined using NAM guidance for weekly weight gain in the third trimester [20]. Univariate and multivariable linear regression were used to examine the association between GDM diagnosis and the change in each outcome variable between 27^{+0} and 28^{+6} weeks' gestation and 34 and 36 weeks' gestation. Models were adjusted for maternal BMI, ethnicity and neonatal sex. To identify whether intervention allocation was an effect modifier on the association between GDM status and each outcome, an interaction term was added to the linear regression analyses. Likelihood ratio tests were conducted to ascertain the statistical significance of the interaction.

Statistical analyses were performed using Stata version 16.0 (StataCorp LP, College Station, TX, USA).

3. Results

Between March 2009 and June 2014, 1555 women were randomised to either the behavioural intervention or standard antenatal care. The present investigation was limited to those participants who received OGTTs (n = 1031 participants, 66.3%) (Figure 1).

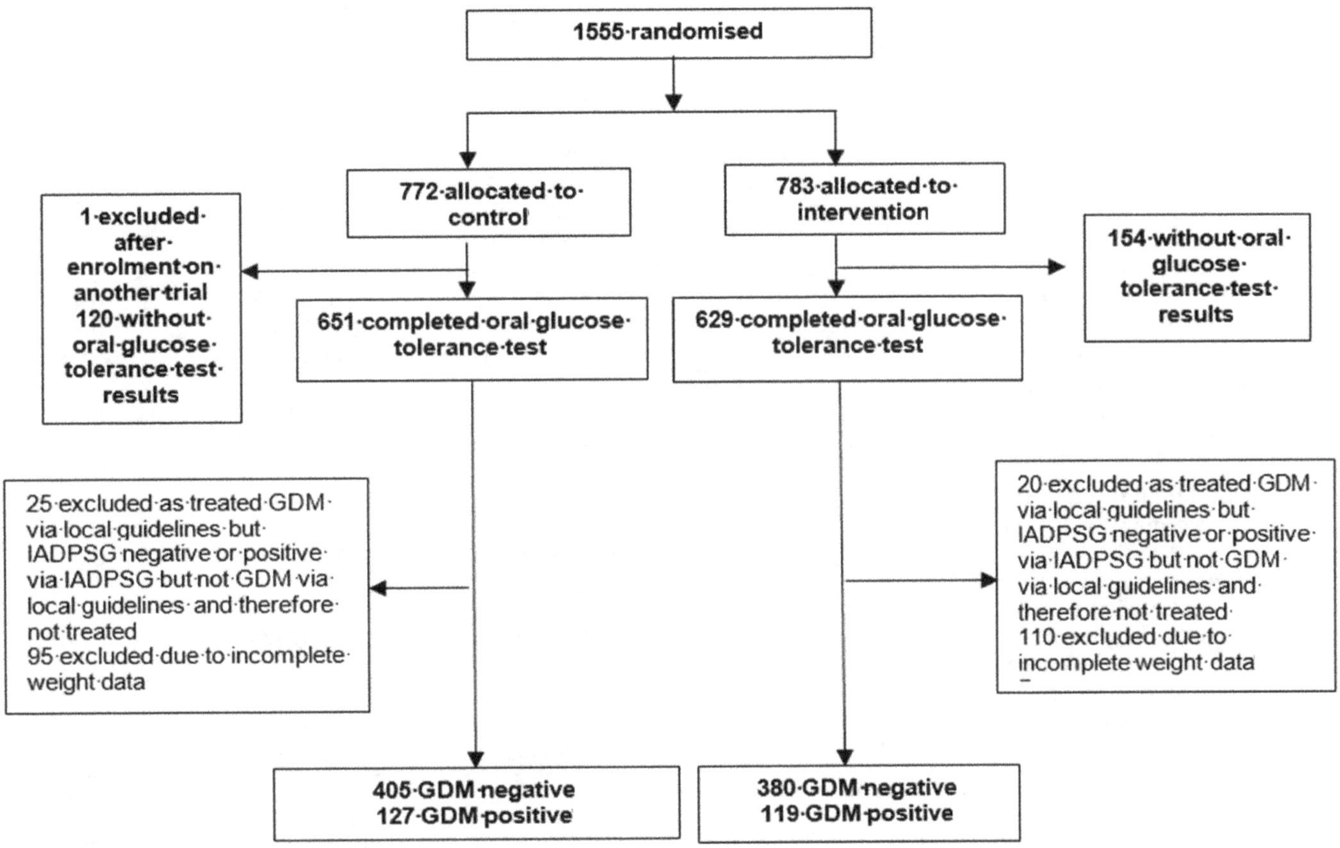

Figure 1. Study profile.

3.1. Study Population

The characteristics of the study population are shown in Table 1. Two hundred and forty-six participants (23.9%) were diagnosed with GDM by OGTT. The non-GDM women were younger at study entry, weighed less, and had a lower BMI than the GDM women (all $p < 0.05$). GDM women were more likely to have a history of GDM. The GDM and non-GDM women were similar in smoking status, ethnicity, parity, education level and IMD quintile. Infants born to GDM women were more likely to be large-for-gestational-age ($p < 0.05$).

Table 1. Characteristics at 15^{+0}–18^{+6} weeks' gestation of the study population who had an oral glucose tolerance test.

	Whole Group n = 1031 (%)	Non-GDM n = 785 (76.1%)	GDM [a] n = 246 (23.9%)	p [d]
Age (years)	30.9 (5.4)	30.4 (5.5)	32.3 (4.9)	<0.001
Ethnicity				
White	688/1031 (66.7)	532/785 (67.8)	156/246 (63.4)	
Black	231/1031 (22.4)	169/785 (21.5)	62/246 (25.2)	0.628
Asian	56/1031 (5.4)	42/785 (5.4)	14/246 (5.7)	
Other	56/1031 (5.4)	42/785 (5.4)	14/246 (5.7)	
Weight (kg)	98.0 (15.0)	97.4 (14.2)	99.9 (17.2)	0.024
BMI (kg/m^2)	35.4 (4.8)	35.2 (4.6)	36.0 (5.3)	0.025
Education [b]				
None or GCSE	202/1031 (19.6)	150/785 (19.1)	52/246 (21.1)	
Vocational qualification	243/1031 (23.6)	175/785 (22.3)	68/246 (27.6)	0.175
A-level (or equivalent)	164/1031 (15.9)	132/785 (16.8)	32/246 (13.0)	
First or higher degree	422/1031 (40.9)	328/785 (41.8)	94/246 (38.2)	
Index of multiple deprivation [c]				
1 (least deprived)	26/820 (3.2)	20/618 (3.2)	6/202 (3.0)	
2	40/820 (4.9)	32/618 (5.2)	8/202 (4.0)	
3	100/820 (12.2)	81/618 (13.1)	19/202 (9.4)	0.118
4	309/820 (37.7)	241/618 (39.0)	68/202 (33.7)	
5 (most deprived)	345/820 (42.1)	244/618 (39.5)	101/202 (50.0)	
Current smoker	62/1031 (6.0)	42/785 (5.4)	20/246 (8.1)	0.460
Multiparous	560/1031 (54.3)	417/785 (53.1)	143/246 (58.1)	0.169
Previous history of GDM	17/560 (3.0)	6/417 (1.4)	11/143 (7.7)	<0.001
Randomised group				
Intervention	499/1031(48.4)	380/785 (48.4)	119/246 (48.4)	0.993
Standard care	532/1031 (51.6)	405/785 (51.6)	127/246 (51.6)	
Neonatal characteristics				
Neonatal sex				
Male	534/1031 (51.8)	410/785 (52.2)	124/246 (50.4)	0.618
Gestational age at delivery (weeks)	39.8 (1.4)	40.1 (1.3)	38.9 (1.2)	<0.001
Birthweight (g)	3482 (493)	3509 (499)	3397 (463)	0.002
Customised birthweight centiles [e]				
≥90th (LGA)	85/1031 (8.2)	55/785 (7.0)	30/246 (12.2)	0.010
≤10th (SGA)	117/1031 (11.4)	95/785 (12.1)	22/246 (8.9)	0.173

Values are mean (standard deviation) or number (%); a GDM, Gestational Diabetes Mellitus; b GCSE, General Certificate of Secondary Education, A-level, General Certificate of Education Advanced level; c Index of multiple deprivation is a measure of relative deprivation. Scores calculated for region of residence by fifths of the population. UK-wide scores were developed from English and Scottish data relating to employment and income domains [17]; d P value comparing the difference between GDM and non-GDM women. Obtained through independent sample t-test for continuous variables and chi-squared for categorical variables; e Large-for-gestational-age (LGA) as >90th customised birthweight centile for gestational age, adjusted for maternal height and weight, ethnic origin, parity, and sex of the baby, and small-for-gestational-age (SGA) as ≤10th customised birthweight centile.

3.2. Gestational Weight Gain

The non-GDM women demonstrated greater total gestational weight gain compared to the GDM women (non-GDM: mean 8.0 kg (SD 4.3) vs. GDM: 5.8 kg (SD 4.5), $p < 0.001$). Following the OGTT at 27^{+0}–28^{+6} weeks' gestation, the change in weight by 34–36 weeks' gestation was greater in the non-GDM women (Table 2 and Figure 2). The non-GDM women gained 1.9 kg (95%CI −2.2, −1.5, $p < 0.001$) more than the GDM women, which was robust to adjustment for confounders (Supplementary Figure S1A). Amongst the non-GDM women, 60.3% ($n = 473$) gained weight above NAM recommendations for third trimester weight gain compared to 26.4% ($n = 65$) of the GDM women. Non-GDM women were also less likely to gain inadequate weight, with 0.6% ($n = 149$) gaining less weight than NAM recommendations, compared to 26.6% ($n = 206$) amongst the GDM women. Although underpowered, no differences in LGA or SGA were noted between the non-GDM women who gained within the NAM guidelines and those who gained above the NAM guidelines (Supplementary Tables S1 and S2).

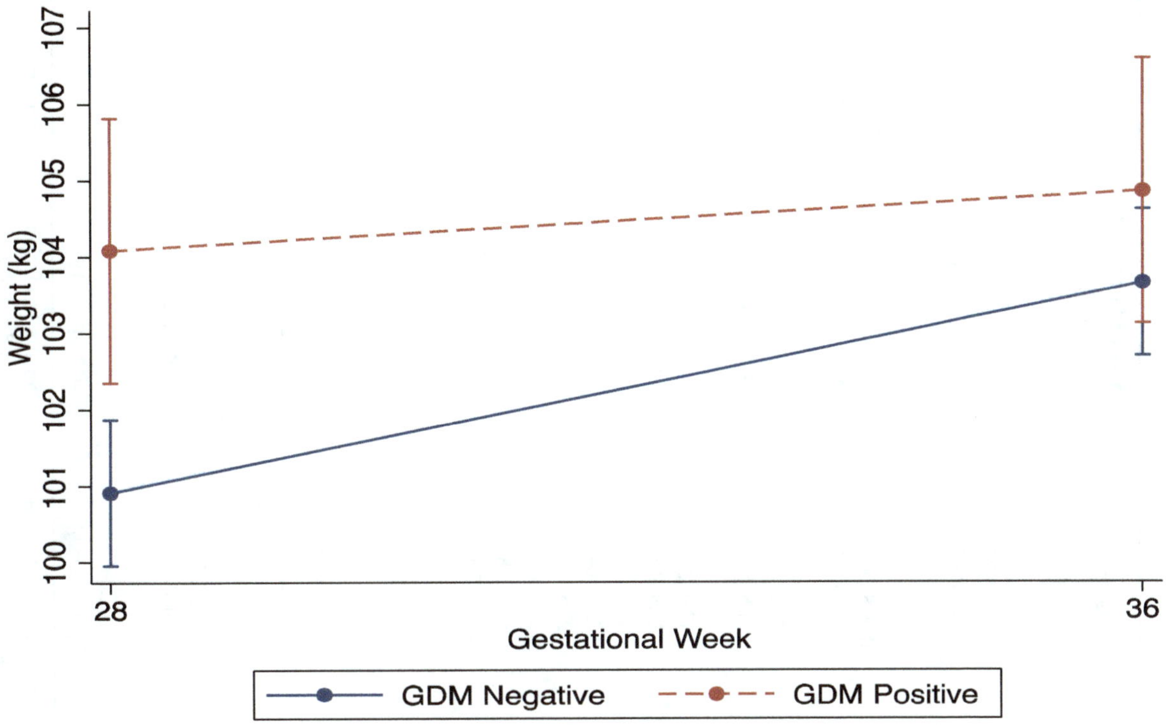

Figure 2. Unadjusted weight (kg) change of GDM and non-GDM women from 27^{+0}–28^{+6} weeks' gestation (28 weeks) to 34–36 weeks' gestation (36 weeks) with 95% confidence intervals.

Table 2. Weight gain, dietary intake and physical activity outcomes for the GDM and non-GDM women by gestational period, and unadjusted and adjusted linear regression models examining the association between GDM diagnosis and change in each outcome variable between 27+0–28+6 weeks' and 34–36 weeks' gestation.

Outcome	Non-GDM	GDM	Unadjusted Coefficient (95% CI)	p	Adjusted Coefficient (95% CI)	p
Weight gain						
Weight (kg)						
27^{+0}–28^{+6} weeks	101.4 (14.1)	103.6 (17.5)				
34–36 weeks	104.1 (14.3)	104.4 (18.0)	−2.0 (−2.3, −1.6)	<0.001	−1.9 (−2.2, −1.5)	<0.001
Dietary intake						
Energy intake (kcal)						
27^{+0}–28^{+6} weeks	1729.9 (527.6)	1809.8 (507.6)				
34–36 weeks	1721.8 (528.4)	1658.8 (499.2)	−142.9 (−241.7, −44.1)	0.005	−142.0 (−242.2, −41.9)	0.006
Total fat intake (%E)						
27^{+0}–28^{+6} weeks	31.0 (5.1)	31.9 (5.0)				
34–36 weeks	31.2 (5.0)	31.6 (5.2)	−0.5 (−1.4, 0.4)	0.253	−0.5 (−1.4, 0.4)	0.318
Saturated fat intake (%E)						
27^{+0}–28^{+6} weeks	12.7 (2.9)	13.0 (2.9)				
34–36 weeks	12.9 (2.8)	12.8 (2.7)	−0.4 (−0.9, 0.1)	0.082	−0.4 (−0.9, 0.1)	0.086
Protein intake (%E)						
27^{+0}–28^{+6} weeks	21.0 (4.3)	22.0 (4.4)				
34–36 weeks	20.5 (4.3)	23.5 (4.8)	1.9 (1.3, 2.6)	<0.001	2.0 (1.3, 2.7)	<0.001
Carbohydrate intake (%E)						
27^{+0}–28^{+6} weeks	48.1 (6.2)	46.1 (6.8)				
34–36 weeks	48.4 (6.5)	45.0 (7.5)	−1.4 (−2.7, −0.2,)	0.021	−1.5 (−2.8, −0.3)	0.016
Glycaemic index						
27^{+0}–28^{+6} weeks	55.8 (4.0)	55.1 (4.2)				
34–36 weeks	56.1 (4.1)	55.0 (4.5)	−0.3 (−1.0, 0.3)	0.279	−0.4 (−1.0, 0.3)	0.272
Glycaemic load						
27^{+0}–28^{+6} weeks	124.7 (46.3)	123.1 (43.1)				
34–36 weeks	125.5 (46.1)	108.8 (36.0)	−15.1 (−23.4, −6.7)	<0.001	−15.2 (−23.6, −6.7)	<0.001
Physical activity						
Moderate or vigorous activity (min/week)						
27^{+0}–28^{+6} weeks	30 (0–240)	15 (0–240)				
34–36 weeks	0 (0–180)	0 (0–180)	−0.02 (−0.4, 0.4)	0.915	−0. 00008 (−0.4, 0.4)	1.0
Walking (min/week)						
27^{+0}–28^{+6} weeks	360 (150–630)	300 (120–630)				
34–36 weeks	300 (140–600)	280 (120–560)	−0.2 (−0.5, 0.1)	0.244	−0.2 (−0.5, 0.1)	0.162

Data are presented as mean (SD) or median (IQR). The weight gain, dietary intake and physical activity estimates (coefficients) were calculated using linear regression and adjusted for BMI at study entry, ethnicity and neonatal sex. The weight gain analyses included 1031 women, of whom 785 did not have GDM and 246 had GDM. There were 653 women included in the dietary intake analysis; 507 did not have GDM and 146 had GDM. The physical activity outcomes were log transformed and the estimates were calculated using linear regression. For the physical activity analyses, 236 women were included in the unadjusted and adjusted analyses; 181 women did not have GDM and 55 had GDM.

3.3. *Dietary Intake*

Changes in dietary intake between the GDM and non-GDM women following the OGTT at 27^{+0}–28^{+6} weeks' gestation to 34–36 weeks' gestation are shown in Table 2 and Figure 3. The GDM women reduced their energy intake by 142kcal (95% CI −242.2, −41.9, $p = 0.006$) more than the non-GDM women. The GDM women also reduced their carbohydrate intake by 1.5%E (95% CI −2.8, 0.3, $p = 0.016$) and their glycaemic load by 15.2%E (95% CI −23.6, −6.7, $P < 0.001$) more than the non-GDM women. The GDM women changed their protein intake by 2%E (95% CI 1.3, 2.7, $p < 0.001$) more than the non-GDM women in the same time period. These associations were robust to adjustment for confounders. Adjusted graphs are presented in Supplementary Figures S1B–E.

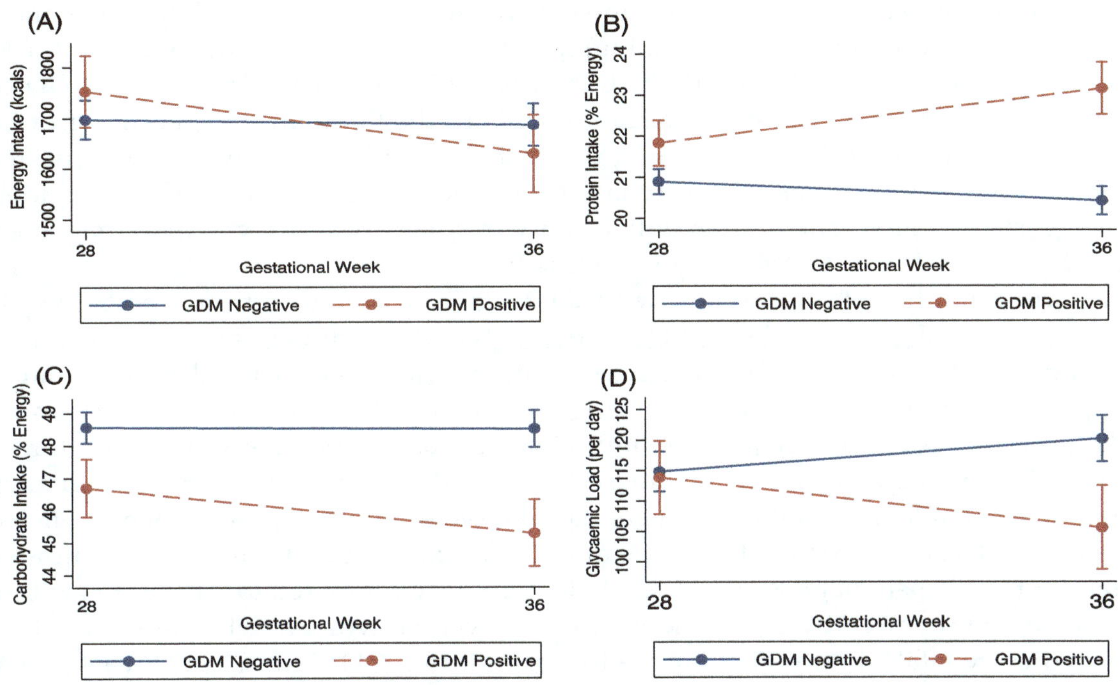

Figure 3. Unadjusted (**A**) energy (kcals), (**B**) protein (% energy), (**C**) carbohydrate (% energy) and (**D**) glycaemic load change of GDM and non-GDM women from 27^{+0}–28^{+6} weeks' gestation (28 weeks) to 34–36 weeks' gestation (36 weeks), with 95% confidence intervals.

There were no differences in change in total fat intake, saturated fat intake or glycaemic index between the GDM and non-GDM women (Table 2).

3.4. *Physical Activity Changes*

There were no differences in change in vigorous and moderate activity and walking between the GDM and non-GDM women (Table 2).

3.5. *Intervention Allocation*

Allocation to either the intervention or control group did not modify the association between GDM status and all outcomes.

4. Discussion

This study found that a higher proportion of pregnant women with obesity who were not diagnosed with GDM gained weight in excess of recommended gestational weight gain in their last trimester of pregnancy. In contrast, the diagnosis and treatment of GDM were associated with lower weight gain and dietary change.

Consistent with our findings, previous studies in women with heterogeneous BMIs assessing weight gain in the interval after GDM screening have found that women without GDM gain more weight than women with GDM [12,14]. In a small US study of 89 women, Chakkalakal et al. reported that women with GDM gained weight at a lower rate than women without GDM (0.30 ± 0.28 kg/week vs. 0.53 ± 0.28 kg/week, $p = 0.001$) [12]. Similarly, women with GDM gained less total weight than women without GDM in a study of 212 Australian women, when weight was assessed in the second and third trimester (GDM: 1.18 kg (1.6%) vs. non-GDM: 4.0 kg (4.8%), $p < 0.001$) [14].

As additionally seen in this study, it is well known that women diagnosed with GDM are more likely to give birth to LGA infants despite dietary changes, physical activity and pharmacological approaches, supporting earlier intervention in such women. Despite a higher prevalence of LGA infants in the GDM group, the finding that a high proportion of obese women without GDM gained weight in excess of the NAM guidelines in the third trimester is of particular concern in a population that already has an increased risk of complications [3]. In the German Programming of Enhanced Adiposity Risk in Childhood–Early Screening (PEACHES) study, excessive third trimester weight gain in women without GDM was related to late-pregnancy dysglycaemia [21]. The evidence from this study suggests that pregnant women with obesity may benefit from weight management advice following OGTT, regardless of GDM diagnostic classification.

In the current study, 26% of women with GDM gained weight which was below the NAM recommendations. Total gestational weight gain below NAM recommendations has been associated with a reduced risk of peripartum complications for pregnant women with obesity but an increased risk of complications in their neonates, including low birth weight, preterm delivery and neonatal mortality [22]. Further research is required to investigate the association between lower third trimester weight gain and pregnancy outcomes in women with GDM who are obese during pregnancy.

Internationally, guidelines for the management of GDM recommend that women be offered dietary advice to improve glycaemic control. This is the most likely explanation for the greater improvement in dietary intake in the women diagnosed with GDM in this study compared to the women without GDM. This contrasts to that reported by Elvebakk et al. in Norwegian women, who showed only marginal differences in dietary intake between women with and without GDM from 18–22 weeks' gestation to 32–36 weeks' gestation [15]. Two cohort studies, in the UK and the US, have reported that women with GDM had lower energy intakes than women without GDM [8,11], similar to the present study. Others have reported that women with GDM had lower intakes of total and saturated fats compared with women without GDM [8,10]. The absence of any changes in total or saturated fat between the groups in the present study may be explained by the focus in the UK on carbohydrate intake to optimise blood glucose control [7]. The difference in weight gain is also likely explained by the management of women with GDM following diagnosis which includes close monitoring of gestational weight gain as well as promotion of dietary change [7,23]. Women with GDM additionally receive regular feedback through the monitoring of blood glucose concentration which can inform dietary choices. Furthermore, they are potentially aware of the risks, particularly to their baby, associated with GDM, which may motivate behaviour change. Women who are not diagnosed with GDM do not have the same motivators; indeed, poor food choices may be positively enforced by apparent lack of disease [24].

There is a paucity of evidence on the association between GDM status and physical activity, with conflicting reports [25,26]. This study identified no differences in physical activity levels between women with and without GDM in the interval following GDM screening. The lack of change in physical activity for both groups aligns with reported barriers to physical activity for such women including a lack of time, pain, fatigue, work and childcare commitments [27].

Whilst it might be hypothesised that randomisation to the intervention arm followed by a diagnosis of GDM might influence the attitude to behavioural change, we found that allocation to a behavioural intervention in early pregnancy did not influence the association between GDM diagnosis and an associated change in diet and physical activity.

This study has several strengths. It is the first to examine the association between GDM status and health behaviours in a cohort of obese pregnant women. The detailed UPBEAT study database provided the opportunity to explore relationships in the interval following GDM screening to late gestation, whereas previous investigations have depended predominantly on cross-sectional data.

Limitations include the collection of dietary intake and physical activity data by self-report questionnaires which may be prone to recall bias [28]. The original trial was not powered to investigate the association between changes in health behaviours and weight gain and pregnancy outcomes. Data were collected in women taking part in a clinical trial, which may have introduced selection bias.

5. Conclusions

Whilst this study confirms that the current guidelines to treat women with GDM are effective in promoting behaviour change and limiting weight gain in obese women diagnosed and treated for GDM, we highlight the unintended consequence of a suboptimal diet and greater weight gain associated with not being diagnosed with GDM. We emphasise the need for strategies to manage dietary intake and gestational weight gain in pregnant women with obesity who receive a negative OGTT result, in order to reduce the risk of adverse health outcomes for mother and child.

Author Contributions: Conceptualisation, S.L.W.; Methodology, S.L.W. and A.C.F.; Formal Analysis, L.A., and S.L.W.; Writing–Original Draft Preparation, L.A., A.C.F. and S.L.W.; Writing–Review and Editing, L.A., L.P., L.H., A.C.F. and S.L.W.; Visualisation, L.A., A.C.F. and S.L.W.; Supervision, L.P., A.C.F. and S.L.W.; Project Administration, L.P., A.C.F. and S.L.W.; Funding Acquisition, L.P. All authors have read and agreed to the published version of the manuscript.

References

1. Baker, C. Obesity Statistics. *Primary Care Clin. Off. Pract.* **2016**, *43*, 121–135.
2. NHS, Digital. *Maternity Services Monthly Statistics*; NHS Digital: Leeds, UK, 2019 January.
3. Poston, L.; Caleyachetty, R.; Cnattingius, S.; Corvalán, C.; Uauy, R.; Herring, S.; Gillman, M.W. Preconceptional and Maternal Obesity: Epidemiology and Health Consequences. *Lancet Diabetes Endocrinol.* **2016**, *4*, 1025–1036. [CrossRef]
4. McIntyre, H.D.; Catalano, P.; Zhang, C.; Desoye, G.; Mathiesen, E.R.; Damm, P. Gestational Diabetes Mellitus. *Nat. Rev. Dis. Prim.* **2019**, *5*. [CrossRef] [PubMed]
5. Marchi, J.; Berg, M.; Dencker, A.; Olander, E.K.; Begley, C. Risks Associated with Obesity in Pregnancy, for the Mother and Baby: A Systematic Review of Reviews. *Obes. Rev.* **2015**, *16*, 621–638. [CrossRef] [PubMed]
6. Zhang, C.; Olsen, S.F.; Hinkle, S.N.; Gore-Langton, R.E.; Vaag, A.; Grunnet, L.G.; Yeung, E.H.; Bao, W.; Bowers, K.; Liu, A.; et al. Diabetes & Women's Health (DWH) Study: An Observational Study of Long-Term Health Consequences of Gestational Diabetes, Their Determinants and Underlying Mechanisms in the USA and Denmark. *BMJ Open* **2019**, *9*, 1–8.
7. National Institute for Health and Care Excellence [NICE]. *Diabetes in Pregnancy: Management from Preconception to the Postnatal Period (NG3)*, 2015; Vol. NG3.
8. Thomas, B.; Ghebremeskel, K.; Lowy, C.; Crawford, M.; Offley-Shore, B. Nutrient Intake of Women with and without Gestational Diabetes with a Specific Focus on Fatty Acids. *Nutrition* **2006**, *22*, 230–236. [CrossRef] [PubMed]
9. Bo, S.; Menato, G.; Lezo, A.; Signorile, A.; Bardelli, C.; De Michieli, F.; Massobrio, M.; Pagano, G. Dietary Fat and Gestational Hyperglycaemia. *Diabetologia* **2001**, *44*, 972–978. [CrossRef]
10. Wang, Y.; Storlien, L.H.; Jenkins, A.B.; Tapsell, L.C.; Jin, Y.; Pan, J.E.; Shao, Y.E.; Calvert, G.D.; Moses, R.G.; Shi, H.L.; et al. Dietary Variables and Glucose Tolerance in Pregnancy. *Diabetes Care* **2000**, *23*, 460–464. [CrossRef]
11. Tepper, B.J.; Seldner, A.C. Sweet Taste and Intake of Sweet Foods in Normal Pregnancy and Pregnancy Complicated by Gestational Diabetes Mellitus. *Am. J. Clin. Nutr.* **1999**, *70*, 277–284. [CrossRef]

12. Chakkalakal, R.J.; Hackstadt, A.J.; Trochez, R.; Gregory, R.; Elasy, T.A. Gestational Diabetes and Maternal Weight Management During and After Pregnancy. *J. Women's Heal.* **2019**, *28*, 646–653. [CrossRef]
13. Huidobro, A.; Prentice, A.; Fulford, T.; Parodi, C.; Rozowski, J. Gestational Diabetes, Comparison of Women Diagnosed in Second and Third Trimester of Pregnancy with Non GDM Women: Analysis of a Cohort Study. *Rev. Med. Chil.* **2010**, *138*, 316–321. [CrossRef]
14. Stewart, Z.A.; Wallace, E.M.; Allan, C.A. Patterns of Weight Gain in Pregnant Women with and without Gestational Diabetes Mellitus: An Observational Study. *Aust. New Zeal. J. Obstet. Gynaecol.* **2012**, *52*, 433–439. [CrossRef] [PubMed]
15. Elvebakk, T.; Mostad, I.L.; Mørkved, S.; Salvesen, K.; Stafne, S.N. Dietary Intakes and Dietary Quality during Pregnancy in Women with and without Gestational Diabetes Mellitus - a Norwegian Longitudinal Study. *Nutrients* **2018**, *10*, 1–13. [CrossRef] [PubMed]
16. Briley, A.L.; Barr, S.; Badger, S.; Croker, H.; Godfrey, K.M.; Holmes, B.; Kinnunen, T.I.; Nelson, S.M.; Oteng-Ntim, E.; Patel, N.; et al. A Complex Intervention to Improve Pregnancy Outcome in Obese Women; the UPBEAT Randomised Controlled Trial. *BMC Pregnancy Child.* **2014**, *14*, 1–74. [CrossRef]
17. Poston, L.; Bell, R.; Croker, H.; Flynn, A.C.; Godfrey, K.M.; Goff, L.; Hayes, L.; Khazaezadeh, N.; Nelson, S.M.; Oteng-Ntim, E.; et al. Effect of a Behavioural Intervention in Obese Pregnant Women (the UPBEAT Study): A Multicentre, Randomised Controlled Trial. *Lancet Diabetes Endocrinol.* **2015**, *3*, 767–777. [CrossRef]
18. Flynn, A.C.; Seed, P.T.; Patel, N.; Barr, S.; Bell, R.; Briley, A.L.; Godfrey, K.M.; Nelson, S.M.; Oteng-Ntim, E.; Robinson, S.M.; et al. Dietary Patterns in Obese Pregnant Women; Influence of a Behavioral Intervention of Diet and Physical Activity in the UPBEAT Randomized Controlled Trial. *Int. J. Behav. Nutr. Phys. Act.* **2016**, *12*. [CrossRef]
19. Metzger, B.E.; Gabbe, S.G.; Persson, B.; Buchanan, T.A.; Catalano, P.M.; Damm, P.; Dyer, A.R.; de Leiva, A.; Hod, M.; Kitzmiller, J.L.; et al. International Association of Diabetes and Pregnancy Study Groups Recommendations on the Diagnosis and Classification of Hyperglycemia in Pregnancy. *Diabetes Care* **2010**, *33*, 676–682. [CrossRef]
20. Institute of Medicine and National Research Council. *Weight Gain during Pregnancy: Reexamining the Guidelines*; National Academies Press: Washington, DC, USA, 2010.
21. Gomes, D.; von Kries, R.; Delius, M.; Mansmann, U.; Nast, M.; Stubert, M.; Langhammer, L.; Haas, N.A.; Netz, H.; Obermeier, V.; et al. Late-Pregnancy Dysglycemia in Obese Pregnancies after Negative Testing for Gestational Diabetes and Risk of Future Childhood Overweight: An Interim Analysis from a Longitudinal Mother–Child Cohort Study. *PLoS Med.* **2018**, *15*, 1–21. [CrossRef]
22. Thompson, A.M.; Thompson, J.A. An Evaluation of Whether a Gestational Weight Gain of 5 to 9 Kg for Obese Women Optimizes Maternal and Neonatal Health Risks. *BMC Pregnancy Child.* **2019**, *19*. [CrossRef]
23. Johns, E.C.; Denison, F.C.; Norman, J.E.; Reynolds, R.M. Gestational Diabetes Mellitus: Mechanisms, Treatment, and Complications. *Trends Endocrinol. Metab.* **2018**, *29*, 743–754. [CrossRef]
24. Bennett, W.L.; Liu, S.H.; Yeh, H.C.; Nicholson, W.K.; Gunderson, E.P.; Lewis, C.E.; Clark, J.M. Changes in Weight and Health Behaviors after Pregnancies Complicated by Gestational Diabetes Mellitus: The CARDIA Study. *Obesity* **2013**, *21*, 1269–1275. [CrossRef] [PubMed]
25. Gao, F.; Luo, H.; Jones, K.; Nicholson, W.; Bell, R.A. Gestational Diabetes and Health Behaviors Among Women: National Health and Nutrition Examination Survey, 2007–2014. *Prev. Chronic Dis.* **2018**, *15*. [CrossRef] [PubMed]
26. Anjana, R.M.; Sudha, V.; Lakshmipriya, N.; Anitha, C.; Unnikrishnan, R.; Bhavadharini, B.; Mahalakshmi, M.M.; Maheswari, K.; Kayal, A.; Ram, U.; et al. Physical Activity Patterns and Gestational Diabetes Outcomes - The Wings Project. *Diabetes Res. Clin. Pract.* **2016**, *116*, 253–262. [CrossRef] [PubMed]
27. Flannery, C.; McHugh, S.; Anaba, A.E.; Clifford, E.; O'Riordan, M.; Kenny, L.C.; McAuliffe, F.M.; Kearney, P.M.; Byrne, M. Enablers and Barriers to Physical Activity in Overweight and Obese Pregnant Women: An Analysis Informed by the Theoretical Domains Framework and COM-B Model. *BMC Pregnancy Child.* **2018**, *18*, 178. [CrossRef]
28. Shim, J.-S.; Oh, K.; Kim, H.C. Epidemiology and Health Dietary Assessment Methods in Epidemiologic Studies. *Epidemiol. Health* **2014**, *36*, 1–8.

12

Methylglyoxal, Glycated Albumin, PAF and TNF-α: Possible Inflammatory and Metabolic Biomarkers for Management of Gestational Diabetes

Gabriele Piuri [1], Katia Basello [2], Gabriele Rossi [3], Chiara Maria Soldavini [3], Silvia Duiella [3], Giulia Privitera [3], Angela Spadafranca [3], Andrea Costanzi [2], Emiliana Tognon [2], Mattia Cappelletti [1], Paola Antonia Corsetto [4], Angela Maria Rizzo [4], Attilio Francesco Speciani [1,2,*] and Enrico Ferrazzi [1,3,5]

1 Inflammation Society, 18 Woodlands Park, Bexley DA52EL, UK; gabriele.piuri@me.com (G.P.); m.cappelletti@me.com (M.C.); enrico.ferrazzi@unimi.it (E.F.)

2 GEK lab–Cryolab, University of Rome Tor Vergata, Via Montpellier, 1—00133 Rome, Italy; katia.basello@gek-group.com (K.B.); andrea.costanzi@gek-group.com (A.C.); emiliana.tognon@gek-group.com (E.T.)

3 Obstetrical Unit, Woman-Child-Newborn Department, Fondazione IRCCS Ca' Granda, Ospedale Maggiore Policlinico, 20122 Milan, Italy; gabriele.rossi@policlinico.mi.it (G.R.); chiaramaria.soldavini@gmail.com (C.M.S.); silvia.duiella@policlinico.mi.it (S.D.); giulia.privitera@policlinico.mi.it (G.P.); angela.spadafranca@gmail.com (A.S.)

4 Department of Pharmacological and Biomolecular Sciences, Università degli Studi di Milano, 20133 Milano, Italy; paola.corsetto@unimi.it (P.A.C.); angelamaria.rizzo@unimi.it (A.M.R.)

5 Fondazione IRCCS Cà Granda, Ospedale Maggiore Policlinico, Department of Clinical Sciences and Community Health, Università degli Studi di Milano, 20122 Milan, Italy

* Correspondence: attilio.speciani@me.com

Abstract: Background: In gestational diabetes mellitus (GDM), pancreatic β-cell breakdown can result from a proinflammatory imbalance created by a sustained level of cytokines. In this study, we investigated the role of specific cytokines, such as B-cell activating factor (BAFF), tumor necrosis factor α (TNF-α), and platelet-activating factor (PAF), together with methylglyoxal (MGO) and glycated albumin (GA) in pregnant women affected by GDM. Methods: We enrolled 30 women whose inflammation and metabolic markers were measured at recruitment and after 12 weeks of strict dietetic therapy. We compared these data to the data obtained from 53 randomly selected healthy nonpregnant subjects without diabetes, hyperglycemia, or any condition that can affect glycemic metabolism. Results: In pregnant women affected by GDM, PAF levels increased from 26.3 (17.4–47.5) ng/mL to 40.1 (30.5–80.5) ng/mL ($p < 0.001$). Their TNF-α levels increased from 3.0 (2.8–3.5) pg/mL to 3.4 (3.1–5.8) pg/mL ($p < 0.001$). The levels of methylglyoxal were significantly higher in the women with GDM ($p < 0.001$), both at diagnosis and after 12 weeks (0.64 (0.46–0.90) μg/mL; 0.71 (0.47–0.93) μg/mL, respectively) compared to general population (0.25 (0.19–0.28) μg/mL). Levels of glycated albumin were significantly higher in women with GDM ($p < 0.001$) only after 12 weeks from diagnosis (1.51 (0.88–2.03) nmol/mL) compared to general population (0.95 (0.63–1.4) nmol/mL). Conclusion: These findings support the involvement of new inflammatory and metabolic biomarkers in the mechanisms related to GDM complications and prompt deeper exploration into the vicious cycle connecting inflammation, oxidative stress, and metabolic results.

Keywords: gestational diabetes; platelet-activating factor; tumor necrosis factor α; methylglyoxal; glycated albumin

---

1. Introduction

The definition of gestational diabetes (GDM) is related to high blood glucose levels that appear for the first time during gestation. In the latter stages of gestation, a pancreatic response to progressive insulin resistance occurs, and GDM is the failure of the pancreas to appropriately increase the β-cell mass and the connected insulin secretion. Around 4% to 10% of all pregnant women develop GDM [1,2]. The predisposition to developing GDM depends on different diagnostic criteria, including individual history of obesity and maternal age at first pregnancy. GDM is also associated with a highly and significantly increased risk of maternal and neonatal morbidity [2]. Among the long-term complications, there is an increased risk of developing type two diabetes in adult life, and GDM can negatively influence epigenetic programming in the fetus and newborn development, increasing their cardiovascular and metabolic risks [3].

Several reports have shown that the systemic inflammatory response is more pronounced in women with GDM [4]. Several inflammatory mediators may play an essential role in GDM pathogenesis. Therefore, knowing the levels of these mediators and their effects during gestation may create new opportunities for improving diagnosis and cures for GDM and preventing GDM complications.

The placenta physiologically contributes to inflammation and insulin resistance by secreting proinflammatory cytokines. In GDM, pancreatic β-cell breakdown can result from the proinflammatory imbalance created by a sustained level of cytokines [5]. In this study, we investigated the role of specific cytokines, such as B-cell activating factor (BAFF), tumor necrosis factor α (TNF-α), and platelet-activating factor (PAF), together with some markers of oxidative stress, in pregnant women affected by GDM. It has already been observed that those signaling cytokines and inflammatory molecules have a role in the mechanisms of insulin resistance and may result in pregnancy complications such as maternal hypertension [6–9].

BAFF plays a role in determining insulin resistance [10–12] and has been implicated in GDM. BAFF is an essential immune regulator that was recently reported to be secreted by the placenta [6,13].

High levels of TNF-α reduce insulin sensitivity by disrupting the translocation of glucose transport GLUT-4 channels and insulin signal transduction [14]. The expression of TNF-α in the placenta is thought to contribute to the insulin resistance associated with pregnancy. However, this TNF-α increase is controversial [15] and is possibly linked to body mass index (BMI) before pregnancy [16].

PAF is another important mediator of inflammation, and its highly unstable molecules could contribute to the pathogenesis of pre-eclampsia [17]. However, no studies have investigated its possible role in GDM.

In GDM, hyperglycemia induces the overproduction of methylglyoxal (MGO), a circulating toxic intermediate metabolite that enters the fetal circulation and crosses cell membranes [18,19]. MGO is an oxidizing substance, and its concentration is directly correlated with blood sugar levels. MGO is controlled via an enzymatic system, which detoxifies the organism by converting 99% of the MGO into less reactive products. An excessive accumulation of MGO results in the addition of this molecule to proteins and DNA, leading to oxidative stress, cellular aging, DNA mutations, and pro-apoptotic effect. Krishnasam et al. also demonstrated that the concentrations of MGO are significantly higher in GDM women compared to MGO in normal pregnant women [20]. Chang and Chan found that MGO has harmful effects on early-stage oocyte maturation and fertilization [21]. Besides its direct effects, MGO is a precursor to advanced glycation end-products (AGEs), which, in turn, are teratogenic. AGEs are formed either directly via a nonenzymatic reaction between glucose and the N-terminal part of proteins, or indirectly through α-oxoaldehydes.

Approximately 60–70% of total serum proteins are represented by human serum albumin, which is the most abundant extracellular protein in plasma. Human serum albumin is a multifunctional protein, and interest has increased in its activity as a biomarker of hyperglycemia due to its high sensitivity to glycation. Several differences exist between HbA1c and albumin, and the latter has a rate of nonenzymatic glycation that is approximately 10-fold higher than that of hemoglobin [22]. The higher susceptibility to glycation of albumin and other plasma proteins compared to intracellular proteins like hemoglobin induces some specific effects. The blood levels of glycated albumin exhibit a broader fluctuation than those of HbA1c, allowing earlier detection of rapid changes in blood glucose [23,24]. Few studies have investigated the association between glycated albumin in diabetic pregnant women, and the results about the complications in their children have been conflicting [25–27].

This study aimed at investigating the longitudinal trends of these inflammatory and metabolic molecules during pregnancy to demonstrate new pathogenetic markers of GDM. The secondary aim of this study was evaluating the possible correlation between these data to routine metabolic analyses and anthropometric measurements of mothers and newborns.

2. Materials and Methods

2.1. *Study Design and Subjects*

We conducted this observational study on a cohort of Caucasian pregnant women with GDM, recruited at the Department of Obstetrics and Gynecology, Fondazione IRCCS Ca' Granda, Ospedale Maggiore Policlinico, Milan, Italy. A two-hour, 75-g oral glucose tolerance test (OGTT), performed at 24–28 weeks according to the International Association of Diabetes and Pregnancy Study Groups (IADPSG) criteria [28], was used to confirm the diagnosis of GDM. Exclusion criteria were chronic gastrointestinal diseases; pre-pregnancy diabetes; celiac disease; a history of eating disorders, such as anorexia or bulimia; vegan, vegetarian, or macrobiotic regimens; and non-Caucasian ethnicity. The institutional board reviewed and approved the study procedures and each subject provided written informed consent. We conducted the study following the Declaration of Helsinki. The local ethical committee approved the study protocol (Clinical Trial Center Fondazione IRCCS Ca' Granda Ospedale Maggiore Policlinico, project identification code 4004, approval number 126_2018 on 28 March 2018). For the general population, we present data obtained from 53 randomly selected healthy nonpregnant subjects, matched to GDM women for age, without diabetes, hyperglycemia, or any condition that can affect glycemic metabolism. The data of this group were derived from an internal database related to healthy nonpregnant subjects who released informed consent for scientific purpose. We collected samples using a finger prick and analyzed the total albumin, GA, and MGO.

We recorded anthropometric measures and fasting blood sample collection to measure serum inflammatory markers (BAFF, PAF, TNF-α, MGO, and GA) during the recruitment visit three days after the OGTT and 12 weeks after GDM diagnosis. All subjects had to present complete medical histories and undergo a physical examination, anthropometric assessment and routine laboratory tests including fasting blood glucose, postprandial blood glucose, glycated hemoglobin, insulin, cortisol at 08:00, total cholesterol, HDL cholesterol, LDL cholesterol, triglycerides, CRP, creatinine, and ferritin. Maternal venous blood was obtained from peripheral venipuncture, and the serum was stored at −80 °C. In this observational study, all OGTT were performed in the same analysis laboratory (Fondazione IRCCS Ca' Granda, Ospedale Maggiore Policlinico, Milan, Italy). All the women whose OGTT levels were positive for a diagnosis of GDM were called by the physician to invite them to participate in this observational study.

2.2. *Anthropometry*

The same operator recorded the anthropometric measurements at the recruitment visit according to standard criteria and measuring procedures [29]. The pregnant women wore only underwear. The operator measured their weight (to the nearest 0.1 kg) and their standing height (SH; to the nearest 0.1 cm) using the same calibrated scale, which had a telescopic vertical steel stadiometer (SECA 711, seca Deutschland, Hamburg, Germany). We calculated the BMI as weight (kg)/stature^2 (m^2). We also calculated pre-pregnancy BMI using the self-reported body weight before pregnancy. Biceps, triceps, and subscapular skinfolds were measured using a Tanner–Whitehouse caliper (Holtain Ltd., Crosswell, U.K.), measuring each skinfold three times and using the mean value for analysis.

2.3. Dietary Intervention

All women received a dietary program to control their glucose metabolism and weight gain. If necessary, their diets were hypocaloric to provide at least the resting energy expenditure estimated by the Harris–Benedict formula considering the pre-pregnant weight and energy surplus linked to gestational age following the Recommended Assumption Levels of Energy and Nutrients for the Italian Population (LARN) [30].

The proposed nutritional pattern agreed with the Healthy Eating Plate proposed by Harvard School of Public Health [31]. The daily total energy intake was distributed across three main meals (breakfast, lunch, and dinner) and two snacks.

The macronutrient composition was balanced as follows: 45% of the total energy from carbohydrates, of which simple sugars comprised less than 12%; 25–35% of total energy from fat, of which less than 7% was from saturated fat and 10% from polyunsaturated fatty acids (PUFAs). The protein intake satisfied the pregnancy requirements, as indicated in the LARN, with 50% derived from vegetable sources and 50% from animal sources. The quality of protein intake was regulated by the following frequencies of consumption: Meat, preferably white, 2 times/week; fish 2–3 times/week, with a preference for blue fish for optimal intake of omega-3 fatty acids; legumes 3–4 times/week; eggs 2 times/week, cheese 1–2 times/week; ham 1 time/week; and nuts 20–30 g every day. Food with a high glycemic index were prohibited. Two servings of fruit and three servings of vegetables were advised to be consumed daily. Olive oil was indicated as the main culinary lipid. Dietary cholesterol was lower than 200 mg/day and fiber intake was about 30 g, in agreement with the Guidelines for Healthy Nutrition.

In order to assess the adherence to the diet and the effect on glycemic profile, every woman was invited to fill a daily food diary and to monitor their glycemic profile twice a day via the use of a glucometer. Fasting glycemic cutoff was 95 mg/dL, while 2h postprandial glucose cutoff was 120 mg/dL. Every two weeks, a meeting with the dietitian and the gynecologist was proposed to evaluate the health status of the fetus and maternal body weight and fat mass. Clinical dietitians were responsible for providing dietary counseling for GDM women.

Subjects included in the control group did not receive any dietary counseling.

2.4. Enzyme-Linked Immunosorbent Assay (ELISA)

Human glycated albumin (GA) and total albumin (TA) concentrations in the plasma samples were determined using a Human Glycated Albumin ELISA Kit (lower range of detection 19.53 pmol/mL, sensitivity <11.719 pmol/mL, Catalog No. abx252493, Abbexa Ltd., Cambridge Science Park, Cambridge, U.K.) and a Human Albumin Immunoperoxidase Assay for the Determination of Albumin kit (lower range of detection 0 ng/ml, Human Samples, Catalog No. E-80AL, Immunology Consultants Laboratory, Portland, OR, USA), respectively. The levels of GA and serum albumin are expressed as a percentage to exclude the influence of serum albumin. We calculated the GA% using the following formula: GA% = GA (μmol/mL)/Total Albumin (μmol/mL) × 100.

MGO was measured using the OxiSelect™ Methylglyoxal Competitive ELISA Kit (lower range of detection 0 μg/mL, Catalog No. STA-811, Cell Biolabs, San Diego, CA, USA), which is an enzyme immunoassay developed for the detection and quantization of protein adducts of methylglyoxal-hydro-imidazoline (MG-H1).

The serum TNF-α, B-cell Activating factor (BAFF), and Human Platelet Activating Factor (PAF) were measured via commercial ELISA kits (Human TNF-a Ultrasensitive ELISA Kit, lower range of detection 0 pg/mL, sensitivity < 0.09 pg/mL, Catalog Number KHC3014, Invitrogen, ThermoFisher Scientific, Carlsbad, CA, USA; Human BAFF/BLyS/TNFSF13B Immunoassay Quantikine®ELISA, lower range of detection 0 pg/mL sensitivity 2.68 pg/mL, Catalog Number PDBLYS0B, R&D Systems Inc, Minneapolis, MN, USA; Human Platelet Activating Factor ELISA Kit, lower range of detection 0.313 ng/mL, sensitivity 0.188 ng/mL, Catalog Number E-EL-H2199, Elabscience Houston, TX, USA, respectively) using the Biomek 4000 ELISA microplate liquid reagent dispensing automation tool

(Beckman Coulter, Brea, CA, USA) and the EL405LS ELISA microplate automated washing system (BioTek Instruments, Winooski, VT, USA). The absorbance of each well was read at a wavelength of 450 nm with a Multiskan FC plate reader (Thermo Scientific, Waltham, MA, USA). The average zero standard optical density was subtracted from all absorbances, and a standard curve was generated using a four-parameter logistic (4-PL) curve fit. The concentration in the test sample was calculated through interpolation along the standard curve by multiplying the result by the dilution factor.

2.5. Statistical Analysis

Statistical analysis of the data was performed using GraphPad Prism 8 for macOS (GraphPad Software, San Diego, CA, USA. Version 8.3.0 (328), 16 October 2019). The median and interquartile range (IQR) were calculated for each variable. The medians were compared using the Mann–Whitney test. The linear correlations were studied using Spearman's rank correlation coefficient. A p-value < 0.05 was used as the limit of statistical significance.

3. Results

We enrolled 30 women whose mean maternal age at recruitment was 34.0 (32.7–38.5) years. Their mean gestational age at recruitment with a positive OGTT was 26 weeks ±6 days (25+4 – 27+4). Tables 1 and 2 provide the anthropometric and metabolic data of the enrolled patients at recruitment and after 12 weeks of dietetic treatment, respectively. Body weight and waist circumference significantly increased as expected, while fat mass, measured by skinfolds, reduced. The median fasting and postprandial plasma glucose levels were within normal ranges both at T0 and after 12 weeks. Table 1 provides more details about delivery and newborns (53% females). Two newborns had a birth weight percentile higher than the 90th. The vast majority of the enrolled population did not experience any complications during delivery and in postpartum except for a case of third-degree laceration and a case of diastasis episiorrhaphy.

Table 1. Anthropometric data of the enrolled women before and during pregnancy and details related to delivery and newborns.

Anthropometric Data	Before Pregnancy		p
Height (cm)	163 (160–168)		-
Pre-gestational weight (kg)	62.8 (55.6–69.6)		-
Pre-gestational BMI (kg/m^2)	23.3 (21.0–26.3)		-
	At diagnosis	**After 12 weeks of diet**	
Weight (kg)	71.0 (63.5–78.5)	78.0 (64.6–82.8)	<0.001
Arm circumference (cm)	29.0 (26.9–30.1)	28.8 (28.0–31.3)	ns
Wrist circumference (cm)	15.0 (14.3–16.0)	15 (14.3–16.0)	ns
Waist circumference (cm)	96.0 (87.5–100.0)	104.0 (97.9–107.1)	<0.001
Bicipital skinfold (mm)	9.0 (7.8–13.3)	10.7 (7.2–12.8)	0.05
Tricipital skinfold (mm)	21.6 (18.0–28.7)	20.1 (16.8–25.8)	0.001
Subscapular skinfold (mm)	18.40 (13.40–25.20)	14.4 (12.3–24.0)	0.02
	Delivery and newborn details		
Gestational age at birth (weeks+days)	39+5 (39+0–39+6)		-
Birth weight (g)	3170 (3040–3460)		-
Birth weight centile	41.5 (22.5–67.8)		-
APGAR 1′	9 (9–9)		-
APGAR 5′	10 (10–10)		-

We measured weight, circumferences, and skinfolds at diagnosis of gestational diabetes mellitus (GDM) and after 12 weeks of diet. Data are expressed as the median and interquartile range.

Table 2. Metabolic data of enrolled women at diagnosis of gestational diabetes mellitus and after 12 weeks of diet.

Metabolic Data	At Diagnosis	After 12 Weeks of Diet	*p*
Fasting blood glucose (mg/dL)	85.4 (79.4–90.8)	80.0 (73.0–90.0)	ns
Post prandial blood glucose (mg/dL)	94.4 (88.4–103.9)	97.1 (92.7–100.7)	ns
Glycated hemoglobin (mmol/mol)	30.5 (28.8–32.0)	33.0 (31.8–35.3)	<0.001
Insulin (μU/mL)	9.3 (5.5–14.3)	9.7 (7.4–15.3)	ns
HOMA index	1.54 (0.88–2.31)	1.45 (0.70–2.30)	ns
Cortisol at 08:00 (μg/dL)	27.6 (21.1–30.9)	27.0 (23.0–32.4)	ns
Total cholesterol (mg/dL)	258 (221–279)	267 (232–301)	ns
HDL cholesterol (mg/dL)	79 (65–87)	75 (66–87)	ns
LDL cholesterol (mg/dL)	142 (109–167)	146 (114–164)	ns
Triglycerides (mg/dL)	185 (150–208)	227 (221–282)	<0.001
CRP (mg/dL)	0.42 (0.17–0.63)	0.35 (0.23–0.60)	ns
Creatinine (mg/dl)	0.47 (0.42–0.62)	0.56 (0.50–0.67)	ns
Ferritin (ng/ml)	18 (12–35)	23 (16–32)	ns

Data are expressed as the median and interquartile range. HOMA index, homeostatic model assessment index; HDL cholesterol, high-density lipoprotein cholesterol; LDL cholesterol, low-density lipoprotein cholesterol; CRP, C-reactive protein.

Inflammation markers were measured at recruitment and after 12 weeks of strict dietetic therapy. PAF levels increased from 26.3 (17.4–47.5) ng/mL to 40.1 (30.5–80.5) ng/mL ($p < 0.001$). TNF-α levels increased from 3.0 (2.8–3.5) pg/mL to 3.4 (3.1–5.8) pg/mL ($p < 0.001$). No significant changes were observed in the levels of BAFF, methylglyoxal, and glycated albumin, and in the ratio of glycated albumin to total albumin (Figure 1).

In the general population (age: 36.2 (31.1–39.3) years), the fasting blood glucose was 85.1 (80.3–92.5) mg/dL, and glycated hemoglobin was 33.1 (29.9–34.1) mmol/mol (as median (IQR), *p* ns compared to GDM group). As shown in Table 3, the levels of MGO were significantly higher in women with GDM ($p < 0.001$), both at diagnosis and after 12 weeks (0.64 (0.46–0.90) μg/mL; 0.71 (0.47–0.93) μg/mL, respectively) compared with general population at 0.25 (0.19–0.28) μg/mL. Levels of glycated albumin were significantly higher in women with GDM ($p < 0.001$) only after 12 weeks of diagnosis (1.51 (0.88–2.03) nmol/mL) compared with general population (0.95 (0.63–1.4) nmol/mL). We found no differences in the ratio of glycated albumin to total albumin.

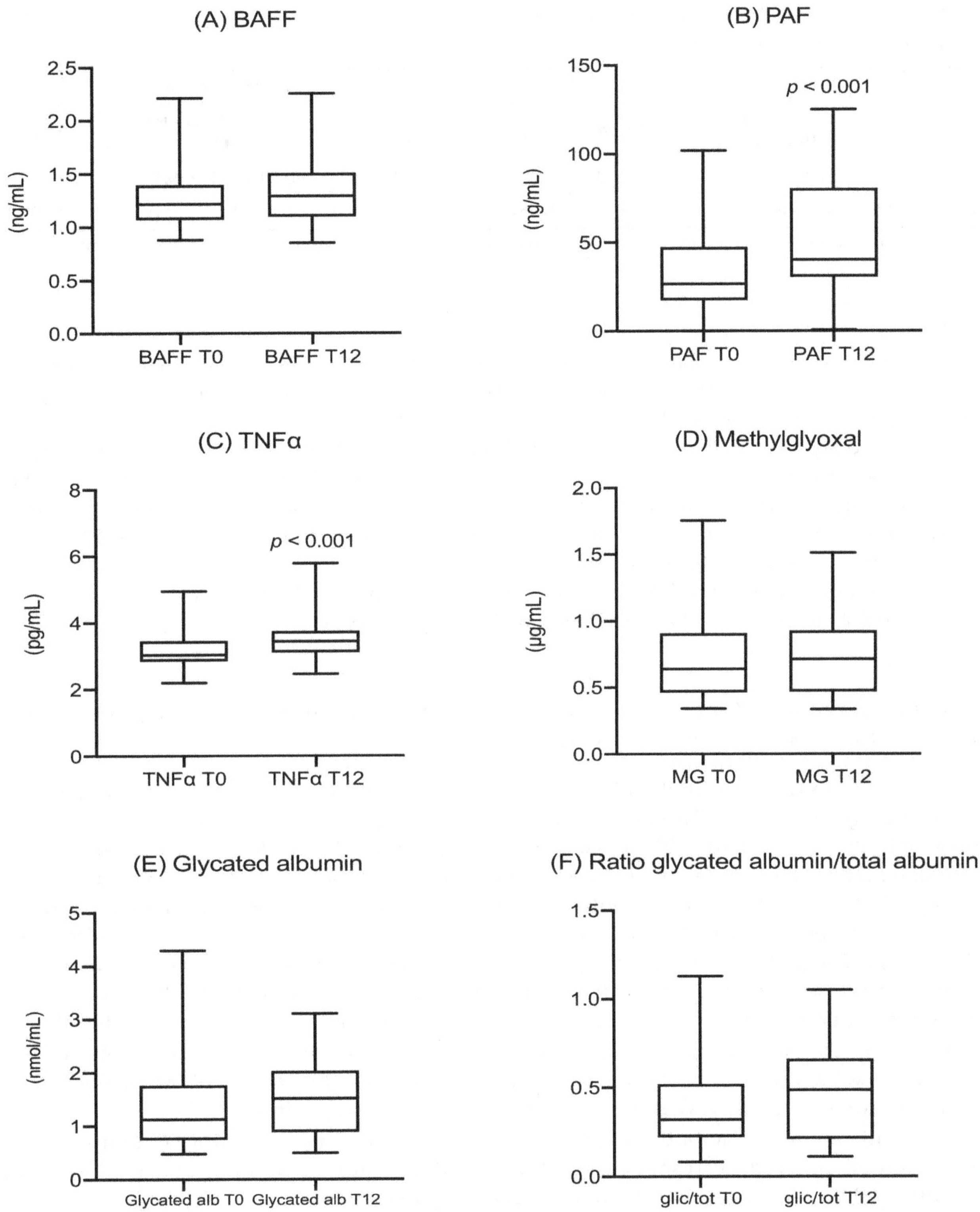

Figure 1. Longitudinal trend of inflammatory and metabolic markers in women with GDM at the time of diagnosis (T0) and after 12 weeks (T12): (**A**) BAFF, (**B**) PAF, (**C**) TNF-α, (**D**) methylglyoxal, (**E**) glycated albumin, (**F**) ratio of glycated albumin to total albumin. BAFF, B-cell activating factor; PAF, platelet-activating factor; TNF-α, tumor necrosis factor α; MG, methylglyoxal; GA, glycated albumin; glic/tot, ratio of glycated albumin to total albumin.

Table 3. Comparison between MGO and GA in general population and women with GDM at the diagnosis and after 12 weeks of diet.

		GDM Women		GDM Women	
	General Population	**At Diagnosis**	p	**After 12 Weeks of Diet**	p
MGO (μg/mL)	0.25 (0.19–0.28)	0.64 (0.46–0.90)	<0.001	0.71 (0.47–0.93)	<0.001
GA (nmol/mL)	0.95 (0.63–1.4)	1.12 (0.74–1.76)	ns	1.51 (0.88–2.03)	<0.001

Data are expressed as the median and interquartile range. MG, methylglyoxal; GA, glycated albumin.

Correlations

PAF levels at diagnosis and after 12 weeks were positively correlated with glycated hemoglobin levels ($r = 0.394$, $p = 0.031$; $r = 0.364$, $p = 0.048$, respectively) and the HOMA index ($r = 0.479$, $p = 0.018$ and $r = 0.422$, $p = 0.040$, respectively).

We observed a positive correlation between MGO levels and HbA1c both at diagnosis ($r = 0.401$, $p = 0.028$) and after 12 weeks ($r = 0.458$, $p = 0.011$). MGO was significantly correlated with the HOMA index only at diagnosis ($r = 0.440$, $p =$ 0. 031). MGO levels were positively correlated with both the pre-pregnancy weight ($r = 0.400$, $p = 0.028$) at GDM diagnosis and after 12 weeks ($r = 0.406$, $p = 0.026$), and with the birth weight ($r = 0.438$, $p = 0.032$).

Glycated albumin levels at GDM diagnosis were positively correlated with pre-pregnancy weight and BMI ($r = 0.388$, $p = 0.037$ and $r = 0.417$, $p = 0.024$, respectively).

4. Discussion

After the enrollment of pregnant women diagnosed with positive OGTT at a gestational age of around 26 weeks, we observed the following:

(1) After the diagnosis, the metabolic parameters of the women following the suggested diet substantially stabilized. The median values of fasting and postprandial glucose levels were normal both at T0 and after 12 weeks, while HbA1c showed a modest increase, but their values remained within the normal range. The same was observed for MGO and GA, which both showed a slight increase in their values but without any statistical significance. The only significant increase was observed in the triglycerides values, confirming the results already shown in literature [32,33]. Despite the stability of the standard glycemic parameters, this increase could reflect an obesogenic pathway [34] due to an inflammatory and metabolic effect on insulin resistance of PAF, TNF-alfa [35], MGO [36], and GA [37], that needs further investigation.

(2) Maternal body weight increased after 12 weeks, while fat mass reduced. This result, also associated with a correct evaluation of the food diaries, suggests an excellent dietetic adherence and a positive effect of the dietary intervention on body composition.

(3) Despite this metabolic stability, a significant increase of two inflammatory cytokines (PAF and TNF-α) was observed, corresponding to the proinflammatory conditions of gestational diabetes mellitus (GDM), acting even without metabolic impairment.

(4) Despite normal HbA1c and fasting glycaemia levels, the metabolic biomarkers MGO and GA were significantly different compared with the general population. For MGO, this difference was evident since the time of diagnosis at around 26 weeks.

(5) Some positive correlations were observed among inflammatory markers, metabolic parameters, and the anthropometric analysis. For example, a strict correlation between MGO and fetal overgrowth was evident, and a correlation between PAF, MGO, and the HOMA index was also observed.

Overall, this evidence indicates the possibility of using these biomarkers to better understand how to prevent possible future GDM complications for mothers and their children.

Pregnancy is one of the most rapidly stressful metabolic events in the life of a woman. Women with a genetic and metabolic predisposition to GDM, even at a young age, can develop GDM, which lasts only during pregnancy due to its metabolic burden. The appearance of this disease is often a prediction of future development of type 2 diabetes, for which age, weight, and other metabolic factors can determine similar conditions of stress, metabolic burden, and oxidative or inflammatory overload.

Until present, the diagnosis of GDM has been based on the OGTT, which is useful for identification of the disease but cannot be used to predict future complications or precise phenotypic correlations like BMI before pregnancy and fetal overgrowth. The use of markers like GA may not be suitable for the diagnosis and the management of GDM due to the reduced duration of episodes of hyperglycemia. According to a longitudinal study of the concentration of MGO and GA, we hypothesize that MGO could be useful for the identification of women with a high risk of GDM and, with the support of OGTT, the diagnosis and prediction of complications (in particular for the prediction of fetal overgrowth). However, GA may not be useful for an accurate diagnosis, but could be used as an excellent metabolic biomarker to evaluate glycemic control in GDM women, similar to how HbA1c is now used in diabetic patients. The identification of new markers for metabolic distress in GDM could lead to a better follow-up for GDM women.

The development of GDM could also be induced by an increase in the inflammatory conditions connected to the TNF-α and PAF pathways, to oxidative stress due to the glycation of many proteins, or due to the production of oxidative substances like MGO. To the best of our knowledge, this is the first time in which inflammatory biomarkers like PAF and TNF-α have been studied longitudinally during GDM pregnancies. The increase in PAF and TNF-α 12 weeks after the diagnosis of GDM could be useful in the future for monitoring this condition and potentially help to explain the hidden mechanisms behind metabolic and inflammatory interactions in GDM.

Limitations

The population analyzed was too small to define precise future guidelines, and further studies with a larger cohort are needed for a better definition. The general population used for the comparison of metabolic values was nonidentical to the GDM-affected women in this study. In future studies, healthy pregnant women should be compared with those who are affected by GDM. However, according to Krishnasam [20], the concentrations of MGO are already known to be significantly higher in GDM women compared with the MGO values in normal pregnant women. In that study, the reported absolute values differed compared to ours, although this may be ascribed to differences in the method, as Krishnaman et al. employed a diverse commercial ELISA methodology [20]. Our study population was represented only by Caucasian women due to the usual referrals to the hospital involved.

5. Conclusions

The aim of this study was to investigate the longitudinal trends of these inflammatory and metabolic molecules to demonstrate new pathogenetic markers of GDM. A specific diet in women with GDM is a crucial factor for the correct management of GDM itself. However, the increase of specific inflammatory biomarkers could exert a role that is potentially related to metabolic impairment.

This study supports the involvement of new inflammatory and metabolic biomarkers in the mechanisms related to the complications of GDM and prompts a deeper exploration into the vicious cycle connecting inflammation, oxidative stress, and metabolic results.

Author Contributions: Conceptualization, G.P. (Gabriele Piuri), G.R., A.M.R., A.F.S. and E.F.; methodology, G.P. (Gabriele Piuri), K.B., G.R., A.M.R., A.F.S. and E.F.; software, G.P. (Gabriele Piuri), K.B. and A.C.; validation, K.B., G.R., C.M.S., S.D., G.P. (Giulia Privitera), A.S., A.C. and P.A.C.; formal analysis, G.P. (Gabriele Piuri) and K.B.;

investigation, K.B., G.R., C.M.S, S.D., G.P. (Giulia Privitera), A.S., A.C. and P.A.C.; resources, K.B., G.R., C.M.S, S.D., G.P. (Giulia Privitera), A.S., A.C. and P.A.C.; data curation, G.P. (Gabriele Piuri), K.B., G.R., C.M.S., S.D., G.P. (Giulia Privitera), A.S. and A.C; writing—original draft preparation, G.P. (Gabriele Piuri), K.B., A.S., A.C., E.T., A.F.S. and E.F.; writing—review and editing, G.P. (Gabriele Piuri), K.B., G.R., A.S., A.C., E.T., M.C., P.A.C, A.M.R., A.F.S. and E.F.; visualization, G.P. (Gabriele Piuri), A.F.S. and E.F.; supervision, G.P. (Gabriele Piuri), G.R., A.F.S. and E.F.; project administration, G.P. (Gabriele Piuri), G.R., A.M.R., A.F.S. and E.F. All authors have read and agreed to the published version of the manuscript.

References

1. Kalter-Leibovici, O.; Freedman, L.S.; Olmer, L.; Liebermann, N.; Heymann, A.; Tal, O.; Lerner-Geva, L.; Melamed, N.; Hod, M. Screening and diagnosis of gestational diabetes mellitus: Critical appraisal of the new International Association of Diabetes in Pregnancy Study Group recommendations on a national level. *Diabetes Care* **2012**, *35*, 1894–1896. [CrossRef] [PubMed]
2. Gümüş, P.; Özçaka, Ö.; Ceyhan-Öztürk, B.; Akcali, A.; Lappin, D.F.; Buduneli, N. Evaluation of biochemical parameters and local and systemic levels of osteoactive and B-cell stimulatory factors in gestational diabetes in the presence or absence of gingivitis. *J. Periodontol.* **2015**, *86*, 387–397. [CrossRef] [PubMed]
3. Harrison, C.L.; Lombard, C.B.; East, C.; Boyle, J.; Teede, H.J. Risk stratification in early pregnancy for women at increased risk of gestational diabetes. *Diabetes Res. Clin. Pract.* **2015**, *107*, 61–68. [CrossRef] [PubMed]
4. Briana, D.D.; Malamitsi-Puchner, A. Reviews: Adipocytokines in normal and complicated pregnancies. *Reprod. Sci.* **2009**, *16*, 921–937. [CrossRef]
5. Cieślak, M.; Wojtczak, A.; Cieślak, M. Role of pro-inflammatory cytokines of pancreatic islets and prospects of elaboration of new methods for the diabetes treatment. *Acta Biochim. Pol.* **2015**, *62*, 15–21. [CrossRef]
6. Stohl, H.E.; Lee, R.H.; Manetta, J.; Kikly, K.; Korst, L.M.; Stohl, W. Maternal Serum B-Cell Activating Factor Levels: Candidate Early Biomarker for Hypertensive Disorders of Pregnancy. *Hypertension* **2017**, *70*, 1007–1013. [CrossRef]
7. Tay, J.; Costanzi, A.; Basello, K.; Piuri, G.; Ferrazzi, E.; Speciani, A.F.; Lees, C.C. Maternal Serum B Cell activating factor in hypertensive and normotensive pregnancies. *Pregnancy Hypertens.* **2018**, *13*, 58–61. [CrossRef]
8. Sankaralingam, S.; Xu, H.; Jiang, Y.; Sawamura, T.; Davidge, S.T. Evidence for increased methylglyoxal in the vasculature of women with preeclampsia: Role in upregulation of LOX-1 and arginase. *Hypertension* **2009**, *54*, 897–904. [CrossRef]
9. Uysal, K.T.; Wiesbrock, S.M.; Marino, M.W.; Hotamisligil, G.S. Protection from obesity-induced insulin resistance in mice lacking TNF-alpha function. *Nature* **1997**, *389*, 610–614. [CrossRef]
10. Kim, Y.-H.; Choi, B.-H.; Cheon, H.-G.; Do, M.-S. B cell activation factor (BAFF) is a novel adipokine that links obesity and inflammation. *Exp. Mol. Med.* **2009**, *41*, 208–216. [CrossRef]
11. Hamada, M.; Abe, M.; Miyake, T.; Kawasaki, K.; Tada, F.; Furukawa, S.; Matsuura, B.; Hiasa, Y.; Onji, M. B cell-activating factor controls the production of adipokines and induces insulin resistance. *Obesity* **2011**, *19*, 1915–1922. [CrossRef] [PubMed]
12. Kim, M.-Y.; Kim, D.-H.; Do, M.-S. B-cell-activating factor is a regulator of adipokines and a possible mediator between adipocytes and macrophages. *Exp. Mol. Med.* **2013**, *45*, e4. [CrossRef] [PubMed]
13. Lundell, A.-C.; Nordström, I.; Andersson, K.; Lundqvist, C.; Telemo, E.; Nava, S.; Kaipe, H.; Rudin, A. IFN type I and II induce BAFF secretion from human decidual stromal cells. *Sci. Rep.* **2017**, *7*, 39904–39913. [CrossRef] [PubMed]
14. Stephens, J.M.; Lee, J.; Pilch, P.F. Tumor necrosis factor-alpha-induced insulin resistance in 3T3-L1 adipocytes is accompanied by a loss of insulin receptor substrate-1 and GLUT4 expression without a loss of insulin receptor-mediated signal transduction. *J. Biol. Chem.* **1997**, *272*, 971–976. [CrossRef] [PubMed]
15. Georgiou, H.M.; Lappas, M.; Georgiou, G.M.; Marita, A.; Bryant, V.J.; Hiscock, R.; Permezel, M.; Khalil, Z.; Rice, G.E. Screening for biomarkers predictive of gestational diabetes mellitus. *Acta Diabetol.* **2008**, *45*, 157–165. [CrossRef] [PubMed]
16. Kinalski, M.; Telejko, B.; Kuźmicki, M.; Krętowski, A.; Kinalska, I. Tumor necrosis factor alpha system and plasma adiponectin concentration in women with gestational diabetes. *Horm. Metab. Res.* **2005**, *37*, 450–454. [CrossRef]

17. Fan, P.; Liu, X.-H.; He, G.-L.; Zhang, S.; Zhang, J.-X.; Bai, H. Maternal and fetal plasma platelet-activating factor acetylhydrolase activity and distribution in pre-eclampsia. *Pediatr. Res.* **2012**, *72*, 426–431. [CrossRef]
18. Mericq, V.; Piccardo, C.; Cai, W.; Chen, X.; Zhu, L.; Striker, G.E.; Vlassara, H.; Uribarri, J. Maternally transmitted and food-derived glycotoxins: A factor preconditioning the young to diabetes? *Diabetes Care* **2010**, *33*, 2232–2237. [CrossRef]
19. Yang, G.; Cancino, G.I.; Zahr, S.K.; Guskjolen, A.; Voronova, A.; Gallagher, D.; Frankland, P.W.; Kaplan, D.R.; Miller, F.D. A Glo1-Methylglyoxal Pathway that Is Perturbed in Maternal Diabetes Regulates Embryonic and Adult Neural Stem Cell Pools in Murine Offspring. *Cell Rep.* **2016**, *17*, 1022–1036. [CrossRef]
20. Krishnasamy, S.; Rajaraman, B.; Ravi, V.; Rajagopal, R.; Ganeshprasad, A.; Kuppuswamy, A.A.; Pathak, A.; Dhevasena, C.S.; Swaminathan, K.; Sundaresan, M.; et al. Association of advanced glycation end products (AGEs) with endothelial dysfunction, oxidative stress in gestational diabetes mellitus (GDM). *Int. J. Diabetes Dev. Ctries.* **2019**, *52*, 707. [CrossRef]
21. Chang, Y.-J.; Chan, W.-H. Methylglyoxal has injurious effects on maturation of mouse oocytes, fertilization, and fetal development, via apoptosis. *Toxicol. Lett.* **2010**, *193*, 217–223. [CrossRef] [PubMed]
22. Garlick, R.L.; Mazer, J.S. The principal site of nonenzymatic glycosylation of human serum albumin in vivo. *J. Biol. Chem.* **1983**, *258*, 6142–6146. [PubMed]
23. Rondeau, P.; Bourdon, E. The glycation of albumin: Structural and functional impacts. *Biochimie* **2011**, *93*, 645–658. [CrossRef] [PubMed]
24. Danese, E.; Montagnana, M.; Nouvenne, A.; Lippi, G. Advantages and pitfalls of fructosamine and glycated albumin in the diagnosis and treatment of diabetes. *J. Diabetes Sci. Technol.* **2015**, *9*, 169–176. [CrossRef] [PubMed]
25. Sugawara, D.; Maruyama, A.; Imanishi, T.; Sugiyama, Y.; Ichihashi, K. Complications in Infants of Diabetic Mothers Related to Glycated Albumin and Hemoglobin Levels During Pregnancy. *Pediatr. Neonatol.* **2016**, *57*, 496–500. [CrossRef]
26. Shimizu, I.; Hiramatsu, Y.; Omori, Y.; Nakabayashi, M. JGA (Japan Glycated Albumin) Study Group Comparison of HbA1c and glycated albumin as a control marker for newborn complications in diabetic women in a multicentre study in Japan (Japan glycated albumin study group: Study 2). *Ann. Clin. Biochem.* **2018**, *55*, 639–646. [CrossRef]
27. Sugawara, D.; Sato, H.; Ichihashi, K.; Nagai, K.; Kawano, A. Glycated albumin level during late pregnancy as a predictive factor for neonatal outcomes of women with diabetes. *J. Matern. Fetal Neonatal Med.* **2018**, *31*, 2007–2012. [CrossRef]
28. International Association of Diabetes and Pregnancy Study Groups Consensus Panel; Metzger, B.E.; Gabbe, S.G.; Persson, B.; Buchanan, T.A.; Catalano, P.A.; Damm, P.; Dyer, A.R.; de Leiva, A.; Hod, M.; et al. International association of diabetes and pregnancy study groups recommendations on the diagnosis and classification of hyperglycemia in pregnancy. *Diabetes Care* **2010**, *33*, 676–682.
29. Lohman, T.G.; Roche, A.F.; Martorell, R. *Anthropometric Standardization Reference Manual*; Human Kinetics: Stanningley, UK, 1991.
30. Società Italiana di Nutrizione (SINU). *Recommended Assumption Levels of Energy and Nutrients for Italian Population—Livelli di Assunzione Raccomandata di Nutrienti per la Popolazione Italiana (L.A.R.N)*, 4th ed.; SICS Editore: Rome, Italy, 2014.
31. Healthy Eating Plate. Available online: https://www.hsph.harvard.edu/nutritionsource/healthy-eating-plate/ (accessed on 17 December 2019).
32. Liang, Z.; Wu, Y.; Zhu, X.; Fang, Q.; Chen, D. Insulin resistance and lipid profile during an oral glucose tolerance test in women with and without gestational diabetes mellitus. *J. Obstet. Gynaecol.* **2016**, *36*, 337–339. [CrossRef]
33. Barbour, L.A.; Hernandez, T.L. Maternal Non-Glycemic Contributors to Fetal Growth in Obesity and Gestational Diabetes: Spotlight on Lipids. *Curr. Diabetes Rep.* **2018**, *18*, 37. [CrossRef]
34. O'Malley, E.G.; Reynolds, C.M.E.; Killalea, A.; O'Kelly, R.; Sheehan, S.R.; Turner, M.J. Maternal obesity and dyslipidemia associated with gestational diabetes mellitus (GDM). *Eur. J. Obstet. Gynecol. Reprod. Biol.* **2020**, *246*, 67–71. [CrossRef] [PubMed]

35. Khosrowbeygi, A.; Rezvanfar, M.R.; Ahmadvand, H. Tumor necrosis factor- α, adiponectin and their ratio in gestational diabetes mellitus. *Casp. J. Intern. Med.* **2018**, *9*, 71–79.
36. Rodrigues, T.; Matafome, P.; Sereno, J.; Almeida, J.; Castelhano, J.; Gamas, L.; Neves, C.; Gonçalves, S.; Carvalho, C.; Arslanagic, A.; et al. Methylglyoxal-induced glycation changes adipose tissue vascular architecture, flow and expansion, leading to insulin resistance. *Sci. Rep.* **2017**, *7*, 1698–1713. [CrossRef] [PubMed]
37. Koga, M.; Murai, J.; Saito, H.; Mukai, M.; Kasayama, S. Serum glycated albumin, but not glycated hemoglobin, is low in relation to glycemia in men with hypertriglyceridemia. *J. Diabetes Investig.* **2010**, *1*, 202–207. [CrossRef] [PubMed]

13

Leptin and Nutrition in Gestational Diabetes

Antonio Pérez-Pérez [1,*], Teresa Vilariño-García [1], Pilar Guadix [2], José L. Dueñas [2] and Víctor Sánchez-Margalet [1,*]

1 Department of Medical Biochemistry and Molecular Biology, and Immnology, School of Medicine, Virgen Macarena University Hospital, 41009 Seville, Spain; tvgarcia@gmail.com
2 Obstetrics and Gynecology Service, Virgen Macarena University Hospital, 41009 Seville, Spain; pilarguadix@gmail.com (P.G.); jlduenas@us.es (J.L.D.)
* Correspondence: antonioresi@gmail.com (A.P.-P.); margalet@us.es (V.S.-M.)

Abstract: Leptin is highly expressed in the placenta, mainly by trophoblastic cells, where it has an important autocrine trophic effect. Moreover, increased leptin levels are found in the most frequent pathology of pregnancy: gestational diabetes, where leptin may mediate the increased size of the placenta and the fetus, which becomes macrosomic. In fact, leptin mediates the increased protein synthesis, as observed in trophoblasts from gestational diabetic subjects. In addition, leptin seems to facilitate nutrients transport to the fetus in gestational diabetes by increasing the expression of the glycerol transporter aquaporin-9. The high plasma leptin levels found in gestational diabetes may be potentiated by leptin resistance at a central level, and obesity-associated inflammation plays a role in this leptin resistance. Therefore, the importance of anti-inflammatory nutrients to modify the pathology of pregnancy is clear. In fact, nutritional intervention is the first-line approach for the treatment of gestational diabetes mellitus. However, more nutritional intervention studies with nutraceuticals, such as polyphenols or polyunsaturated fatty acids, or nutritional supplementation with micronutrients or probiotics in pregnant women, are needed in order to achieve a high level of evidence. In this context, the Mediterranean diet has been recently found to reduce the risk of gestational diabetes in a multicenter randomized trial. This review will focus on the impact of maternal obesity on placental inflammation and nutrients transport, considering the mechanisms by which leptin may influence maternal and fetal health in this setting, as well as its role in pregnancy pathologies.

Keywords: nutrition; polyphenolic compounds; bioactive compounds; leptin resistance; obesity; inflammation; gestational diabetes mellitus; Mediterranean diet

---

1. Introduction

Gestational diabetes (GDM) is a hyperglycemic state that is recognized for the first time during pregnancy [1], and its pathophysiology is not fully clarified yet. GDM is one of the most common complications in pregnancy, affecting 3–8% of all pregnancies [2]. This prevalence has increased in recent decades (≥20% of pregnancies in some parts of the world), both in developed and developing countries, due to increased average age of pregnant women and increased obesity [3], one of the greatest public health challenges of the 21st century. Although the GDM phenotype is highly heterogeneous [4], half of its prevalence can be explained by overweight and obesity [5]. Indeed, obese women have an increased risk of GDM compared to women of normal weight [4]. Moreover, in women with GDM, pre-pregnancy obesity, excessive gestational weight gain and poor glycemic control are also linked with others pregnancy complications, such as gestational hypertension and preeclampsia [6]. It has even been reported that excessive gestational weight gain was the variable with the greatest effect on the probability of a newborn with macrosomia (a conditions associated with an increased risk of perinatal mortality and neonatal morbidity). GDM also increases, in turn, the risk, in both mother and offspring, of developing type 2 diabetes, metabolic syndrome and obesity [7,8]. Therefore, obesity during pregnancy is an important risk factor for adverse health outcomes both in the mother and offspring, and imposes substantial economic burdens. Therefore, prevention of obesity would be directly related to a lower risk of GDM. Impaired glucose homeostasis in GDM is also related to higher production of reactive oxygen species (ROS), consequently depleting the anti-oxidative status. This is why, to restrain the spread of epidemic excess weight, women must receive a comprehensive intervention before, during, and after pregnancy. Lifestyle changes, including nutrition initiated during early pregnancy, have been unsuccessful overall in preventing GDM in at-risk obese women [9]. Now, there is a consensus regarding the need for effective interventions targeting obesity and lifestyle that reduce the metabolic burden earlier in life, well before motherhood, and it underlines that such interventions may benefit both the mother and the future offspring. Although energy restriction leading to weight loss is a successful dietary intervention for improving obesity-associated metabolic disorders, other dietary interventions, such as those leading to a reduction in adipose tissue inflammation regardless of weight loss, have not been explored in detail. In this sense, leptin, produced by adipocytes, is a key regulator of appetite and is present in elevated concentrations in obesity [10]. Therefore, new research into nutritional mechanisms that restore leptin metabolism and signals of energy homeostasis may inspire new treatment options for obesity-related disorders such as GDM. In this review, we wanted to address the current insights and emerging concepts on potentially valuable nutrients and food components to modulate leptin metabolism. Moreover, obesity is associated with a chronic low-grade inflammation in the adipose tissue [11], and several dietary food components, such as phenols, peptides, and vitamins, are able to decrease the grade of inflammation and improve leptin sensitivity by up- or down-regulation of leptin-related genes. Others food components, such as saturated fatty acids should be avoided, since they may worsen chronic inflammation, subsequently increasing the risk for pathological complications. Finally, given the crucial role that the placenta plays in mediating pregnancy outcomes, it is important to consider the impact of micronutrient supplementation on the mechanisms associated with placental function, as well as maternal and fetal homeostasis.

2. Leptin

The hormone leptin, discovered in 1994 [12], critically regulates body weight and metabolism at central level in the brain [13], and disruption of leptin/leptin receptor (LEPR) signaling results in morbid obesity and severe metabolic disease [14,15]. In individuals of normal weight, the brain responds to increased plasma leptin levels by reducing food intake and increasing energy expenditure [16,17]. Leptin and leptin receptors are highly expressed in the preoptic area (POA), in the arcuate nucleus (ARC) of the hypothalamus as well as in other regions, such as the lateral hypothalamus, ventromedial hypothalamus and dorsomedial hypothalamus (DMH) [18]. There, it regulates energy homoeostasis and the neuroendocrine function, among other functions [19]. In these regions, leptin signaling is mediated by the JAK2/Stat3 pathway, in which several negative regulators of JAK2, including SOCS3 and PTP1B, have been reported to promote obesity [20,21], supporting the notion that JAK2 inhibitory molecules increase risk for leptin resistance and obesity. Therefore, hyperleptinemia and hypothalamic inflammation in diet-induced obesity may activate a common negative regulator of leptin signaling, SOCS3 or PTP1B, and contribute to central leptin resistance. In fact, up-regulation of SOCS3 in proopiomelanocortin (POMC) neurons leads to impairment of STAT3 signaling, with consequential leptin resistance and obesity, as well as glucose intolerance [22]. It has also been reported that mice with whole body or neuron-specific deletion of PTP1B are hypersensitive to leptin, and are resistant to diet-induced obesity [23]. Importantly, obesity is associated with impaired adipose sympathetic nerve transmissions [24,25], but the underlying mechanism is poorly understood. In this context, the leptin resistance at a central level may prevent negative feedback on the anti-inflammatory action of the sympathetic nervous system (SNS) [15,26]. That is why leptin is now considered one of the adipokines responsible for the inflammatory state found in obesity that could predispose to GDM. Surprisingly, Sh2b1 (an SH2 and PH domain-containing adaptor protein) [27,28] has emerged as an endogenous sensitizer for leptin action on the sympathetic nervous system (SNS) and energy expenditure, perhaps by enhancing JAK2 activation [29]. In this way, the LepR Sh2b1 neuron mediates leptin stimulation of the SNS and supports the preservation of adipose SNS against degeneration [30].

Apart from the JAK-2/Stat-3 pathway, activation of the MC4R signaling pathway by proopiomelanocortin (POMC)-derived melanocyte stimulating hormone (MSH) peptides also represents a critical convergence point in the control of body weight. The leptin–melanocortin pathway (MC4R pathway) integrates parallel inputs from the orexigenic peptides ghrelin, neuropeptide Y (NPY) and agouti-related peptide (AgRP), and activation of the MC4R pathway dominantly counteracts these orexigens. Limited efficacy of lifestyle intervention in individuals with mutations in gene-encoding components of this pathway demonstrates its importance in the control of body weight homeostasis [31,32].

Therefore, leptin can act as metabolic switch connecting the nutritional status of the body to high energy-consuming processes. This is especially important in pregnancy, where leptin not only modulates satiety and energy homoeostasis in the mother [13,33], but it is also produced by the placenta, which responds to the environment attempting to maintain fetal viability. This placental production of leptin is one of the major sources of higher levels of maternal circulating leptin other than maternal gain of fat mass [34]. Thus, the effects of placental leptin on the mother may contribute to endocrine-mediated alterations in energy balance, such as the mobilization of maternal fat, which could further aggravate the insulin resistance associated with pregnancy and the onset of GDM [35,36]. In fact, obese pregnant women have significantly elevated plasma leptin concentrations compared with nonobese pregnant women throughout pregnancy [1]. Moreover, maternal obesity is also associated with changes in the placental function and structure, which likely impact fetal growth and development. For example, obesity has been associated with several changes related mainly with placental size, hypervascularization, higher branching capillaries of the villi (chorangiosis) [37,38] and increased glycogen deposits, among others. Increased macrophage infiltration is also evident in the placenta of obese women, suggesting an exaggeration of the inflammatory state which occurs in normal pregnancy [39]. However, it is unclear which histological changes are due to the pathophysiology and which are compensatory adaptations to this disease. Regardless, alterations in placental nutrient and hormone transporter capacity have been demonstrated in human and animal models of obesity, and are hypothesized as a mechanism leading to an accelerated fetal growth trajectory and macrosomia [1]. In this sense, we have demonstrated that the increased expression of aquaporin-9 (AQP9) (or others aquaglyceroporins) observed in placentas from obese women with GDM could be mediated by hyperleptinemia, suggesting an increase in the transport of glycerol to the fetus and thus contributing to the increased energy intake requirements in the macrosomic fetus in GDM [40]. Leptin has also been identified as a critical trophic factor that influences the development of the hypothalamic projections [40]. Alterations in the pattern of leptin secretion (premature peak, excess, or deficiency) during neonatal life could have significant adverse effects on hypothalamic development and metabolic phenotype [41] (Figure 1).

Finally, one of the peripheral functions of leptin is a regulatory role in the interplay between energy metabolism and the immune system, which is, in part, responsible for the inflammatory state associated to obesity [42]. Several inflammatory mediators produced by inflammatory cells also regulate leptin expression and promote the development of chronic inflammation [43]. In this regard, leptin effects include the inflammation and the modulation of innate and adaptive immunity [44,45]. Therefore, proinflammatory leptin actions might also have significant implications in the pathogenesis of GDM [29,46].

Taken all together, since hypothalamic inflammation results in central leptin resistance and hepatic insulin resistance [47], blocking the peripheral and central inflammation induced by a high fat diet could have the potential to treat obesity and GDM. Therefore, novel therapies incorporating effective natural agents (macro and micronutrients), particularly agents with the dual properties of preventing inflammation and controlling body weight by improving leptin sensitivity, might be an alternative intervention targeting obesity and GDM.

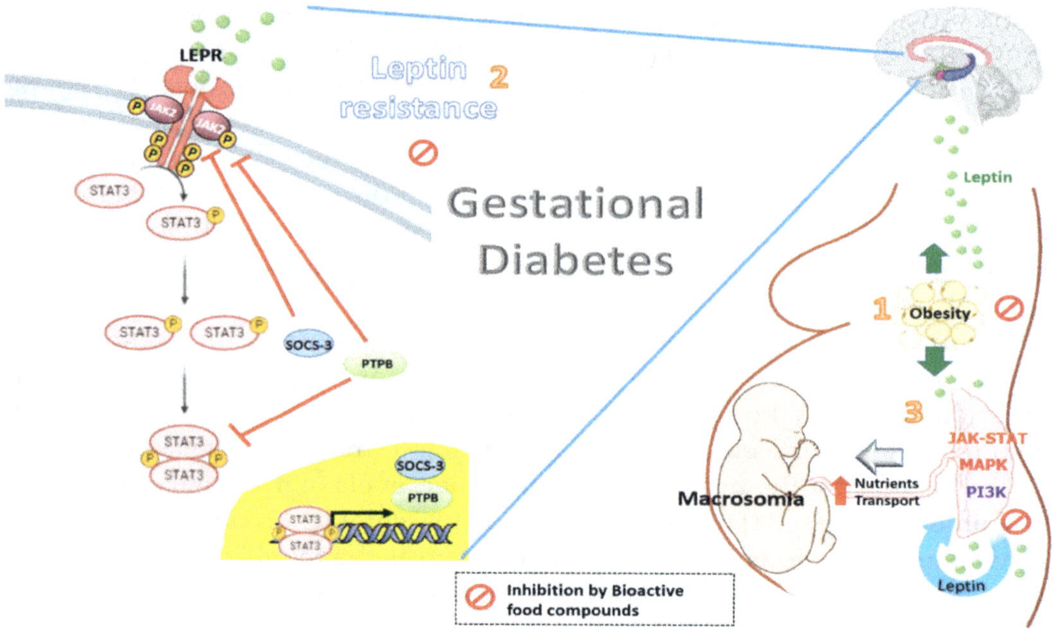

Figure 1. Effects of bioactive food compounds on the leptin resistance associated with obesity and gestational diabetes.

Leptin levels are increased in gestational diabetes with obesity (1). The high plasma leptin levels may be potentiated by leptin resistance at central level, in which SOCS3 and PTPB are induced by leptin and involving in a negative feed-back loop. The resulting effect is a decrease in the leptin-induced activation of the JAK2/STAT-3 signaling, leading to a reduction in the central effects of leptin (2). Leptin also impacts the placenta itself in an autocrine/paracrine fashion. The integration of numerous signaling by intracellular regulatory pathways such as MAPK, PI3K and JAK-STAT has been demonstrated to increase the size of the placenta and to affect placental nutrient transport and fetal growth (macrosomia) (3). Bioactive food compounds such as polyphenols might reduce circulating leptin levels, partly decreasing leptin expression in the placenta from women with GDM. The resulting effect is a decrease in the leptin resistance at a central level and optimal placental nutrients transport.

3. Nutrients and Bioactive Food Components Useful for Counteracting Hyperleptinemia and Leptin Resistance in GDM

Since the landmark Hyperglycemia and Adverse Pregnancy Outcomes (HAPO) study in 2010, an international consensus on diagnostic criteria has not been reached nearly a decade later [47]. However, there is now a consensus regarding the need for effective interventions targeting obesity. In this regard, since first-line medical (pharmaceutical) therapy has recently been called into question [48] and the socioemotional component of nutrition therapy for GDM has a dominant influence on adherence [49], other dietary strategies should be further investigated in detail. For example, since diet plays an important role in inflammation, and both obesity and GDM are considered a state of chronic inflammation, a healthy and active life style, which includes a diet rich in fruits, vegetables, non-sugared foods, non-ultra-processed foods associated with a higher prevention of inflammatory diseases should be incorporated into the diet [50]. However, a high consumption of red, processed meat, saturated or trans-fat, ultra-processed food based on refined ingredients or alcohol associated with pro-inflammatory processes should be avoided [35,36].

Since obese women and women with GDM show high circulating leptin levels and are hence considered leptin-resistant [51,52], we have identified nutritional strategies to counteract leptin resistance in both obesity and GDM. In this context, several micro- and macro-nutrients and bioactive food components might have the ability to increase leptin sensitivity and to reverse leptin resistance in obesity and GDM.

3.1. Polyphenolic Compounds

Polyphenolic compounds such as flavonoids represent an important bioactive component in plants (fruits, vegetables, legumes, tea, etc.) with some specific parts of these foods richer in flavonoids than others (for example the peel of certain fruits) [53]. The accumulation of flavonoids often occurs in plants subjected to abiotic stresses. This fact has made their determination an attractive field in food science and, in recent years, an increased number of studies have analyzed their potential benefits in human health.

As mentioned above, both the impact of nutritional status on the immune system, specially T cells [54,55] and the role of leptin as a mediator of inflammation [42], as well as a link between energy stores and the immune response, have been proposed [56,57]. In this sense, the (poly)phenols might modulate both the leptin effect and circulating leptin levels using different experimental approaches. For example, it has been reported that flavonoids have anti-inflammatory properties and thus have an important role in the control of several immune cells and immune mechanisms that are important in the inflammatory processes. More specifically, certain flavonoids (myricetin, quercetin, procyanidins) can inhibit multiple central kinases that are involved in multiple signaling pathways related to inflammation [58], such as phosphoinositol kinase, protein kinase C (PKC), phosphatidylinositol kinase and tyrosine kinase or cyclin-dependent kinase-4 [59]. Besides, flavonoids can modulate these protein kinases via inhibition of transcription factors (e.g., NF-κB and AP-1) [60]. Intriguingly, both insulin and leptin share several signaling pathways, such as mitogen-activated protein kinase (MAPK) and the phosphatidylinositol 3-kinase (PI3K) pathway, which may also activate several protein kinases involved in signal transduction during the inflammation process, via NF-κB. In this context, our group have demonstrated that the increase in placental leptin expression is mediated by NFκB signaling [61]. Therefore, in GDM, associated with insulin resistance, hyperinsulinemia and hyperleptinemia [62,63], flavonoids might downregulate the synergistic interaction between insulin and leptin signaling in the inflammatory processes. In addition, flavonoids might also decrease leptin expression in the placenta of women with GDM.

It has also been reported that high cAMP levels inhibit leptin expression by human chorionic gonadotropin (hCG), and these increased levels of cAMP have been associated with anti-inflammatory functions [64]. In this sense, flavonoids have also demonstrated the potential to block cAMP degradation and prolong cAMP signaling [65]. Finally, flavonoids may have an impact on cell activation, signaling transduction and cytokine production in several immune cells. For instance, flavonoids have been shown to inhibit maturation of dendritic cells (DCs) by suppressing the expression of CD83 and CD80, which would translate into an inhibitory effect in the secretion of pro-inflammatory cytokines [66,67]. These effects are contrary to leptin, which promotes the switch towards Th1 cell immune responses by increasing interferon-γ (IFN-γ) expression and facilitates Th17 responses. All these findings position flavonoids as modulators of immune response and, very specifically, as inhibitors of transcription factors, involved in the expression of different pro-inflammatory genes such as the leptin gene [60].

On the other hand, it is well known that the imbalance between the oxidative and anti-oxidative systems plays a crucial role in the pathogenesis of several human diseases such as obesity and diabetes, among others [68–70]. In this context, flavonoids are also potent antioxidants that are able to scavenge free radicals and decrease their formation. For example, grape juice by-products are a source of phenolic compounds with demonstrated antioxidant activities [71]. In these, the main phenolic compounds include flavones (luteolin) [71,72], flavonols (myricetin, fisetin, quercetin and kaempferol derivatives) [70,73], anthocyanins (cyanidin-3-glucoside) [74], flavan-3-ols (catechin and epicatechin monomers and proanthocyanidins) [75,76], stilbenes (resveratrol), and phenolic acids [74]. The most studied of these is resveratrol, which has been demonstrated to diminish circulating leptin levels and to reduce intake [77] by increasing phospho-STAT3 content in the hypothalamus, with no changes in SOCS3. This suggest that resveratrol might improve the leptin sensitivity in obesity [78,79]. Proanthocyanidins (PACs), known as condensed tannins, are found in a wide variety of fruits (e.g., berries), in addition to grapes, and other sources such as flowers, seeds of some plants, nuts or barks [80,81]. Plant and food-derived PACs are also attracting attention due to their ability to prevent chronic diseases [82]. For example, PACs from grape seeds and blackberry–blueberry fermented beverages have shown high anti-inflammatory and antioxidant activity in vitro [83] and have shown a broad therapeutic health effect against diabetes mellitus and obesity. In this regard, obesity and related complications such as GDM are linked with higher susceptibility to oxidative stress and the administration of grape seed extracts has shown an improvement in the oxidative status in obese people by inhibiting lipid peroxidation and avoiding ROS production [84]. Moreover, PACs can reduce inflammation by decreasing the oxidative stress or other indirect mechanisms [85]. In this sense, PACs from grape seed extract modulate IL-6, TNF-α and adiponectin gene expression in adipose tissue, thus, reducing the diet-induced low-grade inflammation [86]. PAC-rich extracts have also proved to be involved in obesity modulation (even at low doses) through the suppression of food intake and the increase in energy expenditure [87], possibly by mediating leptin levels. However, the mechanism underlying this effect of grape seed PACs has not been fully elucidated. Finally, grape seed extract improved the insulin resistance index as well as the plasma glucose and insulin levels in diet-induced obese animal models [88], although there are discrepancies in this regard.

Other bioactive food compounds have also been proven to be able to reduce circulating leptin levels in obesity. Myricetin, a bioflavonoid abundant in others fruits (e.g., berries), as well as tea and vegetables, has been shown to reduce hyperleptinemia and to favor insulin action via PI3-kinase pathway activation, and translocation of glucose transporter subtype 4 (GLUT4) to the cell membrane [89]. Accumulating evidence also suggests that propolis extracts (rich in flavonoids and cinnamic acid derivatives) have therapeutic effects on obesity by controlling adipogenesis, adipokine secretion, food intake, and energy expenditure. Particularly, considering the anorectic activity of leptin, propolis has potential to attenuate feeding and subsequently prevent obesity [90]. Moreover, various reports in animal and cellular models have demonstrated that propolis and its derived compounds improve insulin secretion and insulin sensitivity by modulating oxidative stress, the accumulation of advanced glycation end products (AGEs), and adipose tissue inflammation, all of which contribute to insulin resistance or defects in insulin secretion [91,92]. For example, several flavonoids in propolis, such as quercetin, chrysin, luteolin, amentoflavone, luteolin 7-O-glucoside and daidzein, have been found to have therapeutic effects in diabetic animal models by different mechanisms [93,94]. It has also been reported that propolis mitigates metabolic dysfunction through normalization of intestinal microflora [95]. Therefore, propolis intake might have beneficial effects for metabolic disorders such as GDM, attributable to flavonoids and natural phenols. However, propolis might have adverse effects on patients and, therefore, monitoring of biological effects should be carried out.

The polyphenols of olives and olive leaves also have numerous beneficial effects on human health, such as antioxidant capacity, hypoglycemic [96] and anti-inflammatory [97], as well as a coadjuvant role in the treatment of obesity [98]. In this sense, oleuropein, responsible for the bitter taste of olive leaves and drupes, and its derived form, the most abundant phenolic compounds present in olives and olive oils, are well known for their hypoglycemic property; possibly by the potential of affecting glucose-induced insulin release and/or increasing peripheral glucose uptake [99]. This hypoglycemic effect is also attributed, at least in part, to the antioxidant activity of oleuropein [100]. Moreover, it has been reported that oleuropein down-regulates leptin mRNA levels in epididymal adipose tissue and reduces serum leptin levels [101]. That is why the prophylactic use of oleuropein has been proposed in the reduction in complications resulting from oxidative stress in obesity and diabetes [99]. Other major phenolic components present—not only in olive extracts but in fruits (e.g., grapes), such as luteolin and luteolin-4′-O-β-D-glucopyranoside—have been shown to inhibit the formation of AGEs and, thus, might delay the development of diabetic complications [96]. However, these effects have been tested in animals and it is necessary to perform studies in humans in order to confirm the benefits attributed to polyphenols from olives in GDM.

3.2. Polyunsaturated Fatty Acids (PUFAs)

The developing fetus requires substantial amounts of fatty acids to support rapid cellular growth and activity, and especially, metabolic derivatives of the essential fatty acids such as linolenic acid (Ω-3) and linoleic acid (Ω-6) and polyunsaturated fatty acids (PUFAs) are crucial [102]. The most biologically important PUFAs are docosahexaenoic acid (DHA) and eicosapentaenoic acid (EPA) [102]. In this context, DHA appears to be crucial to the fetus and infant for early neural development (brain and visual system) [103]. However, modern dietary trends have led to an imbalance in the consumption of PUFAs, with deficiency in Ω-3 and increasing Ω-6 PUFA intake which far exceeds nutritional requirements, promoting the pathogenesis of many prevalent human diseases including GDM [104].

The placenta may play a key role in the regulation of fatty acid availability via the release of placental-derived leptin, a potent stimulator of lipolysis [105]. In fact, maternal circulating total fatty acid concentrations increase during pregnancy, enhancing placental access to fatty acids. However, as mentioned above, GDM is associated with oxidative stress and placental inflammation [106], and impaired placental fatty acid transport has been reported [107].

Given that PUFAs exhibit both anti-oxidative and anti-inflammatory activities, maternal dietary DHA and EPA supplementation has been proposed as a potential therapeutic intervention for this placenta-related disorder. For example, maternal dietary supplementation with Ω-3 PUFAs during pregnancy exerts beneficial effects such as reduced inflammation by either disrupting proinflammatory eicosanoid generation or promoting the generation of anti-inflammatory forms [108]. Moreover, it has been also reported that dietary supplementation with Ω-3 PUFAs modulates the activity of key transcription factors (peroxisome proliferator-activated receptors (PPARs) and/or nuclear factor κB (NF-κB)) and the G-protein-coupled receptor (GPR120) involved in inflammatory signaling [109–111]. Consequently, dietary supplementation with Ω-3 PUFAs might reduce risk of pregnancy complications [112] as well as the adipose tissue inflammation via GPR120-mediated suppression of macrophage proinflammatory cytokine secretion, including leptin [113]. Indeed, DHA and EPA have been shown to reduce circulating leptin levels activating the adenosine 5′-monophosphate-activated protein kinase (AMPK) pathway [114]. Another beneficial effect of the Ω-3 PUFAs on GPR120 is the increase in the translocation of intracellular vesicles containing GLUT4, which enhances glucose uptake by adipocytes [111]. Oleic acid, a monounsaturated fatty acid (MUFA), also reduces hyperleptinemia via down-regulating PPARγ mRNA levels in abdominal visceral white adipose tissue in obese mice [115]. Through modulation of adipokine secretion, these fatty acids also favor insulin sensitivity [116].

Finally, excessive oxidative stress in utero-placental tissues plays a pivotal role in the development of GDM [106]. In this context, Ω-3 PUFAs could potentially limit oxidative damage by reducing ROS generation [117]. However, it would be important to ascertain the potential risks of excessive dietary PUFA intake given the susceptibility of PUFAs to lipid peroxidation, which may exacerbate cellular damage caused by an oxidative insult [118].

All together, these findings highlight the potential benefit of dietary supplementation with PUFAs to limit oxidative damage and inflammation associated with obesity and GDM, although further research in humans is required to clarify whether these fatty acids can prevent GDM and the potential risks associated if they are used as supplements.

3.3. Terpenes

There is evidences that cafestol and/or its metabolites (kahweol), natural diterpenes extracted from coffee beans, can prevent some chronic diseases such as metabolic disease [119–121]. In this context, it has been demonstrated that cafestol promotes insulin secretion and also increased glucose uptake in muscle cells, similarly to that of antidiabetic rosiglitazone. Moreover, kahweol can activate the AMPK pathway, a central modulator of the metabolism of glucose and lipid that stimulates glucose uptake and inhibits the lipid accumulation. A large number of studies have also shown that cafestol and kahweol have anti-inflammation and antioxidant activity, as well as an inhibitory effect on cell proliferation. More specifically, cafestol blocks the AP-1 pathway to reduce PGE2 production and blocks the PI3K/Akt pathway, promoting apoptosis in tumor cells [122]. All these effects could be beneficial in the placental overgrowth observed in GDM. However, despite the fact that caffeine has been shown to activate STAT-3 via decline of ER stress in the hypothalamus [123], it has been reported that kahweol down-regulated the STAT3 signaling pathway by inhibiting its constitutive phosphorylation and activation [124], which may aggravate the leptin resistance in obesity. Therefore, further research and clinical trials are needed to confirm whether the coffee diterpenes might be used to prevent or treat GDM in humans.

Evidence has been reported regarding the effect of tea preventing obesity and abnormal glucose and lipid metabolism [125]. In this sense, in addition to phenolic components, a major bioactive component of tea extract is teasaponin, a triterpene with significant anti-inflammatory properties. More specifically, teasaponin inhibits proinflammatory cytokines by suppressing NFκB signaling upstream of IKK/IκBα [125]. The anti-inflammatory effects of teasaponin have been associated with an improved glycemic status in animal models. Moreover, teasaponin decreases the expression of hypothalamic proinflammatory cytokines as well as the inflammatory signaling in the mediobasal hypothalamus [125]. This may contribute to improved leptin sensitivity and hypothalamic leptin signaling via p-STAT3. In fact, teasaponin significantly decreases the level of SOCS3, a negative regulator of central leptin signaling in the hypothalamus of high-fat diet-induced obese mice. Therefore, teasaponin has important effects in improving glucose tolerance, central leptin sensitivity, and hypothalamic leptin signaling [125], and it might be a potential candidate as therapeutic intervention for obesity and GDM.

3.4. Probiotics

Early reports of experimental and human studies regarding the role of gut microbiota promoting gut barrier functions and controlling inflammatory responses have attracted scientific interest. The gut microbiota is highly sensitive to the diet and may be involved in fat accumulation, favoring hydrolysis and absorption of indigestible polysaccharides and, thus, excessive storage of nutrients [126,127]. In fact, a distinctive gut microbiota composition in obesity has been reported in humans [127]. For example, a lower fiber intake has been reported to be associated with reduced gut microbiota diversity and richness, greater abundance of genus associated with type 2 diabetes mellitus [128,129], and genus with known pro-inflammatory capacity [34]. Physiological weight gain during pregnancy [130,131] also influences the gut microbiota composition in parallel with weight gain, favoring a higher number of *Bifidobacterium* spp and a lower proportion of *Staphylococcus* spp [132]. These shift in microbial composition are more pronounced in obese pregnancy and women with overweight gain during pregnancy [130–133]. Therefore, a reasonable strategy to fight GDM might be based on specific probiotics, which might counteract excessive absorption and storage of nutrients by modification of the gut microbiota composition. Probiotics in GDM might balance the effect of aberrant indigenous microbiota and normalize the increased intestinal permeability, as well as the secretion of proinflammatory mediators, including leptin. Therefore, as mentioned in a clinical trial [134], specific probiotics or probiotic foods might be used as dietary adjuncts to reduce the risk of diseases associated with aberrant gut microbiota composition, increased intestinal permeability or altered immunological or metabolic balance such as GDM. In fact, the impact of probiotics on GDM might be more pronounced in a high-risk population (e.g., obesity). Moreover, probiotics supplementation would not only affect the maternal metabolic state, but would also modulate fetal physiology and might have a long-term programming effect on child health [135–137]. However, current knowledge about gut microbiota and diet response in pregnancy complicated by GDM is limited and future studies that integrate genetics and clinical variables should be taken into account.

3.5. Others Bioactive Compounds

Lycopene is a lipophilic carotenoid which is responsible for the red color in various vegetables and fruits, and is commonly found in tomatoes [138,139]. This carotenoid is known for its antioxidant and anti-inflammatory effects [140], and has been reported to improve diseases with chronic inflammatory backgrounds such as obesity. As mentioned above, hyperleptinemia is associated with pro-inflammatory responses and with the chronic subinflammatory state observed in obesity [141]. In this context, it has been suggested that lycopene supplementation may attenuate the inflammatory response in obesity, at least in part, by minimizing hyperleptinemia [142,143]. Other bioactive compounds of many cruciferous vegetables (e.g., watercress and broccoli) are isothiocyanates (ITCs), characterized by the presence of thiol-reactive chemicals that can modify critical cysteine residues on a variety of cellular proteins [144–146]. As mentioned above, accumulating evidence suggests that PTP1B could be involved in the pathways leading to leptin resistance as a major negative regulator of leptin and insulin signaling. In this sense, ITCs have been found to inactivate PTP1B [147,148], which has a reactive cysteine residue at the catalytic center [147]. Particularly, phenethyl isothiocyanate (PEITC), a relatively nontoxic constituent, in addition to inhibiting cellular PTP1B activity, has been demonstrated to enhance phosphorylation of LEPRb, JAK2, and STAT3 in the hypothalamus, resulting in the stimulation of leptin signaling and significantly reduced food intake [149].

3.6. Micronutrients

Micronutrients include numerous minerals and vitamins derived from the diet that are essential for cellular metabolism and optimal tissue function. It has been reported that an adequate supply of micronutrients during pregnancy may significantly reduce the risk of developing disorders of pregnancy, including GDM [150]. Throughout the course of pregnancy, there may be increased risk of micronutrient deficiency in response to the requirements of the growing fetus [151]. Therefore, although a healthy diet would be the ideal way to cover the micronutrient requirements, it is possible that the physiological challenge of pregnancy might require additional nutritional support of micronutrients [152]. The majority of supplements on the market contain a wide variety of vitamins (B group vitamins, vitamins C, D, E and folate) and minerals (iron, copper, zinc, iodine, selenium [153]. However, despite the benefits of micronutrients in supporting maternal, placental, and fetal homeostasis during pregnancy [152,154], insignificant evidence and varied results have been noted upon randomized trials of supplementation [155]. Such variability may be linked to variations in specific micronutrient supplement preparations and population contexts [155]. Therefore, the possibility that micronutrients supplementation could prevent complications of pregnancy warrants further investigation with larger trials in this field [151].

4. Mediterranean Diet

Despite the publication of numerous randomized trials on diet and lifestyle interventions in pregnancy [156], as mentioned above, no clear dietary recommendations have emerged to improve pregnancy outcomes for women with metabolic risk factors, particularly GDM. This can be attributed to the lack of robust evidence on effectiveness of the diet [157]. The traditional diet, "Mediterranean diet", has long been associated with preventive activity against chronic inflammation-associated diseases, which are supported by observational and epidemiological data. The Mediterranean-style diet includes components such as a high intake of nuts, extra virgin olive oil, fruit, vegetables, non-refined grains, legumes and micronutrients, as well as moderate to high consumption of fish and low consumption of processed meat, sugary drinks, fast food, and food rich in animal fat [158]. These key components of this diet might help to control the activity of obesity and GDM as well as other inflammatory pathologies. In fact, the Mediterranean diet has been recently found to reduce the risk of GDM in a multicenter randomized trial [159]. It is possible that this beneficial effect on GDM could be due to the high intake of dietary polyphenols and micronutrients found in key components of the Mediterranean diet, such as extra virgin olive oil, grapes and nuts, which together activate insulin receptors, increase the uptake of glucose in the insulin-sensitive tissues, stimulate insulin secretion, and reduce insulin and leptin resistance. However, it should be stressed that the Mediterranean diet is a complex matrix of compounds and its biological activity cannot be attributable only to polyphenols and micronutrients. In fact, it is very likely that compounds of this diet could have not only additive, but also synergic or complementary activities to phenolic components. With the growing incidence of obesity and GDM, health effects of the Mediterranean diet and its multiple bioactive components will be of relevance not only in the treatment of obesity and GDM but, perhaps more importantly, also in their prevention. Therefore, a simple, individualized, Mediterranean-style diet in pregnancy could have the potential to reduce gestational weight gain and the risk of GDM. Figure 2 summarizes the 442 preventive effects of nutrients from the Mediterranean diet on leptin resistance.

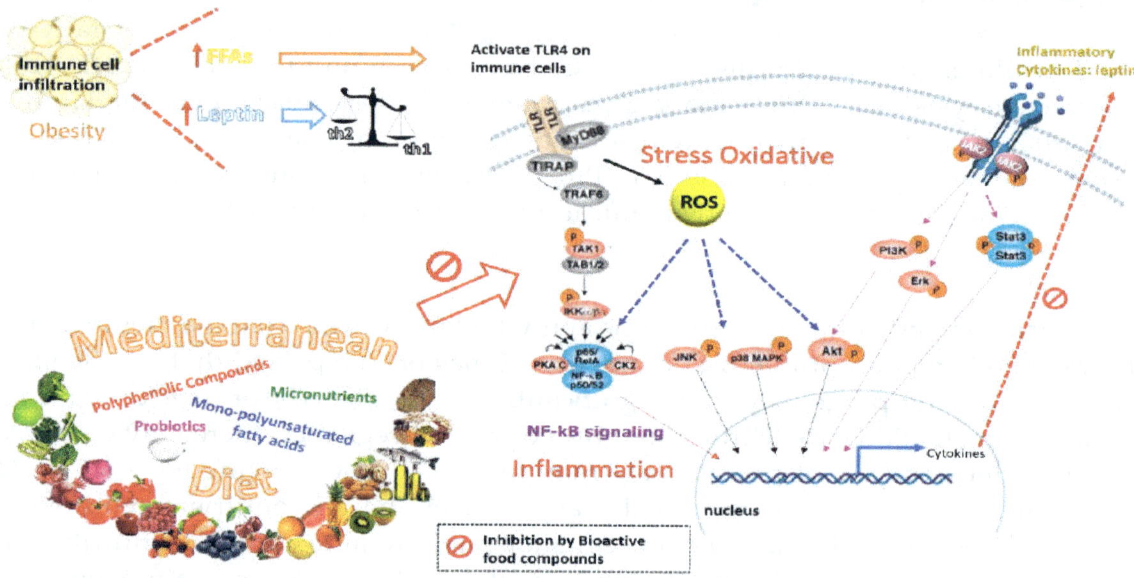

Figure 2. Effects of the Mediterranean diet on the oxidative stress and inflammation associated with obesity and gestational diabetes. Obesity and GDM are linked with higher susceptibility to oxidative stress and inflammation. Adipocyte hypertrophy results in elevated circulation of free fatty acids (FFAs) and increased secretion of leptin, which drives T cells toward a pro-inflammatory phenotype (Th1). These in turn result in immune cell infiltration and the activation of pro-inflammatory signaling pathways. Bioactive food compounds in the Mediterranean diet such as polyphenols exert their anti-inflammatory activity by inhibiting ROS production and inhibiting multiple central kinases that are involved in multiple signaling pathways related to inflammation, such as NF-κB, MAPKs and PI3/Akt signaling pathways.

5. Conclusions

The high social and economic impact of the growing incidence of obesity and GDM have strongly motivated original investigations and the search for novel and rational preventive strategies. Data reported in the literature, and gathered in this review, show that there is scientific evidence supporting the anti-obesity effect of several bioactive compounds present in the Mediterranean diet. In parallel with the reduction in body fat accumulation, other features which are typical of pregnancy with obesity, such as GDM, increased leptin and insulin resistance, stress oxidative and low-grade inflammation, are also improved by these bioactive compounds. Some of the mechanisms of action underlying these effects have been revealed by preclinical studies. Particularly, the leptin sensitivity effect of polyphenolic compounds (one of the most interesting group of bioactive compounds), as well as the improvement of several comorbidities observed in GDM, has also been detailed. However, despite the publication of numerous studies on diet and lifestyle interventions in pregnancy, no clear dietary recommendations have emerged to improve pregnancy outcomes for women with metabolic risk factors. In this regard, observational evidence on the Mediterranean-style diet intervention in pregnancy and potential reductions in weight gain and the risk of gestational diabetes should be taken into account. The key components of this diet include, at the very least, a high intake of polyphenolic and other bioactive compounds. It addresses some important benefits by using additional non-pharmacological therapy that is based on natural compounds and, moreover, it would be feasible to implement in pregnant women. It should be pointed out that future studies should investigate which bioactive compounds present in the Mediterranean diet are responsible for their effects, as well as the potential synergies between them. This strategy would be helpful to find new therapeutic interventions to prevent or treat GDM.

Acknowledgments: The present work was partly funded by grants from the Instituto de Salud Carlos III (ISCIII), PS12/00117, and PI15/01535, funded in part by FEDER Funds, to Víctor Sánchez-Margalet.

References

1. Yan, B.; Yu, Y.; Lin, M.; Li, Z.; Wang, L.; Huang, P.; Song, H.; Shi, X.; Yang, S.; Li, X.; et al. High, but stable, trend in the prevalence of gestational diabetes mellitus: A population-based study in Xiamen, China. *J. Diabetes Investig.* **2019**, *10*, 1358–1364. [CrossRef] [PubMed]
2. Uzelac, P.S.; Li, X.; Lin, J.; Neese, L.D.; Lin, L.; Nakajima, S.T.; Bohler, H.; Lei, Z. Dysregulation of leptin and testosterone production and their receptor expression in the human placenta with gestational diabetes mellitus. *Placenta* **2010**, *31*, 581–588. [CrossRef] [PubMed]
3. Ferrara, A. Increasing prevalence of gestational diabetes mellitus: A public health perspective. *Diabetes Care* **2007**, *30*, S141–S146. [CrossRef] [PubMed]
4. Powe, C.E.; Allard, C.; Battista, M.-C.; Doyon, M.; Bouchard, L.; Ecker, J.L.; Perron, P.; Florez, J.C.; Thadhani, R.; Hivert, M.-F. Heterogeneous contribution of insulin sensitivity and secretion defects to gestational diabetes mellitus. *Diabetes Care* **2016**, *39*, 1052–1055. [CrossRef]
5. Kim, S.Y.; England, L.; Wilson, H.G.; Bish, C.; Satten, G.A.; Dietz, P. Percentage of gestational diabetes mellitus attributable to overweight and obesity. *Am. J. Public Health* **2010**, *100*, 1047–1052. [CrossRef]
6. Weissgerber, T.L.; Mudd, L.M. Preeclampsia and diabetes. *Curr. Diab. Rep.* **2015**, *15*, 9. [CrossRef]
7. Lee, A.J.; Hiscock, R.J.; Wein, P.; Walker, S.P.; Permezel, M. Gestational diabetes mellitus: Clinical predictors and long-term risk of developing type 2 diabetes: A retrospective cohort study using survival analysis. *Diabetes Care* **2007**, *30*, 878–883. [CrossRef]
8. Thadhani, R.; Powe, C.E.; Tjoa, M.L.; Khankin, E.; Ye, J.; Ecker, J.; Schneyer, A.; Karumanchi, S.A. First-trimester follistatin-like-3 levels in pregnancies complicated by subsequent gestational diabetes mellitus. *Diabetes Care* **2010**, *33*, 664–669. [CrossRef]
9. Poston, L.; Bell, R.; Croker, H.; Flynn, A.C.; Godfrey, K.M.; Goff, L.; Hayes, L.; Khazaezadeh, N.; Nelson, S.M.; Oteng-Ntim, E.; et al. Effect of a behavioural intervention in obese pregnant women (the UPBEAT study): A multicentre, randomised controlled trial. *Lancet Diabetes Endocrinol.* **2015**, *3*, 767–777. [CrossRef]
10. Singla, P.; Bardoloi, A.; Parkash, A.A. Metabolic effects of obesity: A review. *World J. Diabetes* **2010**, *1*, 76–88. [CrossRef]
11. Wellen, K.E.; Hotamisligil, G.S. Inflammation, stress, and diabetes. *J. Clin. Invest.* **2005**, *115*, 1111–1119. [CrossRef] [PubMed]
12. Zhang, Y.; Proenca, R.; Maffei, M.; Barone, M.; Leopold, L.; Friedman, J.M. Positional cloning of the mouse obese gene and its human homologue. *Nature* **1994**, *372*, 425–432. [CrossRef] [PubMed]
13. Friedman, J.M.; Halaas, J.L. Leptin and the regulation of body weight in mammals. *Nature* **1998**, *395*, 763–770. [CrossRef] [PubMed]
14. Zhang, Y.; Chua, S. Leptin function and regulation. *Compr. Physiol.* **2018**, *8*, 351–369. [CrossRef]
15. Zhou, Y.; Rui, L. Leptin signaling and leptin resistance. *Front. Med.* **2013**, *7*, 207–222. [CrossRef]
16. Harris, R.B.S.; Apolzan, J.W. Changes in glucose tolerance and leptin responsiveness of rats offered a choice of lard, sucrose, and chow. *Am. J. Physiol. Regul. Integr. Comp. Physiol.* **2012**, *302*, R1327–R1339. [CrossRef]

17. van den Heuvel, J.K.; Eggels, L.; van Rozen, A.J.; Luijendijk, M.C.M.; Fliers, E.; Kalsbeek, A.; Adan, R.A.H.; la Fleur, S.E. Neuropeptide Y and leptin sensitivity is dependent on diet composition. *J. Neuroendocrinol.* **2014**, *26*, 377–385. [CrossRef]
18. Håkansson, M.L.; Brown, H.; Ghilardi, N.; Skoda, R.C.; Meister, B. Leptin receptor immunoreactivity in chemically defined target neurons of the hypothalamus. *J. Neurosci.* **1998**, *18*, 559–572. [CrossRef]
19. Park, H.K.; Ahima, R.S. Leptin signaling. *F1000Prime Rep.* **2014**, *6*, 73. [CrossRef]
20. Matarazzo, V.; Schaller, F.; Nédélec, E.; Benani, A.; Pénicaud, L.; Muscatelli, F.; Moyse, E.; Bauer, S. Inactivation of Socs3 in the hypothalamus enhances the hindbrain response to endogenous satiety signals via oxytocin signaling. *J. Neurosci.* **2012**, *32*, 17097–17107. [CrossRef]
21. Cheng, A.; Uetani, N.; Simoncic, P.D.; Chaubey, V.P.; Lee-Loy, A.; McGlade, C.J.; Kennedy, B.P.; Tremblay, M.L. Attenuation of leptin action and regulation of obesity by protein tyrosine phosphatase 1B. *Dev. Cell* **2002**, *2*, 497–503. [CrossRef]
22. Reed, A.S.; Unger, E.K.; Olofsson, L.E.; Piper, M.L.; Myers, M.G.; Xu, A.W. Functional role of suppressor of cytokine signaling 3 upregulation in hypothalamic leptin resistance and long-term energy homeostasis. *Diabetes* **2010**, *59*, 894–906. [CrossRef] [PubMed]
23. Bence, K.K.; Delibegovic, M.; Xue, B.; Gorgun, C.Z.; Hotamisligil, G.S.; Neel, B.G.; Kahn, B.B. Neuronal PTP1B regulates body weight, adiposity and leptin action. *Nat. Med.* **2006**, *12*, 917–924. [CrossRef]
24. Dodt, C.; Lönnroth, P.; Fehm, H.L.; Elam, M. The subcutaneous lipolytic response to regional neural stimulation is reduced in obese women. *Diabetes* **2000**, *49*, 1875–1879. [CrossRef]
25. Coppack, S.W.; Horowitz, J.F.; Paramore, D.S.; Cryer, P.E.; Royal, H.D.; Klein, S. Whole body, adipose tissue, and forearm norepinephrine kinetics in lean and obese women. *Am. J. Physiol. Endocrinol. Metab.* **1998**, *275*. [CrossRef]
26. Morris, D.L.; Rui, L. Recent advances in understanding leptin signaling and leptin resistance. *Am. J. Physiol. Endocrinol. Metab.* **2009**, *297*, E1247–E1259. [CrossRef]
27. Li, Z.; Zhou, Y.; Carter-Su, C.; Myers, M.G.; Rui, L. SH2B1 enhances leptin signaling by both janus kinase 2 Tyr813 phosphorylation-dependent and -independent mechanisms. *Mol. Endocrinol.* **2007**, *21*, 2270–2281. [CrossRef] [PubMed]
28. Duan, C.; Li, M.; Rui, L. SH2-B promotes insulin receptor substrate 1 (IRS1)- and IRS2-mediated activation of the phosphatidylinositol 3-kinase pathway in response to leptin. *J. Biol. Chem.* **2004**, *279*, 43684–43691. [CrossRef]
29. Pérez-Pérez, A.; Toro, A.; Vilariño-García, T.; Maymó, J.; Guadix, P.; Dueñas, J.L.; Fernández-Sánchez, M.; Varone, C.; Sánchez-Margalet, V. Leptin action in normal and pathological pregnancies. *J. Cell. Mol. Med.* **2018**, *22*, 716–727. [CrossRef]
30. Jiang, L.; Su, H.; Wu, X.; Shen, H.; Kim, M.H.; Li, Y.; Myers, M.G.; Owyang, C.; Rui, L. Leptin receptor-expressing neuron Sh2b1 supports sympathetic nervous system and protects against obesity and metabolic disease. *Nat. Commun.* **2020**, *11*. [CrossRef]
31. Farooqi, I.S.; O'Rahilly, S. 20 years of leptin: Human disorders of leptin action. *J. Endocrinol.* **2014**, *223*, T63–T70. [CrossRef] [PubMed]
32. Krishna, R.; Gumbiner, B.; Stevens, C.; Musser, B.; Mallick, M.; Suryawanshi, S.; Maganti, L.; Zhu, H.; Han, T.H.; Scherer, L.; et al. Potent and selective agonism of the melanocortin receptor 4 with MK-0493 does not induce weight loss in obese human subjects: Energy intake predicts lack of weight loss efficacy. *Clin. Pharmacol. Ther.* **2009**, *86*, 659–666. [CrossRef] [PubMed]
33. Houseknecht, K.L.; Portocarrero, C.P. Leptin and its receptors: Regulators of whole-body energy homeostasis. *Domest. Anim. Endocrinol.* **1998**, *15*, 457–475. [CrossRef]
34. Lin, K.C. Increase of maternal plasma leptin concentrations during pregnancy: Comparison with nonpregnant women. *Kaohsiung J. Med. Sci.* **1999**, *15*, 640–645. [PubMed]
35. Grivennikov, S.I.; Greten, F.R.; Karin, M. Immunity, inflammation, and cancer. *Cell* **2010**, *140*, 883–899. [CrossRef] [PubMed]
36. Bouvard, V.; Loomis, D.; Guyton, K.Z.; Grosse, Y.; Ghissassi, F.E.; Benbrahim-Tallaa, L.; Guha, N.; Mattock, H.; Straif, K.; Stewart, B.W.; et al. Carcinogenicity of consumption of red and processed meat. *Lancet Oncol.* **2015**, *16*, 1599–1600. [CrossRef]
37. Higgins, M.; Felle, P.; Mooney, E.E.; Bannigan, J.; McAuliffe, F.M. Stereology of the placenta in type 1 and type 2 diabetes. *Placenta* **2011**, *32*, 564–569. [CrossRef]

38. Jirkovská, M.; Kučera, T.; Kaláb, J.; Jadrníček, M.; Niedobová, V.; Janáček, J.; Kubínová, L.; Moravcová, M.; Zižka, Z.; Krejčí, V. The branching pattern of villous capillaries and structural changes of placental terminal villi in type 1 diabetes mellitus. *Placenta* **2012**, *33*, 343–351. [CrossRef]
39. Roberts, K.A.; Riley, S.C.; Reynolds, R.M.; Barr, S.; Evans, M.; Statham, A.; Hor, K.; Jabbour, H.N.; Norman, J.E.; Denison, F.C. Placental structure and inflammation in pregnancies associated with obesity. *Placenta* **2011**, *32*, 247–254. [CrossRef]
40. Vilariño-García, T.; Pérez-Pérez, A.; Dietrich, V.; Fernández-Sánchez, M.; Guadix, P.; Dueñas, J.L.; Varone, C.L.; Damiano, A.E.; Sánchez-Margalet, V. Increased expression of aquaporin 9 in trophoblast from gestational diabetic patients. *Horm. Metab. Res.* **2016**, *48*, 535–539. [CrossRef]
41. Yura, S.; Itoh, H.; Sagawa, N.; Yamamoto, H.; Masuzaki, H.; Nakao, K.; Kawamura, M.; Takemura, M.; Kakui, K.; Ogawa, Y.; et al. Role of premature leptin surge in obesity resulting from intrauterine undernutrition. *Cell Metab.* **2005**, *1*, 371–378. [CrossRef] [PubMed]
42. Pérez-Pérez, A.; Vilariño-García, T.; Fernández-Riejos, P.; Martín-González, J.; Segura-Egea, J.J.; Sánchez-Margalet, V. Role of leptin as a link between metabolism and the immune system. *Cytokine Growth Factor Rev.* **2017**, *35*, 71–84. [CrossRef] [PubMed]
43. Lago, F.; Dieguez, C.; Gómez-Reino, J.; Gualillo, O. The emerging role of adipokines as mediators of inflammation and immune responses. *Cytokine Growth Factor Rev.* **2007**, *18*, 313–325. [CrossRef] [PubMed]
44. Sánchez-Margalet, V.; Martín-Romero, C.; Santos-Alvarez, J.; Goberna, R.; Najib, S.; Gonzalez-Yanes, C. Role of leptin as an immunomodulator of blood mononuclear cells: Mechanisms of action. *Clin. Exp. Immunol.* **2003**, *133*, 11–19. [CrossRef]
45. Martín-Romero, C.; Santos-Alvarez, J.; Goberna, R.; Sánchez-Margalet, V. Human leptin enhances activation and proliferation of human circulating T lymphocytes. *Cell. Immunol.* **2000**, *199*, 15–24. [CrossRef]
46. Qiu, C.; Williams, M.A.; Vadachkoria, S.; Frederick, I.O.; Luthy, D.A. Increased maternal plasma leptin in early pregnancy and risk of gestational diabetes mellitus. *Obstet. Gynecol.* **2004**, *103*, 519–525. [CrossRef]
47. Cai, D.; Liu, T. Hypothalamic inflammation: A double-edged sword to nutritional diseases. *Ann. N. Y. Acad. Sci.* **2011**, *1243*, E1–E39. [CrossRef]
48. SMFM Statement: Pharmacological treatment of gestational diabetes SMFM Publications Committee. *Am. J. Obstet. Gynecol.* **2018**, *218*, B2–B4. [CrossRef]
49. Ge, L.; Wikby, K.; Rask, M. Is gestational diabetes a severe illness? Exploring beliefs and self-care behaviour among women with gestational diabetes living in a rural area of the south east of China. *Aust. J. Rural Health* **2016**, *24*, 378–384. [CrossRef]
50. Schwingshackl, L.; Chaimani, A.; Hoffmann, G.; Schwedhelm, C.; Boeing, H. A network meta-analysis on the comparative efficacy of different dietary approaches on glycaemic control in patients with type 2 diabetes mellitus. *Eur. J. Epidemiol.* **2018**, *33*, 157–170. [CrossRef]
51. Münzberg, H.; Flier, J.S.; Bjørbæk, C. Region-specific leptin resistance within the hypothalamus of diet-induced obese mice. *Endocrinology* **2004**, *145*, 4880–4889. [CrossRef]
52. Scarpace, P.J.; Matheny, M.; Tümer, N.; Cheng, K.Y.; Zhang, Y. Leptin resistance exacerbates diet-induced obesity and is associated with diminished maximal leptin signalling capacity in rats. *Diabetologia* **2005**, *48*, 1075–1083. [CrossRef] [PubMed]
53. Li, X.; Wang, T.; Zhou, B.; Gao, W.; Cao, J.; Huang, L. Chemical composition and antioxidant and anti-inflammatory potential of peels and flesh from 10 different pear varieties (*Pyrus* spp.). *Food Chem.* **2014**, *152*, 531–538. [CrossRef]
54. Cohen, S.; Danzaki, K.; MacIver, N.J. Nutritional effects on T-cell immunometabolism. *Eur. J. Immunol.* **2017**, *47*, 225–235. [CrossRef]
55. Alwarawrah, Y.; Kiernan, K.; MacIver, N.J. Changes in nutritional status impact immune cell metabolism and function. *Front. Immunol.* **2018**, *9*, 1055. [CrossRef] [PubMed]
56. Faggioni, R.; Feingold, K.R.; Grunfeld, C. Leptin regulation of the immune response and the immunodeficiency of malnutrition. *FASEB J.* **2001**, *15*, 2565–2571. [CrossRef] [PubMed]
57. Lord, G.M.; Matarese, G.; Howard, J.K.; Baker, R.J.; Bloom, S.R.; Lechler, R.I. Leptin modulates the T-cell immune response and reverses starvation-induced immunosuppression. *Nature* **1998**, *394*, 897–901. [CrossRef]
58. Hou, D.X.; Kumamoto, T. Flavonoids as protein kinase inhibitors for cancer chemoprevention: Direct binding and molecular modeling. *Antioxid. Redox Signal.* **2010**, *13*, 691–719. [CrossRef]

59. Yokoyama, T.; Kosaka, Y.; Mizuguchi, M. Structural insight into the interactions between death-associated protein kinase 1 and natural flavonoids. *J. Med. Chem.* **2015**, *58*, 7400–7408. [CrossRef] [PubMed]
60. Lin, Y.; Bai, L.; Chen, W.; Xu, S. The NF-κB activation pathways, emerging molecular targets for cancer prevention and therapy. *Expert Opin. Ther. Targets* **2010**, *14*, 45–55. [CrossRef]
61. Schanton, M.; Pérez-Pérez, A.; Gambino, Y.; Maskin, B.; Sánchez-Margalet, V.; Varone, C. Placental leptin expression is mediated by NFκB signaling. *Placenta* **2018**, *62*, 79. [CrossRef] [PubMed]
62. Araújo, J.R.; Keating, E.; Martel, F. Impact of gestational diabetes mellitus in the maternal-to-fetal transport of nutrients. *Curr. Diab. Rep.* **2015**, *15*, 569. [CrossRef]
63. Desoye, G.; Hauguel-De Mouzon, S. The human placenta in gestational diabetes mellitus: The insulin and cytokine network. *Diabetes Care* **2007**, *30*. [CrossRef] [PubMed]
64. Maymó, J.L.; Pérez Pérez, A.; Dueñas, J.L.; Calvo, J.C.; Sánchez-Margalet, V.; Varone, C.L. Regulation of placental leptin expression by cyclic adenosine 5′-monophosphate involves cross talk between protein kinase A and mitogen-activated protein kinase signaling pathways. *Endocrinology* **2010**, *151*, 3738–3751. [CrossRef] [PubMed]
65. Wahlang, B.; McClain, C.; Barve, S.; Gobejishvili, L. Role of cAMP and phosphodiesterase signaling in liver health and disease. *Cell. Signal.* **2018**, *49*, 105–115. [CrossRef]
66. Masilamani, M.; Wei, J.; Bhatt, S.; Paul, M.; Yakir, S.; Sampson, H.A. Soybean isoflavones regulate dendritic cell function and suppress allergic sensitization to peanut. *J. Allergy Clin. Immunol.* **2011**, *128*, 1242–1250.e1. [CrossRef]
67. Lin, W.; Wang, W.; Wang, D.; Ling, W. Quercetin protects against atherosclerosis by inhibiting dendritic cell activation. *Mol. Nutr. Food Res.* **2017**, *61*. [CrossRef]
68. D'Ambrosio, D.; Panina-Bordignon, P.; Sinigaglia, F. Chemokine receptors in inflammation: An overview. *J. Immunol. Methods* **2003**, *273*, 3–13. [CrossRef]
69. Shen, Y.C.; Chiou, W.F.; Chou, Y.C.; Chen, C.F. Mechanisms in mediating the anti-inflammatory effects of baicalin and baicalein in human leukocytes. *Eur. J. Pharmacol.* **2003**, *465*, 171–181. [CrossRef]
70. Feldmann, M. Development of anti-TNF therapy for rheumatoid arthritis. *Nat. Rev. Immunol.* **2002**, *2*, 364–371. [CrossRef]
71. Andreakos, E.T.; Foxwell, B.M.; Brennan, F.M.; Maini, R.N.; Feldmann, M. Cytokines and anti-cytokine biologicals in autoimmunity: Present and future. *Cytokine Growth Factor Rev.* **2000**, *13*, 299–313. [CrossRef]
72. Di Carlo, G.; Mascolo, N.; Izzo, A.A.; Capasso, F. Flavonoids: Old and new aspects of a class of natural therapeutic drugs. *Life Sci.* **1999**, *65*, 337–353. [CrossRef]
73. Middleton, E. Effect of plant flavonoids on immune and inflammatory cell function. *Adv. Exp. Med. Biol.* **1998**, *439*, 175–182. [CrossRef] [PubMed]
74. Habtemariam, S. Natural inhibitors of tumour necrosis factor-alpha production, secretion and function. *Planta Med.* **2000**, *66*, 303–313. [CrossRef] [PubMed]
75. Kotanidou, A.; Xagorari, A.; Bagli, E.; Kitsanta, P.; Fotsis, T.; Papapetropoulos, A.; Roussos, C. Luteolin reduces lipopolysaccharide-induced lethal toxicity and expression of proinflammatory molecules in mice. *Am. J. Respir. Crit. Care Med.* **2002**, *165*, 818–823. [CrossRef]
76. Xagorari, A.; Papapetropoulos, A.; Mauromatis, A.; Economou, M.; Fotsis, T.; Roussos, C. Luteolin inhibits an endotoxin-stimulated phosphorylation cascade and proinflammatory cytokine production in macrophages. *J. Pharmacol. Exp. Ther.* **2001**, *296*, 181–187.
77. Franco, J.G.; Dias-Rocha, C.P.; Fernandes, T.P.; Albuquerque Maia, L.; Lisboa, P.C.; Moura, E.G.; Pazos-Moura, C.C.; Trevenzoli, I.H. Resveratrol treatment rescues hyperleptinemia and improves hypothalamic leptin signaling programmed by maternal high-fat diet in rats. *Eur. J. Nutr.* **2016**, *55*, 601–610. [CrossRef]
78. Ardid-Ruiz, A.; Ibars, M.; Mena, P.; Del Rio, D.; Muguerza, B.; Bladé, C.; Arola, L.; Aragonès, G.; Suárez, M. Potential involvement of peripheral leptin/STAT3 signaling in the effects of resveratrol and its metabolites on reducing body fat accumulation. *Nutrients* **2018**, *10*. [CrossRef]
79. Ibars, M.; Ardid-Ruiz, A.; Suárez, M.; Muguerza, B.; Bladé, C.; Aragonès, G. Proanthocyanidins potentiate hypothalamic leptin/STAT3 signalling and Pomc gene expression in rats with diet-induced obesity. *Int. J. Obes.* **2017**, *41*, 129–136. [CrossRef]
80. Zhu, F. Proanthocyanidins in cereals and pseudocereals. *Crit. Rev. Food Sci. Nutr.* **2019**, *59*, 1521–1533. [CrossRef]

81. Neilson, A.P.; O'Keefe, S.F.; Bolling, B.W. High-molecular-weight proanthocyanidins in foods: Overcoming analytical challenges in pursuit of novel dietary bioactive components. *Annu. Rev. Food Sci. Technol.* **2016**, *7*, 43–64. [CrossRef] [PubMed]
82. Nie, Y.; Stürzenbaum, S.R. Proanthocyanidins of natural origin: Molecular mechanisms and implications for lipid disorder and aging-associated diseases. *Adv. Nutr.* **2019**, *10*, 464–478. [CrossRef] [PubMed]
83. Hopmans, T.E.P.; van Houten, C.; Kasius, A.; Kouznetsova, O.I.; Nguyen, L.A.; Rooijmans, S.V.; Voormolen, D.N.; van Vliet, E.O.G.; Franx, A.; Koster, M.P.H.W. Increased risk of type II diabetes mellitus and cardiovascular disease after gestational diabetes mellitus: A systematic review. *Ned. Tijdschr. Geneeskd.* **2015**, *159*, A8043. [PubMed]
84. Thiruchenduran, M.; Vijayan, N.A.; Sawaminathan, J.K.; Devaraj, S.N. Protective effect of grape seed proanthocyanidins against cholesterol cholic acid diet-induced hypercholesterolemia in rats. *Cardiovasc. Pathol.* **2011**, *20*, 361–368. [CrossRef] [PubMed]
85. Weseler, A.R.; Bast, A. Masquelier's grape seed extract: From basic flavonoid research to a well-characterized food supplement with health benefits. *Nutr. J.* **2017**, *16*, 5. [CrossRef] [PubMed]
86. Terra, X.; Montagut, G.; Bustos, M.; Llopiz, N.; Ardèvol, A.; Bladé, C.; Fernández-Larrea, J.; Pujadas, G.; Salvadó, J.; Arola, L.; et al. Grape-seed procyanidins prevent low-grade inflammation by modulating cytokine expression in rats fed a high-fat diet. *J. Nutr. Biochem.* **2009**, *20*, 210–218. [CrossRef] [PubMed]
87. Chen, F.; Wang, H.; Zhao, J.; Yan, J.; Meng, H.; Zhan, H.; Chen, L.; Yuan, L. Grape seed proanthocyanidin inhibits monocrotaline-induced pulmonary arterial hypertension via attenuating inflammation: In vivo and in vitro studies. *J. Nutr. Biochem.* **2019**, *67*, 72–77. [CrossRef]
88. Pascual-Serrano, A.; Arola-Arnal, A.; Suárez-García, S.; Bravo, F.I.; Suárez, M.; Arola, L.; Bladé, C. Grape seed proanthocyanidin supplementation reduces adipocyte size and increases adipocyte number in obese rats. *Int. J. Obes.* **2017**, *41*, 1246–1255. [CrossRef]
89. Choi, H.N.; Kang, M.J.; Lee, S.J.; Kim, J.I. Ameliorative effect of myricetin on insulin resistance in mice fed a high-fat, high-Sucrose diet. *Nutr. Res. Pract.* **2014**, *8*, 544–549. [CrossRef]
90. Washio, K.; Shimamoto, Y.; Kitamura, H. Brazilian propolis extract increases leptin expression in mouse adipocytes. *Biomed. Res.* **2015**, *36*, 343–346. [CrossRef]
91. Hotamisligil, G.S.; Peraldi, P.; Budavari, A.; Ellis, R.; White, M.F.; Spiegelman, B.M. IRS-1-mediated inhibition of insulin receptor tyrosine kinase activity in TNF-α- and obesity-induced insulin resistance. *Science* **1996**, *271*, 665–670. [CrossRef]
92. Bachiega, T.F.; Orsatti, C.L.; Pagliarone, A.C.; Sforcin, J.M. The effects of propolis and its isolated compounds on cytokine production by murine macrophages. *Phyther. Res.* **2012**, *26*, 1308–1313. [CrossRef] [PubMed]
93. Kim, J.S.; Kwon, C.S.; Son, K.H. Inhibition of alpha-glucosidase and amylase by luteolin, a flavonoid. *Biosci. Biotechnol. Biochem.* **2000**, *64*, 2458–2461. [CrossRef] [PubMed]
94. Coskun, O.; Kanter, M.; Korkmaz, A.; Oter, S. Quercetin, a flavonoid antioxidant, prevents and protects streptozotocin-induced oxidative stress and β-cell damage in rat pancreas. *Pharmacol. Res.* **2005**, *51*, 117–123. [CrossRef] [PubMed]
95. Nakajima, M.; Arimatsu, K.; Minagawa, T.; Matsuda, Y.; Sato, K.; Takahashi, N.; Nakajima, T.; Yamazaki, K. Brazilian propolis mitigates impaired glucose and lipid metabolism in experimental periodontitis in mice. *BMC Complement. Altern. Med.* **2016**, *16*, 329. [CrossRef]
96. Kontogianni, V.G.; Charisiadis, P.; Margianni, E.; Lamari, F.N.; Gerothanassis, I.P.; Tzakos, A.G. Olive leaf extracts are a natural source of advanced glycation end product inhibitors. *J. Med. Food* **2013**, *16*, 817–822. [CrossRef]
97. Khalatbary, A.R.; Zarrinjoei, G.R. Anti-inflammatory effect of oleuropein in experimental Rat Spinal cord trauma. *Iran. Red Crescent Med. J.* **2012**, *14*, 229–234.
98. Santiago-Mora, R.; Casado-Díaz, A.; De Castro, M.D.; Quesada-Gómez, J.M. Oleuropein enhances osteoblastogenesis and inhibits adipogenesis: The effect on differentiation in stem cells derived from bone marrow. *Osteoporos. Int.* **2011**, *22*, 675–684. [CrossRef]
99. Al-Azzawie, H.F.; Alhamdani, M.S.S. Hypoglycemic and antioxidant effect of oleuropein in alloxan-diabetic rabbits. *Life Sci.* **2006**, *78*, 1371–1377. [CrossRef]
100. Sato, H.; Genet, C.; Strehle, A.; Thomas, C.; Lobstein, A.; Wagner, A.; Mioskowski, C.; Auwerx, J.; Saladin, R. Anti-hyperglycemic activity of a TGR5 agonist isolated from Olea europaea. *Biochem. Biophys. Res. Commun.* **2007**, *362*, 793–798. [CrossRef]

101. Hoek-van den Hil, E.F.; van Schothorst, E.M.; van der Stelt, I.; Swarts, H.J.M.; van Vliet, M.; Amolo, T.; Vervoort, J.J.M.; Venema, D.; Hollman, P.C.H.; Rietjens, I.M.C.M.; et al. Direct comparison of metabolic health effects of the flavonoids quercetin, hesperetin, epicatechin, apigenin and anthocyanins in high-fat-diet-fed mice. *Genes Nutr.* **2015**, *10*. [CrossRef] [PubMed]
102. Haggarty, P. Fatty acid supply to the human fetus. *Annu. Rev. Nutr.* **2010**, *30*, 237–255. [CrossRef] [PubMed]
103. Rogers, L.K.; Valentine, C.J.; Keim, S.A. DHA supplementation: Current implications in pregnancy and childhood. *Pharmacol. Res.* **2013**, *70*, 13–19. [CrossRef] [PubMed]
104. Simopoulos, A.P. Importance of the omega-6/omega-3 balance in health and disease: Evolutionary aspects of diet. *World Rev. Nutr. Diet.* **2011**, *102*, 10–21. [CrossRef]
105. Haggarty, P. Effect of placental function in fatty acid requirements during pregnancy. *Eur. J. Clin. Nutr.* **2004**, *58*, 1559–1570. [CrossRef]
106. Burton, G.J.; Jauniaux, E. Oxidative stress. *Best Pract. Res. Clin. Obstet. Gynaecol.* **2011**, *25*, 287–299. [CrossRef]
107. Magnusson, A.L.; Waterman, I.J.; Wennergren, M.; Jansson, T.; Powell, T.L. Triglyceride hydrolase activities and expression of fatty acid binding proteins in the human placenta in pregnancies complicated by intrauterine growth restriction and diabetes. *J. Clin. Endocrinol. Metab.* **2004**, *89*, 4607–4614. [CrossRef]
108. Prescott, S.L.; Barden, A.E.; Mori, T.A.; Dunstan, J.A. Maternal fish oil supplementation in pregnancy modifies neonatal leukotriene production by cord-blood-derived neutrophils. *Clin. Sci. (Lond.)* **2007**, *113*, 409–416. [CrossRef]
109. Calder, P.C. Fatty acids and inflammation: The cutting edge between food and pharma. *Eur. J. Pharmacol.* **2011**, *668* (Suppl. 1), S50–S58. [CrossRef]
110. Jawerbaum, A.; Capobianco, E. Review: Effects of PPAR activation in the placenta and the fetus: Implications in maternal diabetes. *Placenta* **2011**, *32* (Suppl. 2), S212–S217. [CrossRef]
111. Oh, D.Y.; Talukdar, S.; Bae, E.J.; Imamura, T.; Morinaga, H.; Fan, W.; Li, P.; Lu, W.J.; Watkins, S.M.; Olefsky, J.M. GPR120 is an omega-3 fatty acid receptor mediating potent anti-inflammatory and insulin-sensitizing effects. *Cell* **2010**, *142*, 687–698. [CrossRef] [PubMed]
112. Oken, E.; Ning, Y.; Rifas-Shiman, S.L.; Rich-Edwards, J.W.; Olsen, S.F.; Gillman, M.W. Diet during pregnancy and risk of preeclampsia or gestational hypertension. *Ann. Epidemiol.* **2007**, *17*, 663–668. [CrossRef]
113. Jones, M.L.; Mark, P.J.; Mori, T.A.; Keelan, J.A.; Waddell, B.J. Maternal dietary omega-3 fatty acid supplementation reduces placental oxidative stress and increases fetal and placental growth in the rat. *Biol. Reprod.* **2013**, *88*. [CrossRef] [PubMed]
114. Flachs, P.; Mohamed-Ali, V.; Horakova, O.; Rossmeisl, M.; Hosseinzadeh-Attar, M.J.; Hensler, M.; Ruzickova, J.; Kopecky, J. Polyunsaturated fatty acids of marine origin induce adiponectin in mice fed a high-fat diet. *Diabetologia* **2006**, *49*, 394–397. [CrossRef]
115. El Akoum, S.; Lamontagne, V.; Cloutier, I.; Tanguay, J.F. Nature of fatty acids in high fat diets differentially delineates obesity-linked metabolic syndrome components in male and female C57BL/6J mice. *Diabetol. Metab. Syndr.* **2011**, *3*. [CrossRef] [PubMed]
116. Kalupahana, N.S.; Claycombe, K.J.; Moustaid-Moussa, N. (n-3) Fatty acids alleviate adipose tissue inflammation and insulin resistance: Mechanistic insights. *Adv. Nutr.* **2011**, *2*, 304–316. [CrossRef]
117. Hatakeyama, Y.; Scarpace, P.J. Transcriptional regulation of uncoupling protein-2 gene expression in L6 myotubes. *Int. J. Obes. Relat. Metab. Disord.* **2001**, *25*, 1619–1624. [CrossRef]
118. Al-Gubory, K.H. Mitochondria: Omega-3 in the route of mitochondrial reactive oxygen species. *Int. J. Biochem. Cell Biol.* **2012**, *44*, 1569–1573. [CrossRef]
119. Shang, F.; Li, X.; Jiang, X. Coffee consumption and risk of the metabolic syndrome: A meta-analysis. *Diabetes Metab.* **2016**, *42*, 80–87. [CrossRef]
120. Poole, R.; Kennedy, O.J.; Roderick, P.; Fallowfield, J.A.; Hayes, P.C.; Parkes, J. Coffee consumption and health: Umbrella review of meta-analyses of multiple health outcomes. *BMJ* **2017**, *359*, j5024. [CrossRef]
121. Ding, M.; Bhupathiraju, S.N.; Satija, A.; van Dam, R.M.; Hu, F.B. Long-term coffee consumption and risk of cardiovascular disease: A systematic review and a dose-response meta-analysis of prospective cohort studies. *Circulation* **2014**, *129*, 643–659. [CrossRef]
122. Shen, T.; Park, Y.C.; Kim, S.H.; Lee, J.; Cho, J.Y. Nuclear factor-κB/signal Transducers and activators of transcription-1- mediated inflammatory responses in Lipopolysaccharide-activated macrophages are a major inhibitory target of kahweol, a coffee diterpene. *Biol. Pharm. Bull.* **2010**, *33*, 1159–1164. [CrossRef]

123. Hosoi, T.; Toyoda, K.; Nakatsu, K.; Ozawa, K. Caffeine attenuated ER stress-induced leptin resistance in neurons. *Neurosci. Lett.* **2014**, *569*, 23–26. [CrossRef]
124. Kim, H.G.; Hwang, Y.P.; Jeong, H.G. Kahweol blocks STAT3 phosphorylation and induces apoptosis in human lung adenocarcinoma A549 cells. *Toxicol. Lett.* **2009**, *187*, 28–34. [CrossRef]
125. Yu, Y.; Wu, Y.; Szabo, A.; Wu, Z.; Wang, H.; Li, D.; Huang, X.F. Teasaponin reduces inflammation and central leptin resistance in diet-induced obese male mice. *Endocrinology* **2013**, *154*, 3130–3140. [CrossRef]
126. Zhao, L. The gut microbiota and obesity: From correlation to causality. *Nat. Rev. Microbiol.* **2013**, *11*, 639–647. [CrossRef]
127. Ley, R.E.; Turnbaugh, P.J.; Klein, S.; Gordon, J.I. Microbial ecology: Human gut microbes associated with obesity. *Nature* **2006**, *444*, 1022–1023. [CrossRef]
128. Barrett, H.L.; Gomez-Arango, L.F.; Wilkinson, S.A.; McIntyre, H.D.; Callaway, L.K.; Morrison, M.; Dekker Nitert, M. A vegetarian diet is a major determinant of gut microbiota composition in early pregnancy. *Nutrients* **2018**, *10*. [CrossRef]
129. Gomez-Arango, L.F.; Barrett, H.L.; Wilkinson, S.A.; Callaway, L.K.; McIntyre, H.D.; Morrison, M.; Dekker Nitert, M. Low dietary fiber intake increases Collinsella abundance in the gut microbiota of overweight and obese pregnant women. *Gut Microbes* **2018**, *9*, 189–201. [CrossRef]
130. Collado, M.C.; Isolauri, E.; Laitinen, K.; Salminen, S. Effect of mother's weight on infant's microbiota acquisition, composition, and activity during early infancy: A prospective follow-up study initiated in early pregnancy. *Am. J. Clin. Nutr.* **2010**, *92*, 1023–1030. [CrossRef]
131. Santacruz, A.; Collado, M.C.; García-Valdés, L.; Segura, M.T.; Marítn-Lagos, J.A.; Anjos, T.; Martí-Romero, M.; Lopez, R.M.; Florido, J.; Campoy, C.; et al. Gut microbiota composition is associated with body weight, weight gain and biochemical parameters in pregnant women. *Br. J. Nutr.* **2010**, *104*, 83–92. [CrossRef] [PubMed]
132. Koren, O.; Goodrich, J.K.; Cullender, T.C.; Spor, A.; Laitinen, K.; Kling Bäckhed, H.; Gonzalez, A.; Werner, J.J.; Angenent, L.T.; Knight, R.; et al. Host remodeling of the gut microbiome and metabolic changes during pregnancy. *Cell* **2012**, *150*, 470–480. [CrossRef] [PubMed]
133. Collado, M.C.; Isolauri, E.; Laitinen, K.; Salminen, S. Distinct composition of gut microbiota during pregnancy in overweight and normal-weight women. *Am. J. Clin. Nutr.* **2008**, *88*, 894–899. [CrossRef]
134. Luoto, R.; Laitinen, K.; Nermes, M.; Isolauri, E. Impact of maternal probiotic-supplemented dietary counselling on pregnancy outcome and prenatal and postnatal growth: A double-blind, placebo-controlled study. *Br. J. Nutr.* **2010**, *103*, 1792–1799. [CrossRef]
135. Rautava, S.; Collado, M.C.; Salminen, S.; Isolauri, E. Probiotics modulate host-microbe interaction in the placenta and fetal gut: A randomized, double-blind, placebo-controlled trial. *Neonatology* **2012**, *102*, 178–184. [CrossRef]
136. Rautava, S.; Kainonen, E.; Salminen, S.; Isolauri, E. Maternal probiotic supplementation during pregnancy and breast-feeding reduces the risk of eczema in the infant. *J. Allergy Clin. Immunol.* **2012**, *130*, 1355–1360. [CrossRef]
137. Isolauri, E.; Rautava, S.; Salminen, S. Probiotics in the development and treatment of allergic disease. *Gastroenterol. Clin. North. Am.* **2012**, *41*, 747–762. [CrossRef]
138. Khachik, F.; Carvalho, L.; Bernstein, P.S.; Muir, G.J.; Zhao, D.Y.; Katz, N.B. Chemistry, distribution, and metabolism of tomato carotenoids and their impact on human health. *Exp. Biol. Med.* **2002**, *227*, 845–851. [CrossRef]
139. Mangels, A.R.; Holden, J.M.; Beecher, G.R.; Forman, M.R.; Lanza, E. Carotenoid content of fruits and vegetables: An evaluation of analytic data. *J. Am. Diet. Assoc.* **1993**, *93*, 284–296. [CrossRef]
140. Marcotorchino, J.; Romier, B.; Gouranton, E.; Riollet, C.; Gleize, B.; Malezet-Desmoulins, C.; Landrier, J.F. Lycopene attenuates LPS-induced TNF-α secretion in macrophages and inflammatory markers in adipocytes exposed to macrophage-conditioned media. *Mol. Nutr. Food Res.* **2012**, *56*, 725–732. [CrossRef]
141. Fantuzzi, G. Adipose tissue, adipokines, and inflammation. *J. Allergy Clin. Immunol.* **2005**, *115*, 911–919. [CrossRef]
142. Luvizotto, R.D.A.M.; Nascimento, A.F.; Imaizumi, E.; Pierine, D.T.; Conde, S.J.; Correa, C.R.; Yeum, K.J.; Ferreira, A.L.A. Lycopene supplementation modulates plasma concentrations and epididymal adipose tissue mRNA of leptin, resistin and IL-6 in diet-induced obese rats. *Br. J. Nutr.* **2013**, *110*, 1803–1809. [CrossRef]

143. Saravanan, S.; Pari, L. Role of thymol on hyperglycemia and hyperlipidemia in high fat diet-induced type 2 diabetic C57BL/6J mice. *Eur. J. Pharmacol.* **2015**, *761*, 279–287. [CrossRef]
144. Shibata, T.; Kimura, Y.; Mukai, A.; Mori, H.; Ito, S.; Asaka, Y.; Oe, S.; Tanaka, H.; Takahashi, T.; Uchida, K. Transthiocarbamoylation of proteins by thiolated isothiocyanates. *J. Biol. Chem.* **2011**, *286*, 42150–42161. [CrossRef] [PubMed]
145. Kumari, V.; Dyba, M.A.; Holland, R.J.; Liang, Y.H.; Singh, S.V.; Ji, X. Irreversible inhibition of glutathione S-transferase by phenethyl isothiocyanate (PEITC), a dietary cancer chemopreventive phytochemical. *PLoS ONE* **2016**, *11*. [CrossRef]
146. Cross, J.V.; Foss, F.W.; Rady, J.M.; Macdonald, T.L.; Templeton, D.J. The isothiocyanate class of bioactive nutrients covalently inhibit the MEKK1 protein kinase. *BMC Cancer* **2007**, *7*. [CrossRef]
147. Chiarugi, P.; Cirri, P. Redox regulation of protein tyrosine phosphatases during receptor tyrosine kinase signal transduction. *Trends Biochem. Sci.* **2003**, *28*, 509–514. [CrossRef]
148. Lewis, S.M.; Li, Y.; Catalano, M.J.; Laciak, A.R.; Singh, H.; Seiner, D.R.; Reilly, T.J.; Tanner, J.J.; Gates, K.S. Inactivation of protein tyrosine phosphatases by dietary isothiocyanates. *Bioorg. Med. Chem. Lett.* **2015**, *25*, 4549–4552. [CrossRef] [PubMed]
149. Yagi, M.; Nakatsuji, Y.; Maeda, A.; Ota, H.; Kamikubo, R.; Miyoshi, N.; Nakamura, Y.; Akagawa, M. Phenethyl isothiocyanate activates leptin signaling and decreases food intake. *PLoS ONE* **2018**, *13*. [CrossRef]
150. Scholl, T.O.; Hediger, M.L.; Bendich, A.; Schall, J.I.; Smith, W.K.; Krueger, P.M. Use of multivitamin/mineral prenatal supplements: Influence on the outcome of pregnancy. *Am. J. Epidemiol.* **1997**, *146*, 134–141. [CrossRef]
151. Black, R.E.; Allen, L.H.; Bhutta, Z.A.; Caulfield, L.E.; de Onis, M.; Ezzati, M.; Mathers, C.; Rivera, J. Maternal and child undernutrition: Global and regional exposures and health consequences. *Lancet* **2008**, *371*, 243–260. [CrossRef]
152. Ramakrishnan, U.; Grant, F.; Goldenberg, T.; Zongrone, A.; Martorell, R. Effect of women's nutrition before and during early pregnancy on maternal and infant outcomes: A systematic review. *Paediatr. Perinat. Epidemiol.* **2012**, *26*, 285–301. [CrossRef] [PubMed]
153. Perkins, A.V.; Vanderlelie, J.J. Multiple micronutrient supplementation and birth outcomes: The potential importance of selenium. *Placenta* **2016**, *48*, S61–S65. [CrossRef] [PubMed]
154. Steegers-Theunissen, R.P.M.; Twigt, J.; Pestinger, V.; Sinclair, K.D. The periconceptional period, reproduction and long-term health of offspring: The importance of one-carbon metabolism. *Hum. Reprod. Update* **2013**, *19*, 640–655. [CrossRef]
155. Kawai, K.; Spiegelman, D.; Shankar, A.H.; Fawzi, W.W. Maternal multiple micronutrient supplementation and pregnancy outcomes in developing countries: Meta-analysis and meta-regression. *Bull. World Health Organ.* **2011**, *89*, 402B–411B. [CrossRef]
156. The International Weight Management in Pregnancy (i-WIP) Collaborative Group. Effect of diet and physical activity based interventions in pregnancy on gestational weight gain and pregnancy outcomes: Meta-analysis of individual participant data from randomised trials. *BMJ* **2017**, *358*, j3119. [CrossRef]
157. Rogozińska, E.; Marlin, N.; Jackson, L.; Rayanagoudar, G.; Ruifrok, A.E.; Dodds, J.; Molyneaux, E.; van Poppel, M.N.; Poston, L.; Vinter, C.A.; et al. Effects of antenatal diet and physical activity on maternal and fetal outcomes: Individual patient data meta-analysis and health economic evaluation. *Health Technol. Assess.* **2017**, *21*, 1–158. [CrossRef]
158. Estruch, R.; Ros, E.; Salas-Salvadó, J.; Covas, M.I.; Corella, D.; Arós, F.; Gómez-Gracia, E.; Ruiz-Gutiérrez, V.; Fiol, M.; Lapetra, J.; et al. Primary prevention of cardiovascular disease with a Mediterranean diet. *N. Engl. J. Med.* **2013**, *368*, 1279–1290. [CrossRef]
159. Al Wattar, B.H.; Dodds, J.; Placzek, A.; Beresford, L.; Spyreli, E.; Moore, A.; Gonzalez Carreras, F.J.; Austin, F.; Murugesu, N.; Roseboom, T.J.; et al. Mediterranean-style diet in pregnant women with metabolic risk factors (ESTEEM): A pragmatic multicentre randomised trial. *PLoS Med.* **2019**, *16*, e1002857. [CrossRef]

14

Influence of Diabetes during Pregnancy on Human Milk Composition

Chiara Peila [1,*], Diego Gazzolo [2], Enrico Bertino [1], Francesco Cresi [1] and Alessandra Coscia [1]

1 Complex Structure Neonatology Unit, Department of Public Health and Paediatric, University of Turin, 10100 Turin, Italy; enrico.bertino@unito.it (E.B.); francesco.cresi@unito.it (F.C.); alessandra.coscia@unito.it (A.C.)

2 Department of Maternal, Fetal and Neonatal Health, C. Arrigo Children's Hospital, 15121 Alessandria, Italy; dgazzolo@hotmail.com

* Correspondence: peila.chiara@gmail.com

Abstract: Human milk (HM) is a unique nourishment believed to contain biological factors contributing to both short and long-term benefits. Considering that a mother's own milk is often considered the first choice for nutrition of neonates, an aspect of increased interest is the possible effect of diabetes on the mammary gland and therefore on breast milk composition. This article aims to review the published literature on this topic, and to offer additional insights on the role of this disease on the composition of HM. This review was performed by searching the MEDLINE, EMBASE, CINHAL and Cochrane Library databases. A total of 50 articles were selected, focused specifically on one of the two types of diabetes: gestational diabetes mellitus (21 studies) and insulin-dependent diabetes mellitus (8 studies). Overall, the findings from the literature suggest that diabetes can alter the composition of HM. Nevertheless, the studies in this field are scarce, and the related protocols present some limitations, e.g., evaluating the variability of just a few specific milk biochemical markers in association with this syndrome.

Keywords: human milk; breastfeeding; gestational diabetes mellitus; insulin-dependent diabetes mellitus; preterm newborn

---

1. Introduction

Human milk (HM) is a specie-specific biological dynamic fluid and significantly varies from one woman to another. HM constantly changes during lactation to adapt to the physiological needs of the developing infant [1] and this also comes about because of the gradual maturation of the mammary gland, which depends on the placenta and thus on the progress of the pregnancy. The policy statement of the American Academy of Pediatrics (AAP) regarding breastfeeding affirms that "Breastfeeding and human milk are the normative standards for infant feeding and nutrition" [1]. In addition, the AAP highlights that the mother's own milk, fortified appropriately, should be the primary diet also for the preterm newborns. These recommendations are due also to the fact that breastfeeding has been shown to have beneficial effects on short- and long-term maternal and infant health outcomes [1–3].

It has been proposed that nutrition signals during the early postnatal period may influence metabolic developmental pathways and induce permanent changes to metabolic disease susceptibility [4,5]. In support of these hypotheses, studies have reported that human milk (HM) has a protective effect on obesity and type 2 diabetes later in life [5,6]. Benefits of HM are mediated by specific bioactive substances that transiently regulate tissue activities while the neonate's systems mature [7,8]. Biological active components, such as hormones, immunoglobulins, lysozyme, lactoferrin, saccharides, nucleotides growth factors and enzymes antioxidants, are involved in immunological and metabolic regulation, and it has been hypothesized that they mediate growth and development in infancy [9,10]. Furthermore, HM is a "dynamic" system: the composition changes and is influenced by several conditions, such as term-preterm delivery, maternal diet, metabolic abnormalities and pathologies [11].

Diabetes is a pathological condition of the lactating mother that may preexist (type 2 diabetes, type 1 diabetes or insulin-dependent diabetes mellitus (IDDM)) or appear during the pregnancy. The latter case is identified as gestational diabetes mellitus (GDM) and is a common pregnancy complication. It is defined as a carbohydrate intolerance of variable severity, with onset or first recognition during pregnancy. Diabetes is associated with several short- and long-term complications for the mother and the newborns and it is known that this pathology can delay the onset of lactogenesis II and affect the composition of the human milk [12]. Bearing in mind the important impact of the HM on the development of the newborns and the potential effects of the diabetes on the composition of the milk, several studies were conducted to evaluate the variability of milk biochemical markers in association with this pathology.

A comprehensive review and comparison of the related data on the effects of diabetes conditions on the specific composition of HM of the lactating mother is, to the best of the authors' knowledge, not available in the literature. Our aim is to assess the current knowledge on the interactions between diabetes in pregnancy and the composition of the HM in order to better understand the potential effects of this pathology on the nutrition and development of newborns.

2. Materials and Methods

The literature review was performed by conducting electronic searches of MEDLINE (via PubMed and PubMed Central), EMBASE, CINHAL and the Cochrane Library. The electronic search used the following keywords and MeSH terms: (i) human milk AND (gestational diabetes OR gestational diabetes mellitus OR insulin-dependent diabetes mellitus OR type 2 diabetes); (ii) breastfeeding composition AND (gestational diabetes OR gestational diabetes mellitus OR insulin-dependent diabetes mellitus OR type 2 diabetes); (iii) breast milk AND (gestational diabetes OR gestational diabetes mellitus OR insulin-dependent diabetes mellitus OR type 2 diabetes); (iv) preterm breast milk AND (gestational diabetes OR gestational diabetes mellitus OR insulin-dependent diabetes mellitus OR type 2 diabetes); (v) human milk composition AND (gestational diabetes OR gestational diabetes mellitus OR insulin-dependent diabetes mellitus OR type 2 diabetes); (vi) breast milk composition AND (gestational diabetes OR gestational diabetes mellitus OR insulin-dependent diabetes mellitus OR type 2 diabetes).

No publication date limits were set. For a complete comprehension of the studies, the inclusion criteria were: (i) primary (original) research published in a peer-reviewed journal in the English language and (ii) full text available. For the same reason, case reports, commentaries, letters to the editor, and reviews were excluded. Articles including data related to animal milk were also excluded.

Literature searches were performed in the period between 1 June 2019 and 1 November 2019.

3. Results

A total of 50 articles were found from a combination of the searches, but only 29 fulfilled the inclusion criteria, as shown in the flow diagram below, Figure 1.

The selected literature studies were focused specifically on one of two types of diabetes: GDM or IDDM. In line with this finding, we evaluated the studies separately, based on the diabetes type. Since type 2 diabetes was only referenced in a single article and compared to GDM, it is not discussed separately in our review.

The available literature data on GDM and HM are summarized in Tables 1 and 2, whereas data on IDDM and HM are summarized in Tables 3 and 4.

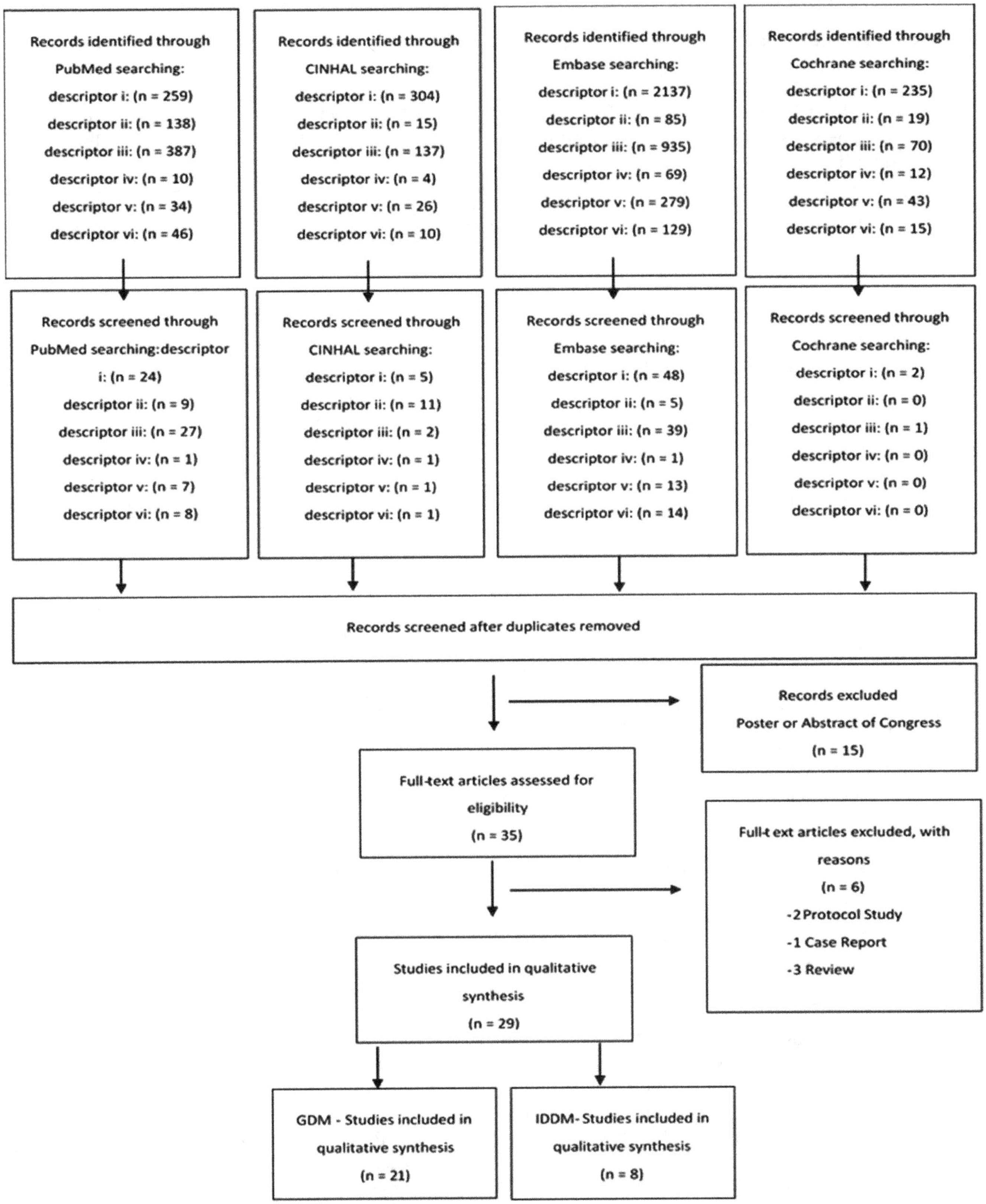

Figure 1. Flow diagram of the different phases of the review.

3.1. Gestational Diabetes Mellitus—GDM

We found 21 articles focused on gestational diabetes mellitus; the related information is summarized in Tables 1 and 2.

Table 1. Materials and methods of the different studies included in the survey regarding gestational diabetes mellitus (GDM) and human milk (HM). (Col: colostrum; Trans: Transitional milk; Mat: Mature milk).

Study	GDM Treatments	Sample Time	Gestational Age	Parameters Analyzed	Sample Size (GDM vs. Control Women)
[13]	Diet	Col: 0–5 days Trans: 6–14 days Mat: >14 days	Preterm	Macronutrients and energy	27 vs. 183
[14]	Diet Other medications	Col: 72 h Trans: 7 days Mat: 14 days	Term	Macronutrients and energy	31 vs. 31
[15]	Not evaluated	Col: 2–4 days	Term	Total proteins Total lipids Triglycerides cholesterol Lactose Glucose Calcium Inorganic phosphorus Electrolytes IgA	20 vs. 20
[16]	Diet	Col: 7 days Mat: 3 months	Term	Adiponectin Insulin	170 women
[17]	Diet Insulin	Col: 3 days Mat: 42–90 days	Term	Leptin insulin ghrelin adiponectin	48 vs. 48
[18]	Not evaluated	Col: 24–48 h Mat: 30 days	N/A	Leptin adiponectin insulin	12 vs. 21
[19]	Diet	Col/Mat	Term	Apelin nefastin-1 ghrelin	10 vs. 10
[20]	Diet	Col: 2 days Mat: 15 days	Term	Ghrelin	14 vs. 12 vs. 3 Pre-GDM
[21]	Not evaluated	Col: 72 h Mat: 6 weeks	Term	Irisin a SREBP-1c	33 vs. 33
[22]	Not evaluated	Col: –5 days Trans: 6–15 days Mat: >15 days	Term	Irisin Adropin Copeptin	15 vs. 15
[23]	Not evaluated	Col: 1 day Trans: 7 days Mat: 20 days	Term	Preptin Salusin Hepcidin	12 vs. 12
[24]	Not evaluated	Trans: 2 weeks	Term	Lactoferrin sIgA oligosaccharides	8 vs. 16
[25]	Diet	Col: 1–5 days Trans: 7–10 days Mat: 15–17 days	Term	Chemerin Dermcidin	26 vs. 27

Table 1. *Cont.*

Study	GDM Treatments	Sample Time	Gestational Age	Parameters Analyzed	Sample Size (GDM vs. Control Women)
[26]	Insulin	Col: First day of secretion and 2 days later	Term	Neutrophil gelatinase-associated lipocalin (NGAL) Complex NGAL/matrix metalloproteinase-9 (MMP-9)	13 vs. 22
[27]	Diet Insulin	Col: within 4 days Mat: 6 weeks	Term	Free amino acids	21 vs. 47
[28]	Diet Insulin Other medications	Col: 1–3 days	Term	Proteome	6 vs. 12
[29]	Not evaluated	Col:1–5 days	Term	Fatty acid composition	29 vs. 34
[30]	Diet insulin	Col: 1–3 day	Term	Sodium	17 vs. 116
[31]	Not evaluated	Col: 1 day	Term Preterm	Alpha-Tocopherol	20 vs. 31
[32]	Not evaluated	Col: 3–5 days Mat: 3 months	Term	MicroRNAs	19 vs. 47
[33]	Not evaluated	Col: 1–3 days Trans: 7–10 days Mat: 4 weeks	Term	Metabolome	90 vs. 94

Table 2. Results of the different studies included in the survey regarding GDM and HM.

Components	Effects	Reference
Energy content	Increase Decrease	Col/Trans/Mat: [13] Mat: [14]
Total protein content	No differences Decrease	Col: [13–15] Trans/mat: [14] Trans/mat: [13]
Insulin	No differences Increase	Col: [16,18] Mat: [18] Col: [17] Mat: [16,17]
Adiponectin	No differences Decrease	Col/Mat: [16,18] Col/Mat: [17]
Ghrelin	No differences Decrease	Trans: [17,19,20] Col/Mat: [17,19,20]
Irisin	Decrease No Differences	Col/Trans: [21,22] Mat: [21] Mat: [22]
Apelins and Nesfatin-1	Increase	Col/Mat: [19]
Copeptin, adropin	No Differences	Col/Trans/Mat: [22]
Preptin	Increase No Differences	Col: [23] Trans/Mat: [23]
Salusin-alpha/-beta	Decrease No Differences	Col: [23] Trans/Mat: [23]

Table 2. *Cont.*

Components	Effects	Reference
Pro-hepcidin and hepcidin-25	Increase No Differences	Col/Trans: [23] Mat: [23]
SREBP1-c	No Differences	Col/Mat: [21]
IgA	No Differences Decrease	Col: [15] Trans: [24]
Lactoferrin	Increase	Trans: [24]
Chemerin and Dermicin	Increase	Col/Trans/Mat: [21]
NGAL NGAL/MMP-9	No differences Increase	Col: [26] Col: [26]
Total saccharides content	No differences Decrease	Col/Trans: [13,14] Mat: [13] Mat: [14]
Glucose	No differences	Col: [15]
Lactose	Decrease	Col: [15]
Oligosaccharides	No differences	Trans: [24]
Total lipid content	No differences	Col: [13,14] Trans: [13,14] Mat: [13]
	Decrease	Col: [15] Mat: [14]
Cholesterols	No differences	Col: [15]
triglycerides	No differences	Col: [15]
Fatty acid composition -γ-linolenic, eicosatrienoic, arachidonic, and docosatetraenoic	No differences Increase	Col: [29] Col: [29]
Potassium, Phosphorus and Calcium	No differences	Col: [15]
Sodium	No differences	Col: [15,30]
Vitamin E	No differences	Col: [31]
Micro RNA	No differences	Col/Mat: [32]

3.1.1. Energy

The energy content of the HM of women diagnosed with GDM was evaluated in two studies, with opposite results: one study showed higher energy content in all phases of lactation with respect to healthy mothers, whereas the other study reported a lower energy content in the mature milk of pathological mothers. Both studies used an MIRIS scanner for the analyses of the samples; the differences only consisted of the methods used to collect and store HM samples [13,14].

3.1.2. Protein Content

The total protein content was investigated in three studies, with similar results concerning the colostrum: no significant differences were found with respect to the control group. Nonetheless, data reported in relation to transitional and mature milk were conflicting: Dritsaku et al. found a reduction in concentration of both types of HM, whereas the results of Saphira et al. showed no differences [13–15].

3.1.3. Hormones

Insulin was evaluated in several studies, both in colostrum and mature milk. Ley et al. used an electrochemiluminescence immunoassay and showed that insulin concentrations in early milk were higher than those in mature milk. They found that maternal prenatal metabolic measures, including higher pre-gravid body mass index (BMI), gravid hyperglycemia, insulin resistance, lower insulin sensitivity and higher serum adiponectin were associated with higher insulin concentrations in mature milk, whereas these factors were not associated with altered insulin concentrations in early milk [16]. Another two studies analyzed the HM samples with an ELISA test, but found opposite results. Yu et al. showed an increase of insulin levels, not only in mature milk, but also in colostrum in women with GDM, especially in those receiving insulin injections [17]. Nunes et al. did not find differences in both types of milk [18].

Adiponectin levels showed similar conflicting results: two studies demonstrated that GDM was not associated with variations of adiponectin levels in HM, whereas Yu et al. observed that women with GDM had lower concentrations of adiponectin in colostrum on day 3 and mature milk on day 90, but no differences on day 42 [16–18].

There is agreement in the Ghrelin data: Ghrelin levels were found to be lower in colostrum and mature milk, but no differences were observed in transitional milk [17,19,20].

Irisin concentrations, analyzed in two studies, were accordingly found to be low in GDM subjects in the colostrum and transitional milk [21,22]. In mature milk, Fatima et al. observed a reduction in concentrations, not confirmed by Aydin et al. [21,22]. In addition, the study by Aydin et al. found Irisin levels to increase from the colostrum to transitional and mature milk in both normal glucose tolerant and GDM patients [22].

Several other biologically active components with hormonal activity are evaluated in one study by the same group of researchers. The study considered only mothers who did not take insulin, with no complications during pregnancy and who had full term deliveries. Instead, the concentrations of Apelins and Nesfatin-1 in HM in GDM lactating women was lower than in the control samples and the concentrations of Apelins and Nesfatin-1 were higher in the mature milk than in colostrum [19]. Copeptin, adropin and polypeptide are hormones implicated in energy homeostasis and diabetes [22]. The authors found that the copeptin concentration was significantly higher in colostrum than transitional milk, and the highest concentration was in mature milk from women with or without GDM [22]. Conversely, the adropin concentrations were significantly lower in the colostrum than in transitional milk, and the lowest concentration was in mature milk from women with or without GDM [22]. Preptin, salusin-alpha and -beta and pro-hepcidin and hepcidin-25 concentrations were evaluated in all phases of breastfeeding [23]. The data demonstrated that women with GDM had significantly higher colostrum preptin and colostrum/transitional pro-hepcidin and hepcidin-25 concentrations than healthy lactating women. Salusin-alpha and -beta levels were lower in colostrum of women with GDM [23]. SREBP1-c profile showed a level reduced from a very low value to an undetectable range in colostrum and mature breast milk, respectively [21].

3.1.4. Anti-Infective Proteins

IgA content was evaluated in the colostrum in one study and in transitional milk in another study [15,24]. No differences were observed in the colostrum, while a decrease of total protein and glycosylation of sIgA was found in transitional milk. Lactoferrin was analyzed only by Smilowitz et al. in transitional milk, observing an increased glycosylation of this protein. The results suggest that maternal glucose dysregulation during pregnancy has lasting consequences that may influence the innate immune protective functions of HM [24].

Ustebay et al. analyzed Chemerin and Dermicin in all phases of lactation and found that these are significantly increased by GDM; moreover, the highest amount was found in the colostrum and the lowest in mature milk [25].

Metallinou et al. evaluated the levels of Neutrophil gelatinase-associated lipocalin (NGAL) and its complex with matrix metalloproteinase-9 (MMP-9) in the colostrum and found that the mean complex concentration was significantly higher in diabetic pregnancies in comparison to normal ones [26].

3.1.5. Proteomics Profile

The proteomics profile was assessed in two studies, using different techniques (high-performance liquid chromatography or high-sensitivity, label-free, semiquantitative mass spectrometry) [27,28]. Klein et al. evaluated the content of 11 free amino acids (FAAs) in the colostrum and mature milk in women with or without GDM. The authors found that the total amount of FAA increased from colostrum to mature milk in all patients. Moreover, the total amount did not significantly differ between groups, as well as the concentrations of each individual amino acid [27].

Grapov et al. determined the proteomic profiling only of colostrum. A total of 601 proteins were identified, of which 260 were quantified. Orthogonal partial least-squares discriminant analysis identified 27 proteins that best predict GDM. The power law global error model, corrected for multiple testing, was used to confirm that 10 of the 27 proteins were also statistically significantly different between women with GDM and those without GDM. The identified changes in protein expression suggest that diabetes mellitus during pregnancy has consequences on human colostral proteins involved in immunity and nutrition [28].

3.1.6. Saccharides

The total saccharides content was evaluated in two studies. Both found no differences between groups in the colostrum and transitional milk, although different results regarding mature milk were reported: Saphira et al. observed a lower concentration in GDM, while Dritsaku et al. did not find differences [13,14].

Lactose and glucose were analyzed only in one study and only in the colostrum; lactose was found to be lower in GDM women, whereas glucose seemed unaltered by this pathological condition [15].

In conclusion, a single study evaluated the oligosaccharides in transitional milk and no differences between groups were found in the results [24].

3.1.7. Lipids

The total lipid content was evaluated in three studies with discordant results. Kaushik et al. analyzed only the colostrum and found a reduction in total content in the GDM group [15]. On the other hand, Dritsaku et al. and Saphira et al. did not show any difference in concentration. Similarly, regarding mature milk, Saphira et al. found a reduction, but Dritsaku et al. did not observe a significant difference. Regarding transitional milk, all studies agreed and found no differences between groups [13,14].

Kaushik et al. also analyzed the concentration of triglycerides and cholesterols in colostrum; in this case no differences in content in GDM HM were identified [15].

Azulay Chertok et al. examined the effect of GDM on colostrum fatty acid composition. Analyses of the fatty acid composition revealed significantly higher concentrations of four essential ω-6 polyunsaturated fatty acids (γ-linolenic, eicosatrienoic, arachidonic, and docosatetraenoic) in the colostrum of GDM women, as compared to non-GDM women [29].

3.1.8. Electrolytes

Sodium was evaluated in two studies in colostrum, and both showed an increase of sodium concentrations in correlation to GDM; moreover Galipau et al. found an increase in relation to insulin use [15,30]. Potassium, phosphorus and calcium were analyzed by Kaushik et al. in the colostrum and no differences were found [15].

3.1.9. Vitamin E

GDM was not associated with changes in α-tocopherol concentration in the colostrum. No correlation was found between the concentration of α-tocopherol in the serum and in the colostrum for control and diabetic groups [31].

3.1.10. MicroRNA

A recent study evaluated the microRNAs levels (let-7a, miRNA-30B and miRNA-378) in HM, all of which are known to participate in adipogenesis. Data showed a significant difference in let-7a and miRNA-378 among the normal group and the GDM group. However, these differences disappeared by controlling maternal pre-pregnancy BMI, because pre-pregnancy BMI was a confounder that was correlated to gestational metabolic complications [32].

3.1.11. Metabolome

Wen et al. determined the human milk metabolome profile of GDM women over the first month of lactation. A total of 187 metabolites were identified in the breast milk, including 4 alkanes, 17 amino acid derivatives, 21 amino acids, 22 saturated fatty acids, 29 unsaturated fatty acids, 8 TCA cycle intermediates, 3 cofactors or vitamins, 3 keto acids and derivatives, 1 glycolytic intermediate, 43 organic acids, and 36 organic compounds. The metabolome composition and differences among the colostrum, transition milk, and mature milk from GDM mothers shared many similarities with those from normal pregnancies. However, there were 28 metabolites that were found to be significantly different between women with normal pregnancies and women with GDM pregnancies in the colostrum, transition milk, and mature milk samples [33].

3.2. Insulin-Dependent Diabetes Mellitus—IDDM

We found eight studies that focused on IDDM and all were published before the 21st century. These articles evaluated the HM of diabetic women with diagnosis and exordium before the pregnancy, with different durations of the pathology and different controls of the therapies. Four studies were conducted based on the same protocol.

The results are summarized and reported in Tables 3 and 4.

Table 3. Materials and Methods of the different studies included in the survey regarding insulin-dependent diabetes mellitus (IDDM) and HM.

Study	Metabolic Control in Pregnancy	Sample Time	Gestational Age	Parameters Analyzed	Sample Size IDDM vs. Control Women
[34]	Moderately controlled	24 h pool of mature milk: 16–90 days	Term	Total nitrogen, lactose, fat, trace minerals, lactoferrin, sIgA, glucose, sodium.	5 vs. 42
[35]	Poorly controlled	3, 4, 5, 6, 7 days	Term	Lipids, glucose, lactose, citrate, sodium, potassium, chloride, calcium, magnesium, total protein	1 vs. 13

Table 3. *Cont.*

Study	Metabolic Control in Pregnancy	Sample Time	Gestational Age	Parameters Analyzed	Sample Size IDDM vs. Control Women
[36]	Tightly controlled with continuous subcutaneous insulin infusion	0, 3, 5, 7, 9, 10, 12, 15, 17, 21, 25, 29, 35 days	Term	Triglycerides, lactose, protein, cholesterol, glucose, myoinositol, fatty acid	6 vs. 5
[37]	Tightly controlled	2, 3, 7, 14, 42, 84 days	Term Preterm	Prolactin	33 vs. 33 and 11 healthy reference women
[38]	Tightly controlled	3, 7, 14, 42, 84 days	Term Preterm	Total lipid, medium-chain fatty acids, saturated and monounsaturated long-chain fatty acid, long chain polyunsaturated fatty acid	33 vs. 33 and 11 healthy reference women
[39]	Tightly controlled	7, 14, 42, 84 days	Term Preterm	Vitamin E	33 vs. 33 and 11 healthy reference women
[40]	Not indicated	8–10 days	Term Preterm	Lactose, citrate and glucose	6 vs. 38
[41]	Tightly controlled	2, 3, 7, 14, 42, 84 days	Term Preterm	Lactose, total nitrogen, conductivity, osmolality	33 vs. 33 and 11 healthy reference women

Table 4. Results of the different studies included in the survey regarding IDDM and HM.

Components	Effects	Reference
Total protein content	No differences	Col/Trans/mat: [34–36]
Lactoferrin	No differences	Mat: [34]
Glucose	No differences Increase	Col/Trans/Mat: [36] Mat: [34]
Lactose	No differences	Col/Trans/Mat: [34–36]
Myoinositol	No differences	Col/Trans/Mat: [36]
Total lipid content	No differences Decrease	Col/Trans/Mat: [34,36,38] Col: [35]
Cholesterols	No differences Decrease	Col/Trans/Mat: [36] Col/Trans/Mat: [36]
Triglycerides	No differences	Col: [36]
Fatty Acid Profile	No differences	Col/Trans/Mat: [36]
medium-chain fatty acid	Decrease No differences	Col: [34] Col/Trans/Mat: [38]
polyunsaturated fatty acids	Increase Decrease	Col: [35] Col/Trans/Mat: [38]

Table 4. *Cont.*

Components	Effects	Reference
oleic acid	Increase	Col: [35]
Potassium, magnesium and calcium	No differences	Col/Mat: [34,35]
Sodium	No differences Increase	Col: [35] Mat: [34]
Phosphorus, zinc, copper, iron	No differences	Mat: [34]
Chlorite and citrate	No differences	Col: [35]
Vitamin E	No differences	Col/Trans/Mat: [39]

3.2.1. Proteins

Three studies did not find a difference in concentrations in total protein content between groups, although several differences were found in the protocol, as shown in Table 3 [34–36].

Only one study evaluated the lactoferrin and secretory IgA and no differences were found between IDDM mothers and healthy mothers [34].

Another study investigated prolactin levels and found that, in the first postnatal week, milk immunoreactive prolactin concentrations were lower for women with IDDM than for the control group [37]. The significantly lower milk prolactin concentration could be related to elevated serum glucose. High postprandial capillary glucose explained much of the variance in HM prolactin measurements for IDDM mothers. The good glycemic control during pregnancy and early postpartum period was associated with higher perinatal milk prolactin values. Moreover, the inverse relationship between lactose and milk prolactin, which was significant at day 2 postpartum for reference women, was delayed until day 14 postpartum for women with IDDM. These data reflect the delay in lactogenesis and in establishment of lactation experience by IDDM mothers [37].

3.2.2. Lipids

Lipids are the nutrients more extensively studied in the relationship between IDDM and HM composition: we found four different studies on this topic. The results are quite discordant: three found no changes in total fat, but the data from Bitman et al. had a mean fat content 1.5 times lower in IDDM [34–37].

The cholesterol level was tested in two studies, with opposite results: one observed five times lower concentration, while the other observed no differences [35,36].

The triglycerides were evaluated in one study and no differences were found [36].

Fatty acid profile was analyzed in three different studies [35–37]. Van Beusekom et al. did not find abnormalities in total fatty acid composition [36]. Bitman et al. demonstrated a decreased medium-chain fatty acid, suggesting impairment of fatty acid synthesis in the mammary gland, and an increased oleic acid and high concentrations of polyunsaturated fatty acids, suggesting increased chain elongation [35]. Ferris et al. reported that medium-chain fatty acids in the group with IDDM were similar to or greater than those of the control and reference groups at all times, and were within normal reported ranges. In addition, HM long-chain polyunsaturated fatty acids were lower in women with IDDM from 14 to 84 days postpartum [38].

3.2.3. Carbohydrates

Three studies evaluated the carbohydrate levels, per se, such as the macronutrients of HM [34–36]. The data agree in terms of lactose levels and no differences were found [34–36]. Results are discordant for the glucose levels: Butte et al. observed that milk glucose was 2.3 times higher in IDDM mothers, whereas Van Beusekom et al. did not find differences [34,36].

In the end, one study analyzed the myoinositol levels and no differences were found [36].

3.2.4. Electrolytes

There were no differences in HM levels of potassium, calcium, magnesium between groups in two different studies. The results of these studies are discordant regarding sodium: Butte et al. reported that sodium was 1.2 times higher, but Bitman et al. did not find differences [34,35].

Moreover, no differences were found between groups for phosphorus, zinc, copper, iron [34] concentrations in one study, and chlorite and citrate levels in another study [35].

3.2.5. Vitamins

Only one vitamin (i.e., alpha tocopherol) was analyzed in one study in IDDM HM. Tocopherol decreased by 50% in all groups between 7–14 days postpartum [39], with no difference between groups.

3.2.6. Markers of Lactogenesis

Neubauer et al. and Arthur et al. evaluated the markers for the onset of milk secretion [40,41]. Arthur et al. reported that the peak in milk lactose occurred significantly later for women with IDDM, suggesting that lactation was delayed. Concentrations of lactose, citrate and glucose increase significantly in milk of IDDM between day 2 and 3. The plateau was reached for all metabolites on day 4 [37]. These data confirm the results by Neubauer et al., finding a significantly lower lactose and higher total nitrogen in the colostrum. Milk lactose increased significantly over time to 42 days postpartum. Breast milk lactose was inversely correlated with breast milk conductivity at 3 days postpartum. Total nitrogen was also inversely correlated with milk lactose for women with IDDM. Conductivity and osmolality did not differ among the three group [40].

4. Discussion

Diabetes is a frequent pathology during pregnancy that potentially determines several complications and is a significant risk factor for newborn morbidity [6,42]. The impact of maternal metabolic abnormalities on early postnatal nutrition and infant metabolic curves is of considerable interest, because the offspring of women, both with preexistent diabetes or GDM, are at increased long-term risk for type 2 diabetes, although epidemiologic evidence has also shown a long-term protective effect of breastfeeding against obesity and type 2 diabetes in offspring [1–3,43]. Based on this strong correlation between maternal and neonatal morbidity, it is important to know the effects of this condition on the composition of HM, especially in relation to the benefits mediated by the HM for newborns [1–3]. In the absence of any clear conclusion about this topic, clinical practice should continue to promote and support breastfeeding, as indicated in recognized international guidelines [1], also for GDM women.

Until now, few studies have been reported in the literature assessing the composition of the human milk of diabetic mothers. The main observation is that GDM and IDDM can alter the composition of HM milk. The effect on HM is present not only in the first day post-partum, but is continued throughout all of the lactating phases. These studies hypothesize that the modification inducted by GDM have a potential role that can be, not only detrimental but also protective for the babies. The data on IDDM highlight that the modification of the composition is related to the control of the pathology.

However, we believe that these studies present some limitations:

(i) Several studies analyzed only one phase of milk and did not consider the variation at different time points during lactation. In addition, the definition of the different phases of lactation are not univocal, i.e., the time of sampling of colostrum ranges between 24 h and 7 days postpartum.

(ii) Some studies do not have a case/control protocol focused on GDM or IDDM, but rather, evaluate the effect of preterm delivery; diabetes is considered in metanalysis as a risk factor.

(iii) Concomitant drug therapies are rarely considered and analyzed.

(iv) The studies focused on IDDM are all published before 21st century, and four have the same protocol study.
(v) No dedicated study focused on type 2 diabetes is present in literature.

5. Conclusions

The number of available studies on this topic is scarce and they evaluate the effects of diabetes on a few specific milk biochemical markers with several and heterogeneous variables. Bearing in mind the previous considerations, it is therefore difficult to quantify the real effect of this pathology on the different components of HM, or on the health benefits mediated by mother's milk for the child. Future studies are needed to obtain a more comprehensive evaluation. Moreover, we believe that the protocols should be assessed with case/control structure, specifically focused on preterm delivery and with a match on gestational age (GA). It will also be important to analyze the effect of different diabetes drugs on HM and their potential interaction on the different biological components. Finally, considering the rising prevalence of type 2 diabetes in association with obesity, we believe it is important to plan future studies to determine possible effects on human milk in this population. These future findings are important to individualize and modify the maternal therapies and supplement the nutrition of the preterm newborns.

Author Contributions: C.P. has made a substantial contribution to the conception, design and drafting of the manuscript. A.C. and D.G. has been involved in drafting the manuscript and revising it critically for its important intellectual content. E.B. and F.C. revised the manuscript critically for its important intellectual content and gave the final approval of the version to be published. All authors have read and agreed to the published version of the manuscript.

Abbreviations

American Academy of Pediatrics	AAP
Body mass index	BMI
Colostrum	Col
Free amino acids	FAAs
Gestational age	GA
Gestational diabetes mellitus	GDM
Human milk	HM
Insulin-dependent diabetes mellitus	IDDM
Mature milk	Mat
Matrix metalloproteinase-9	MMP-9
Neutrophil gelatinase-associated lipocalin	NGAL
Not applicable	N/A
Transitional milk	Trans

References

1. American Academy of Paediatrics. Breastfeeding and use of human milk. *Pediatrics* **2012**, *129*, e827–e841. [CrossRef] [PubMed]
2. World Health Organization. Global Strategies for Infant and Young Child Feeding. Available online: http://www.who.int/child_adolescent_health/documents/9789241595193/en/index.html (accessed on 10 March 2019).
3. Horta, B.L.; Victora, C.G.; World Health Organization. Long-term Effects of Breastfeeding: A Systematic Review. Available online: https://apps.who.int/iris/bitstream/handle/10665/79198/9789241505307_eng.pdf?sequence=1 (accessed on 10 March 2019).
4. Lucas, A.; Fewtrell, M.S.; Cole, T.J. Fetal origins of adult disease—The hypothesis revisited. *Br. Med. J.* **1999**, *319*, 245–249. [CrossRef] [PubMed]

5. Plagemann, A. A matter of insulin: Developmental programming of body weight regulation. *J. Matern. Fetal Neonatal Med.* **2008**, *21*, 143–148. [CrossRef] [PubMed]
6. Owen, C.G.; Martin, R.M.; Whincup, P.H.; Smith, G.D.; Cook, D.G. Does breastfeeding influence risk of type 2 diabetes in later life? A quantitative analysis of published evidence. *Am. J. Clin. Nutr.* **2006**, *84*, 1043–1054. [CrossRef]
7. Hamosh, M. Bioactive factors in human milk. *Pediatr. Clin. N. Am.* **2001**, *48*, 69–86. [CrossRef]
8. Adair, L.S. Methods appropriate for studying the relationship of breastfeeding to obesity. *J. Nutr.* **2009**, *139*, S408–S411. [CrossRef]
9. Hawkes, J.; Bryan, D.L.; Gibson, R. Cells from mature human milk are capable of cytokine production following in vitro stimulation. *Adv. Exp. Med. Biol.* **2004**, *554*, 467–470.
10. McGill, H.C., Jr.; Mott, G.E.; Lewis, D.S.; McMahan, C.A.; Jackson, E.M. Early determinants of adult metabolic regulation: Effects of infant nutrition on adult lipid and lipoprotein metabolism. *Nutr. Rev.* **1996**, *54*, S31–S40. [CrossRef]
11. Ballard, O.; Morrow, A.L. Human Milk Composition: Nutrients and Bioactive Factors. *Pediatr. Clin. N. Am.* **2013**, *60*, 49–74. [CrossRef]
12. Hartmann, P.; Cregan, M. Lactogenesis and the Effects of Insulin-Dependent Diabetes Mellitus and Prematurity. *J. Nutr.* **2001**, *131*, 3016S–3020S. [CrossRef]
13. Dritsakou, K.; Liosis, G.; Valsami, G. The impact of maternal- and neonatal-associated factors on human milk's macronutrients and energy. *J. Matern. Fetal Neonatal Med.* **2017**, *30*, 1302–1308. [CrossRef] [PubMed]
14. Shapira, D.; Mandel, D.; Mimouni, F.B.; Moran-Lev, H.; Morom, R.; Mangel, L.; Lubetzky, R. The effect of gestational diabetes mellitus on human milk macronutrients content. *J. Perinatol.* **2019**, *39*, 820–823. [CrossRef] [PubMed]
15. Kaushik, S.; Trivedi, S.S.; Jain, A.; Bhattacharjee, J. Unusual changes in colostrum composition in lactating indian women having medical complications during pregnancy—A pilot study. *Indian J. Clin. Biochem.* **2002**, *17*, 68–73. [CrossRef] [PubMed]
16. Ley, S.H.; Hanley, A.J.; Sermer, M.; Zinman, B.; O'Connor, D.L. Associations of prenatal metabolic abnormalities with insulin and adiponectin concentrations in human milk. *Am. J. Clin. Nutr.* **2012**, *95*, 867–874. [CrossRef]
17. Yu, X.; Rong, S.S.; Sun, X.; Ding, G.; Wan, W.; Zou, L.; Wu, S.; Li, M.; Wang, D. Associations of breast milk adiponectin, leptin, insulin and ghrelin with maternal characteristics and early infant growth: A longitudinal study. *Br. J. Nutr.* **2018**, *120*, 1380–1387. [CrossRef] [PubMed]
18. Nunes, M.; da Silva, C.H.; Bosa, V.L.; Bernardi, J.R.; Werlang, I.C.R.; Goldani, M.Z.; NESCA Group. Could a remarkable decrease in leptin and insulin levels from colostrum to mature milk contribute to early growth catch-up of SGA infants? *BMC Pregnancy Childbirth* **2017**, *17*, 410. [CrossRef]
19. Aydin, S. The presence of the peptides apelin, ghrelin and nesfatin-1 in the human breast milk, and the lowering of their levels in patients with gestational diabetes mellitus. *Peptides* **2010**, *31*, 2236–2240. [CrossRef]
20. Aydin, S.; Geckil, H.; Karatas, F.; Donder, E.; Kumru, S.; Kavak, E.C.; Colak, R.; Ozkan, Y.; Sahin, I. Milk and blood ghrelin level in diabetics. *Nutrition* **2007**, *23*, 807–811. [CrossRef]
21. Fatimaa, S.S.; Khalidb, E.; Ladakc, A.A.; Ali, S.A. Colostrum and mature breast milk analysis of serum irisin and sterol regulatory element-binding proteins-1c in gestational diabetes mellitus. *J. Matern. Fetal Neonatal Med.* **2019**, *32*, 2993–2999. [CrossRef]
22. Aydin, S.; Kuloglu, T.; Aydin, S. Copeptin, adropin and irisin concentrations in breast milk and plasma of healthy women and those with gestational diabetes mellitus. *Peptides* **2013**, *47*, 66–70. [CrossRef]
23. Aydin, S.; Celik, O.; Gurates, B.; Sahin, I.; Ulas, M.; Yilmaz, M.; Kalayci, M.; Kuloglu, T.; Catak, Z.; Aksoy, A.; et al. Concentrations of preptin, salusins and hepcidins in plasma and milk of lactating women with or without gestational diabetes mellitus. *Peptides* **2019**, *49*, 123–130. [CrossRef]
24. Smilowitz, J.T.; Totten, S.M.; Huang, J.; Grapov, D.; Durham, H.A.; Lammi-Keefe, C.J.; Lebrilla, C.; German, J.B. Human Milk Secretory Immunoglobulin A and Lactoferrin N-Glycans Are Altered in Women with Gestational Diabetes Mellitus. *J. Nutr.* **2013**, *143*, 1906–1912. [CrossRef]
25. Ustebay, S.; Baykus, Y.; Deniz, R.; Ugur, K.; Yavuzkir, S.; Yardim, M.; Kalayci, M.; Çaglar, M.; Aydin, S. Chemerin and Dermcidin in Human Milk and Their Alteration in Gestational Diabetes. *J. Hum. Lact.* **2019**, *35*, 550–558. [CrossRef]

26. Metallinou, D.; Lykeridou, K.; Karampas, G.; Liosis, G.T.; Skevaki, C.; Rizou, M.; Papassotiriou, I.; Rizos, D. Postpartum human breast milk levels of neutrophil gelatinase-associated lipocalin (NGAL) and matrix metalloproteinase-9 (MMP-9)/NGAL complex in normal and pregnancies complicated with insulin-dependent gestational diabetes mellitus. A prospective pilot case-control study. *J. Obstet. Gynaecol.* **2019**, *29*, 1–7.
27. Klein, K.; Bancher-Todesca, D.; Graf, T.; Garo, F.; Roth, E.; Kautzky-Willer, A.; Worda, C. Concentration of free amino acids in human milk of women with gestational diabetes mellitus and healthy women. *Breastfeed. Med.* **2013**, *8*, 111–115. [CrossRef]
28. Grapov, D.; Lemay, D.G.; Weber, D.; Phinney, B.S.; Azulay Chertok, I.R.; Gho, D.S.; German, J.B.; Smilowitz, J.T. The Human Colostrum Whey Proteome Is Altered in Gestational Diabetes Mellitus. *J. Proteome Res.* **2015**, *14*, 512–520. [CrossRef]
29. Azulay Chertok, I.R.; Haile, Z.T.; Eventov-Friedman, S.; Silanikove, N.; Argov-Argaman, N. Influence of gestational diabetes mellitus on fatty acid concentrations in human colostrum. *Nutrition* **2017**, *36*, 17–21. [CrossRef]
30. Galipeau, R.; Goulet, C.; Chagnon, M. Infant and Maternal Factors Influencing Breastmilk Sodium Among Primiparous Mothers. *Breastfeed. Med.* **2012**, *7*, 290–294. [CrossRef]
31. Resende, F.B.S.; Clemente, H.A.; Fernandes Bezerra, D.; Grilo, E.C.; de Melo, L.R.; Bellot, P.E.; Dantas, R.C.; Dimenstein, R. Alpha-tocopherol concentration in serum and colostrum of mothers with gestational diabetes mellitus. *Rev. Paul. Pediatr.* **2014**, *32*, 178–186. [CrossRef]
32. Xi, Y.; Jiang, X.; Li, R.; Chen, M.; Song, W.; Li, X. The levels of human milk microRNAs and their association with maternal weight characteristics. *Eur. J. Clin. Nutr.* **2016**, *70*, 445–449. [CrossRef]
33. Wen, L.; Wu, Y.; Yang, Y.; Han, T.L.; Wang, W.; Fu, H.; Zheng, Y.; Shan, T.; Chen, J.; Xu, P.; et al. Gestational Diabetes Mellitus Changes the Metabolomes of Human Colostrum, Transition Milk and Mature Milk. *Med. Sci. Monit.* **2019**, *25*, 6128–6152. [CrossRef]
34. Butte, N.F.; Garza, C.; Burr, R.; Goldman, A.S.; Kennedy, K.; Kitzmiller, J.L. Milk composition of insulin-dependent diabetic women. *J. Pediatr. Gastroenterol. Nutr.* **1987**, *6*, 936–941. [CrossRef]
35. Bitman, J.; Hamosh, M.; Hamosh, P. Milk composition and volume during the onset of lactation in a diabetic mother. *Am. J. Clin. Nutr.* **1989**, *50*, 1364–1369. [CrossRef] [PubMed]
36. Van Beusekom, C.M.; Zeegers, T.A.; Martini, I.A.; Velvis, H.J.; Visser, G.H.; van Doormaal, J.J.; Muskiet, F.A. Milk of patients with tightly controlled insulin-dependent diabetes mellitus has normal macronutrient and fatty acid composition. *Am. J. Clin. Nutr.* **1993**, *57*, 938–943. [CrossRef]
37. Ostrom, K.M.; Ferris, A.M. Prolactin concentrations in serum and milk of mothers with and without insulin-dependent diabetes. *Am. J. Clin. Nutr.* **1993**, *58*, 49–53. [CrossRef] [PubMed]
38. Jackson, M.B.; Lammi-Keefe, C.J.; Jensen, R.G. Total lipid and fatty acid composition of milk from women with and without insulin-dependent diabetes mellitus. *Am. J. Clin. Nutr.* **1994**, *60*, 353–361. [CrossRef]
39. Lammi-Keefe, C.J.; Jonas, C.R.; Ferris, A.M.; Capacchione, C.M. Vitamin E in plasma and milk of lactating women with insulin-dependent diabetes mellitus. *J. Pediatr. Gastroenterol. Nutr.* **1995**, *20*, 305–309. [CrossRef] [PubMed]
40. Arthur, P.G.; Smith, M.; Hartmann, P.E. Milk lactose, citrate, and glucose as markers oflactogenesis in normal and diabetic women. *J. Pediatr. Gastroenterol. Nutr.* **1989**, *9*, 488–496. [CrossRef] [PubMed]
41. Neubauer, S.H.; Ferris, A.M.; Chase, C.G.; Fanelli, J.; Thompson, C.A.; Lammi-Keefe, C.J.; Clark, R.M.; Jensen, R.G.; Bendel, R.B.; Green, K.W.; et al. Delayed lactogenesis in women with insulin-dependent diabetes. *Am. J. Clin. Nutr.* **1993**, *58*, 54–60. [CrossRef] [PubMed]
42. Arenz, S.; Ruckerl, R.; Koletzko, B.; von Kries, R. Breast-feeding and childhood obesity—A systematic review. *Int. J. Obes. Relat. Metab. Disord.* **2004**, *28*, 1247–1256. [CrossRef]
43. Lucas, A. Long-term programming effects of early nutrition—Implications for the preterm infant. *J. Perinatol.* **2005**, *25*, S2–S6. [CrossRef] [PubMed]

15

Ketonuria Is Associated with Changes to the Abundance of *Roseburia* in the Gut Microbiota of Overweight and Obese Women at 16 Weeks Gestation

Helen Robinson [1,*], Helen Barrett [2], Luisa Gomez-Arango [3], H. David McIntyre [2], Leonie Callaway [4] and Marloes Dekker Nitert [3]

1 Department of Obstetric Medicine, Royal Brisbane and Women's Hospital, Butterfield St, Herston, QLD 4029, Australia
2 Mater Research Institute, The University of Queensland, Brisbane, QLD 4101, Australia
3 School of Chemistry and Molecular Biosciences, The University of Queensland, St Lucia, QLD 4072, Australia
4 Women's and Newborn Services, Royal Brisbane and Women's Hospital, Butterfield St, Herston, QLD 4029, Australia
* Correspondence: robinsonhelenlouise@gmail.com

Abstract: The gut microbiome in pregnancy has been associated with various maternal metabolic and hormonal markers involved in glucose metabolism. Maternal ketones are of particular interest due to the rise in popularity of low-carbohydrate diets. We assessed for differences in the composition of the gut microbiota in pregnant women with and without ketonuria at 16 weeks gestation. Fecal samples were obtained from 11 women with fasting ketonuria and 11 matched controls. The samples were analyzed to assess for differences in gut microbiota composition by 16S rRNA sequencing. Supervised hierarchical clustering analysis showed significantly different beta-diversity between women with and without ketonuria, but no difference in the alpha-diversity. Group comparisons and network analysis showed that ketonuria was associated with an increased abundance of the butyrate-producing genus *Roseburia*. The bacteria that contributed the most to the differences in the composition of the gut microbiota included *Roseburia*, *Methanobrevibacter*, *Uncl. RF39*, and *Dialister* in women with ketonuria and *Eggerthella*, *Phascolarctobacterium*, *Butyricimonas*, and *Uncl. Coriobacteriaceae* in women without ketonuria. This study found that the genus *Roseburia* is more abundant in the gut microbiota of pregnant women with ketonuria. *Roseburia* is a butyrate producing bacterium and may increase serum ketone levels.

Keywords: microbiome; pregnancy; obesity; ketonuria; *Roseburia*

---

1. Introduction

Pregnancy is a time of metabolic and hormonal change. Ketogenesis is accelerated in pregnancy, particularly in the third trimester. Ketones are produced from the breakdown of lipids when the mother's metabolic needs can no longer be met by glucose. The body produces three ketone bodies, beta-hydroxybutyrate, acetoacetate, and acetone. Beta-hydroxybutyrate and acetoacetate can be used as energy sources by the mother and the fetus and occur in a 1:1 ratio. Elevated maternal ketone levels have been associated with adverse fetal and childhood outcomes, particularly with regard to intelligence quotient (IQ), although results of these studies have been inconsistent [1–4].

The role of the gut microbiome in the metabolic changes of pregnancy has been an area of increasing interest. We have reported that the composition of the gut microbiome in pregnancy is associated with various metabolic and hormonal markers involved in glucose metabolism [5]. Whether the gut microbiome actually causes these metabolic changes is yet to be fully determined. However, mice colonized with the microbiome from women in the third trimester of pregnancy develop insulin resistance and increased adiposity, supporting the idea that the gut microbiome itself drives some of the metabolic changes observed in pregnancy [6].

Butyrate is a short-chain fatty acid (SCFA) that is produced by certain bacteria within the microbiome. Known butyrate-producing species include *Faecalibacterium prausnitzii*, *Roseburia* spp., and *Eubacterium rectale* [7]. Butyrate is the main fuel for energy production in colonocytes and studies of metabolism of human and rat colonocytes have shown that butyrate is metabolized to ketone bodies and carbon dioxide [8,9]. In keeping with this finding, mice colonized with *Roseburia* have higher serum levels of the ketone, beta-hydroxybutyrate [10].

There are no studies that have reported an association between the composition of the gut microbiome in pregnancy and maternal ketone levels. We hypothesized that gut microbiome composition is associated with maternal ketone levels and that butyrate-producing bacteria are more abundant in women with higher ketone levels.

2. Materials and Methods

Women enrolled in the Study of Probiotics IN Gestational diabetes (SPRING study) who supplied a stool sample and fasting urine sample at baseline (<16 weeks gestation) were included in this study. Women taking probiotics in pregnancy prior to 16 weeks gestation and sample collection were excluded from enrolment. This study was approved by the human research ethics committee of the Royal Brisbane and Women's Hospital on the 16th January 2012 (HREC/11/QRBW/467) and The University of Queensland on the 25th January 2012 (201200080). All subjects gave their informed consent for inclusion before they participated in the study. The study was conducted in accordance with the Declaration of Helsinki. All women enrolled in the study were either overweight or obese, as defined by pre-pregnancy body mass index (BMI) > 25 kg/m^2. Women collected a stool sample and fasting urine sample within a 24-h time period. Women fasted for between 9.5 and 12 h prior to collection of urine. The stool sample was kept in storage at −80 °C prior to fecal DNA isolation. Urine samples were immediately tested for the presence of ketones. Urine dipstick tests were performed using SIEMENS Multistix 10 SG reagent strips and measured levels of the ketone, acetoacetate. A ketone level of trace, small, moderate, and large corresponded to an acetoacetate level of 0.5 mmol/L, 1.5 mmol/L, 4 mmol/L, and >= 8 mmol/L, respectively. All women provided dietary information from the start of pregnancy by food frequency questionnaire (Cancer Council Victoria's Dietary Questionnaire for Epidemiological Studies (Version (2)).

Women with any level of ketonuria present were matched with women with no ketonuria. The matching was performed on future GDM status, ethnicity, BMI and age. Fecal samples from each group were then analyzed to assess for differences in the gut microbiota between these two groups. Funding for this study was provided by the National Health and Medical Research Committee (NHMRC1028575) of Australia, the Royal Brisbane and Women's Hospital Foundation, the Mater Foundation and the Australian Diabetes in Pregnancy Society. HB is funded by an NHMRC Early Career Fellowship.

2.1. Fecal DNA Extraction

Stored stool samples were thawed at 4 °C before analysis. Aliquots of 250 mg of stool were removed from each sample for DNA extraction using the repeated bead beating and column (RBB + C) protocol. The aliquots were mixed with the RBB + C lysis buffer and sterile zirconia beads (0.1 and 0.5 mm diameter) and homogenized using a Tissue Lyser II (Qiagen, Chadstone VIC, Australia) for 3 min at 30 Hz. Samples underwent DNA purification using Qiagen AllPrep columns [5,11]. The quality and quantity of DNA was analyzed using the Nanodrop ND 1000 spectrophotometer (NanoDrop Technologies, Thermo Scientific, Scoresby, VIC, Australia) system.

2.2. Fecal Bacterial Identification

Bacteria within each sample were identified via 16S rRNA Sequencing. PCR amplification for the V6–V8 hypervariable regions of the bacterial 16S rRNA gene was performed using the 926F forward (50-TCG TCG GCA GCG TCA GAT GTG TAT AAG AGA CAG AAA CTY AAA KGA ATT GRC GG-30) and 1392R reverse (50-GTC TCG TGG GCT CGG AGA TGT GTA TAA GAG ACA GAC GGG CGG TGW GTR C-30) primers. Positive (*E. coli* JM109 DNA) and negative (deionized sterile water) controls were included in each PCR run. Nextera XT V2 index kit Sets A and B were used to barcode PCR products and the AMPure XP bead system (Illumina, San Diego, CA, USA) was used for purification. Barcoded DNA underwent quantification, normalization and pooling to develop sequencing libraries which were then sequenced on the Illumina MiSeq platform (Illumina, San Diego, CA, USA) at the Australian Centre for Ecogenomics at The University of Queensland. The Quantitative insights Into Microbial Ecology (QIIME) v1.9.1 analysis tool was used to join and de-multiplex forward and reverse sequences. Using the Greengenes reference database, the open reference operational taxonomic unit (OTU) picking method was used for taxonomic assignments with a pairwise identity threshold of 97%. Taxonomic units that were present in the negative controls were removed from the analysis along with OTUs with a relative abundance of <0.0001. Prior to downstream analysis, the OTU table was rarefied to 3000 sequences/sample with no samples removed in this step.

2.3. Statistical Analysis

Median and interquartile ranges (IQR) were used to present the data as bacterial abundance was not normally distributed. Non-parametric statistical methods were used and a p value of <0.05 was considered statistically significant. Sample profiles were analyzed via the online Calypso software tool [12] and results are presented at the genus level of taxonomic assignment. Chao1 and Shannon indices were used for comparison of alpha diversity (within sample diversity) and the Bray-Curtis dissimilarity index was used to assess beta diversity (between sample diversity). Network analysis was performed to identify positive and negative correlations between bacterial taxa for both patients with and without ketonuria. Genera associated with samples from women with and without ketonuria were identified using Spearman's rho correlation coefficients with 1000-fold permutations. The strength of the color of the node reflects the significance of the association with either group and results are reported as significant if the false discovery rate (FDR) was <0.05. The size of the node reflects the abundance of the genus. Group comparisons were performed on genus level using the Wilcoxon Rank test, with no genera passing the statistical threshold for multiple testing, which is likely a reflection of the overall number of participants in this sub-study.

3. Results

Eleven women with ketonuria at 16-weeks gestation were matched with 11 women without ketonuria (Table 1). There were no differences in baseline BMI, maternal age, ethnicity, fasting blood glucose levels, future GDM status, or carbohydrate intake between the groups.

Table 1. Participant characteristics.

	Ketonuria	No Ketonuria
N	11	11
Maternal age (years)	33 (29–38)	32 (29–33)
Gestation (weeks)	14 (14–15)	14 (14–15)
Maternal BMI (kg/m^2)		
25–30 (%)	4 (36%)	4 (36%)
30–35 (%)	0 (0%)	0 (0%)
>35 (%)	7 (64%)	7 (64%)

Table 1. *Cont.*

	Ketonuria	No Ketonuria
Ethnicity		
Caucasian (%)	11 (100%)	11 (100%)
Fasting blood glucose (mmol/L)	4.4 (4.3–4.5)	4.2 (4.0–4.4)
Carbohydrate intake (g/day)	137.2 (95.7–171.2)	155.9 (122.0–170.1)
Later developed GDM (%)	1 (9%)	1 (9%)
Level of ketonuria		
Trace	8 (73%)	
Small	1 (9%)	
Moderate	1 (9%)	
Large	1 (9%)	

Data presented as median (IQR). BMI, body mass index; GDM, gestational diabetes mellitus; g, grams.

Comparison of Gut Microbiome Composition

There was no difference in the alpha diversity at genus level (Chao1, Shannon index) between the two groups (see Figure 1A,B). There was also no difference between the two groups in beta diversity at genus level with unsupervised hierarchical clustering principle coordinates analysis (PCoA)(Bray-Curtis dissimilarity index) (See Figure 2A), but with supervised redundancy analysis (RDA) there was a significant difference ($P < 0.0001$; RDA analysis, see Figure 2B). Analysis of the variance in the beta-diversity displayed no significant difference between the groups (see Figure 2C).

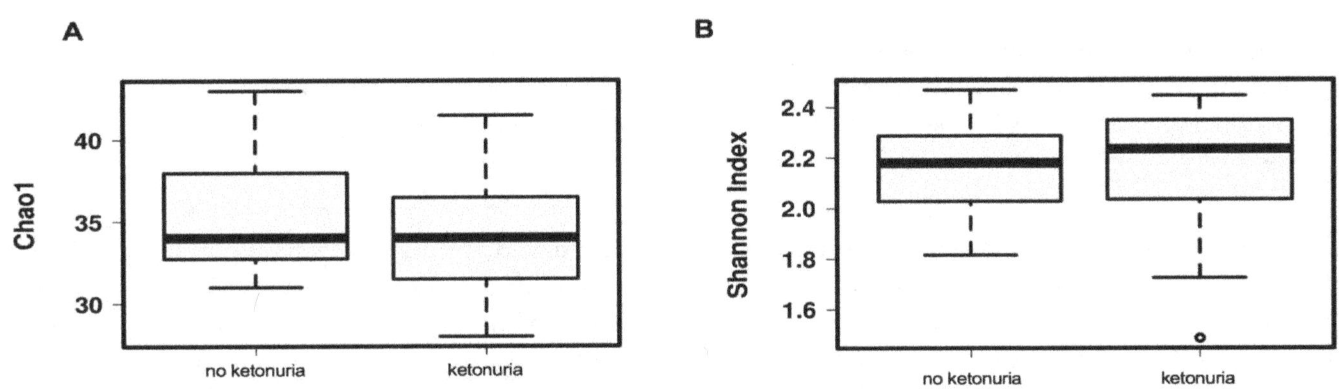

Figure 1. Alpha diversity of the gut microbiota at genus level between women with and without ketonuria. (**A**) Alpha diversity as assessed with the Chao1 index; (**B**) alpha diversity, as assessed with the Shannon index.

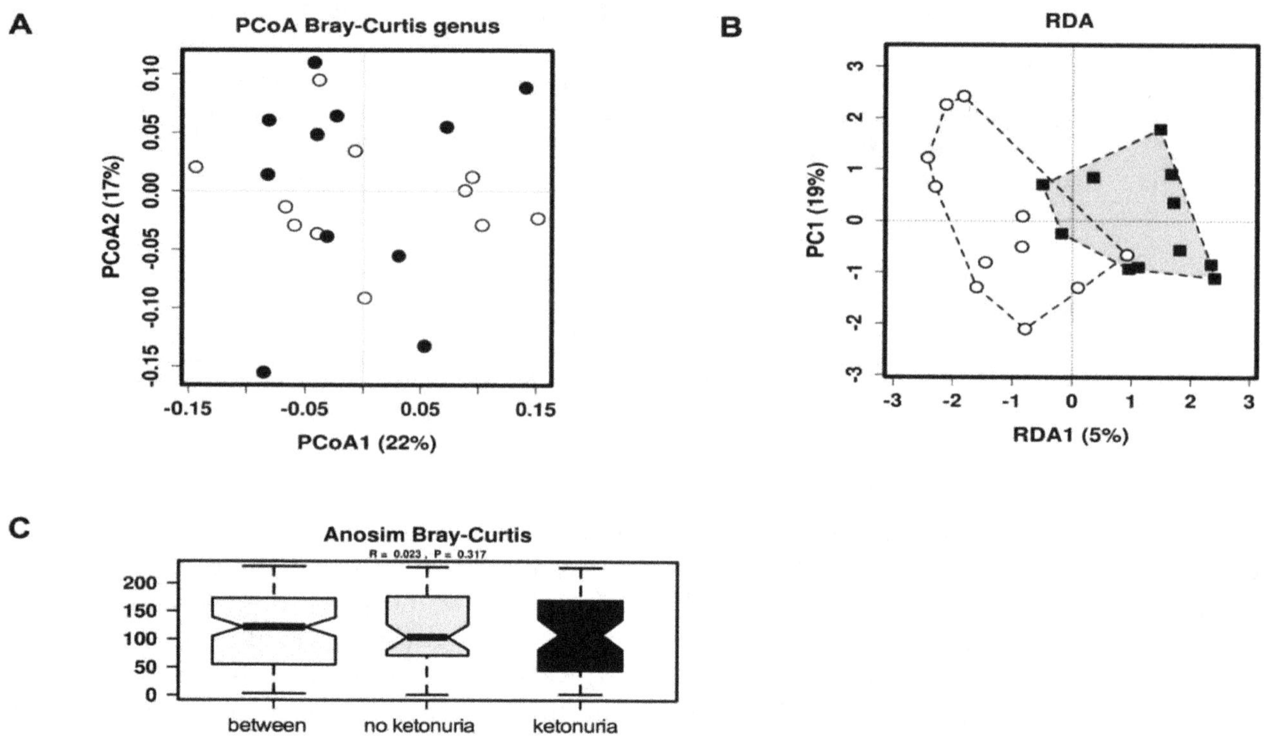

Figure 2. Beta diversity of the gut microbiota at genus level between women with and without ketonuria. (**A**) Unsupervised hierarchical clustering analysis by PCoA; (**B**) supervised clustering analysis by RDA and (**C**) variance analysis by Anosim analysis. Black circles/squares, ketonuria; white circles, no ketonuria.

Presence of urinary ketones was associated with an increased abundance of the butyrate-producing genus *Roseburia* in the network analysis. The brightness of the nodes is related to the level of significance of the association. *Roseburia* is the brightest of the nodes associated with ketonuria (see Figure 3); however, the butyrate-producer *Faecalibacterium* is also associated with ketonuria as is the acetate/propionate producer *Dialister*. In women who did not have ketonuria at 16 weeks, the abundance of *Adlercreutzia, Bifidobacterium, Dorea,* and *Collinsella* was higher (see Figure 3). Group comparisons revealed a statistically significantly higher abundance of *Roseburia* in women with ketonuria (see Figure 4A), and *Dialister* and *Faecalibacterium* abundance tended to be higher in the women with ketonuria ($P = 0.066$ and $P = 0.076$ respectively). In the women without ketonuria, *Adlercreutzia* abundance trended to be higher ($P = 0.066$), but that of *Bifidobacterium, Dorea,* and *Collinsella* was not significantly higher ($P = 0.15$; $P = 0.14$; and $P = 0.17$), respectively.

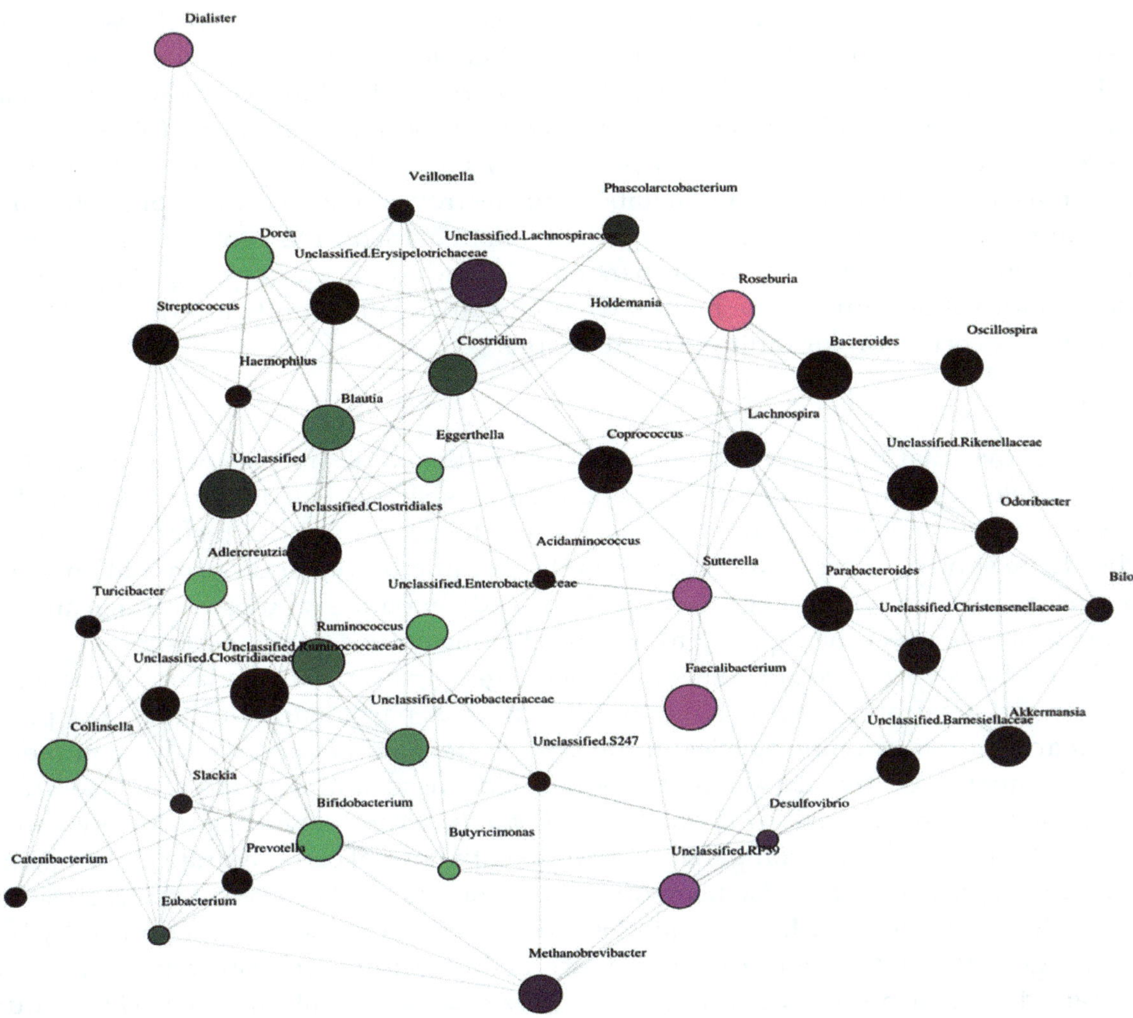

Figure 3. Network analysis of gut microbiota composition between women with and without ketonuria at genus level. Purple circles, ketonuria; green circles, no ketonuria; lines indicate positive correlations between the abundances of the bacteria. The size of the circle indicates the overall abundance of the genus and the brightness of the color indicates the degree to which the genus is associated with the group.

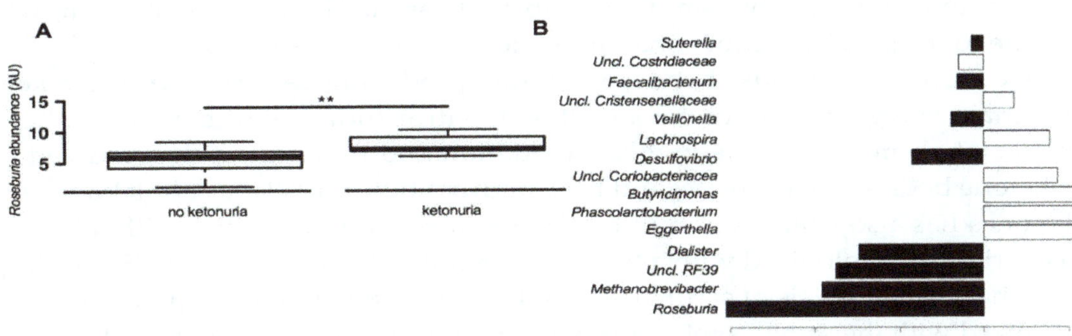

Figure 4. Bacterial genera that are specifically associated with the presence or absence of ketonuria. (**A**) Abundance of *Roseburia* between the groups. (**B**) sPLS-DA analysis of the contribution of bacteria genera to the differences between the gut microbiota between the groups. Black bars, ketonuria; white bars, no ketonuria. ** $p < 0.01$.

The bacteria that contribute the most to the differences in the composition of the gut microbiota include *Roseburia, Methanobrevibacter, Uncl. RF39,* and *Dialister* in the women with ketonuria and

Eggerthella, Phascolarctobacterium, Butyricimonas, and *Uncl. Coriobacteriaceae* in the women without ketonuria (see Figure 4B). Predicted bacterial functions that were increased in women with ketonuria included riboflavin metabolism, lipid biosynthesis, carbon fixation pathways in prokaryotes, zeatin biosynthesis, adipocytokine signaling pathway, biotin metabolism, folate biosynthesis, prenyltransferases, and peroxisome (See Supplementary Figure S1). In women without ketonuria, bacterial functions ascorbate and aldarate metabolism; electron transfer carriers, phosphotransferase system PTS; aminobenzoate degradation, drug metabolism cytochrome P450; limonene and pinene degradation; chlorocyclohexane and chlorobenzene degradation; and styrene degradation were predicted to be more abundant. These results were all statistically significant ($p < 0.05$) on simple testing, but not after correction for multiple comparisons.

4. Discussion

This study shows that *Roseburia* is more abundant in the stool samples of women with fasting ketonuria at 16 weeks gestation. *Faecalibacterium* and *Dialister* species tended higher in the stool samples of women with ketonuria; however, this increased abundance did not reach statistical significance. Other studies have shown an association between the gut microbiota and hormonal and metabolic markers of glucose metabolism in pregnancy [5]. Our study expands on these findings and suggests that the microbiota may affect the capacity to produce ketone bodies during fasting.

Roseburia and *Faecalibacterium* are both genera of obligate gram-positive anaerobic bacteria. These bacteria ferment carbohydrates in the colon to produce SCFAs, particularly butyrate. The presence of both *Roseburia* and *Faecalibacterium* species in the gut has been associated with human metabolism outside of pregnancy. In two large metagenome-wide association studies, concentrations of butyrate-producing bacteria, *Roseburia intestinalis* and *Faecalibacterium prausnitzii* were lower in patients with type 2 diabetes mellitus when compared with those with normal carbohydrate metabolism [13,14]. The abundance of *F. prausnitzii* has also been found to be significantly lower in obese patients when compared with lean subjects [15]. In contrast, *Roseburia* has been found to be significantly higher in patients with higher BMI [16]. *Roseburia* abundance is linked to overall carbohydrate intake with individuals with lower carbohydrate intake having lower *Roseburia* abundance [17]. In our study, carbohydrate intake was not significantly different between women with ketonuria (137.2 (95.7–171.2) g/day) and those without ketonuria (155.9 (122.0–170.1) g/day; $P = 0.46$), but this may be due to the small sample size. *Roseburia* spp. contain genes involved in riboflavin metabolism and folate biosynthesis indicating how the increases in the abundance in the predicted function analysis may be related to increased *Roseburia* abundance. In addition, *Dialister* spp. and *Faecalibacterium* spp. also express genes for riboflavin metabolism, folate biosynthesis, and biotin metabolism, which could further contribute to the predicted functional differences between the groups.

Studies have found various links between butyrate-producing bacteria and serum ketone levels. Butyrate is the main energy source for colonocytes. In vitro studies of human and rat colonic cells show that the metabolism of butyrate involves oxidation and that part of the oxidized butyrate is converted to ketone bodies, acetoacetate, and beta-hydroxybutyrate [8,9]. A link between *Roseburia* and serum ketones has also been seen in mice. When mice were fed a diet with a high content of plant polysaccharides and colonized with a 'core' community of bacterial species including *Roseburia intestinalis*, they had higher levels of serum beta-hydroxybutyrate when compared with mice on the same diet, colonized with the same 'core' community without *Roseburia intestinalis* [10]. It is uncertain as to how these results can be extrapolated to humans, as the human gut microbiota is highly diverse and it is unclear if the presence of a single species would elicit a similarly large effect. Furthermore, dietary intake varies between individuals and across cultures.

A different mechanism for the link between butyrate and ketone levels has been hypothesized. Intraperitoneal administration of butyrate into mice led to increased serum beta-hydroxybutyrate levels and fibroblast growth factor 21 (FGF21) levels [18]. The hormone FGF21 stimulates fatty acid metabolism in the liver leading to increased ketogenesis. The authors postulated that the increase in serum ketone levels was due to butyrate increasing FGF21 levels via induction of FGF21 gene expression in the liver. In humans, FGF21 is also expressed in the liver and is a downstream target of the transcription factor peroxisome proliferator-activated receptor alpha (PPARα). PPARα is a major regulator of lipid metabolism in the liver and is activated by both fasting and by consumption of ketogenic diets [19]. It is not known whether serum butyrate induces FGF21 gene expression in humans and what level of butyrate would be required to do so. In the current study, butyrate levels in the circulation were not measured and it is not clear if the increased abundance of *Roseburia* results in higher levels in the circulation.

Adlercreutzia abundance trended to be higher in those without ketonuria. *Adlercreutzia* is an obligate anaerobic coccobacillus and has been linked to various inflammatory conditions including inflammatory bowel disease, primary sclerosing cholangitis and multiple sclerosis [20–22]. Studies linking *Adlercreutzia* to human metabolism are lacking. One study did find a reduced abundance of *Adlercreutzia* in patients with HIV who developed diabetes compared with those who did not develop diabetes [23]. *Eggerthella, Phascolarctobacterium, Butyricimonas,* and *Uncl. Coriobacteriaceae* were the bacteria that contributed most to the differences in the composition of the gut microbiota in women without ketonuria. In a metagenome-wide association study of GDM, *Phascolarctobacterium* was more abundant in women with GDM whereas *Eggerthella* was more abundant in healthy controls [24]. In the same study, when assessing metagenomic linkage groups, *Methanobrevibacter smithii* was enriched in healthy controls. In our study, *Methanobrevibacter* was one of the bacteria that contributed most to the differences in the composition of the gut microbiota in women with ketonuria.

Maternal ketonuria has been associated with adverse fetal and childhood outcomes, particularly reduced childhood IQ [1,2]. However, these studies had disparate methodologies, with inconsistent results [3,4]. Ketone production occurs more rapidly in pregnancy, particularly in the third trimester [25]. It is felt to be due to increased maternal lipid metabolism and reduced glucose levels due to glucose being transported to the fetus for energy [26,27]. A maternal diet that is low in carbohydrate will also result in increased maternal ketone levels. The fetus utilizes ketones for energy and also as an important precursor for brain tissue [28]. It would therefore appear necessary for the fetus to be exposed to some level of ketones, however whether a high level of ketone exposure *per se* is harmful to the fetus is unclear. Our results suggest that ketone production in pregnancy may be more complex than a simple metabolic switch from glucose to lipid metabolism when maternal glucose supply is low. The gut microbiota may have a role to play via other metabolic pathways.

Limitations of the study included that urine ketone levels were only measured at one time point in the first trimester. Women in the control group may have had ketonuria at other times from when their samples were collected. A strength of the study is that women fasted for at least 9.5 h prior to the collection of the urine and ketogenesis is more pronounced with increased duration of the fasting state. Our sample size was limited which may have reduced the power of the study, particularly in relation to any differences in dietary intake. Lastly, circulating SCFA levels were not measured, which could indicate whether circulating butyrate levels are different in women with and without ketonuria.

5. Conclusions

Roseburia is more abundant in the microbiome of pregnant women with ketonuria. *Roseburia* is a butyrate-producing bacteria and studies have shown a link between both *Roseburia* and butyrate in the colon and elevated serum ketone levels. This study is further evidence of such a link and the first time that this link has been seen in pregnancy. Increased butyrate production by the gut microbiota may alter signaling in the host and thereby contribute to overall metabolic health in pregnancy. Larger studies of the microbiome in pregnant women with and without ketonuria at multiple time points in the pregnancy, with detailed dietary data needs to be done to further understand the relationship between *Roseburia* and maternal metabolism.

Author Contributions: Conceptualisation H.R., M.D.N., H.B., Methodology H.R., M.D.N., H.B., Formal Analysis M.D.N., L.G.-A., Data Curation H.R., Original Draft Preparation H.R., Writing H.R., M.D.N., H.B., L.C., L.G.-A., L.C., H.D.M., Supervision M.D.N., H.B., L.C., Funding Acquisition L.C., H.D.M.

References

1. Churchill, J.A.; Berendes, H.W. Intelligence of children whose mothers had acetonuria during pregnancy. *Perinat. Factors Affect. Hum. Dev.* **1969**, *185*, 30–35.
2. Hamdi, K.; Bastani, P.; Gafarieh, R.; Mozafari, H.; Hashemi, S.H.; Ghotbi, M.H. The influence of maternal ketonuria on fetal well-being tests in postterm pregnancy. *Arch. Iran. Med.* **2006**, *9*, 144–147. [PubMed]
3. Naeye, R.L.; Chez, R.A. Effects of maternal acetonuria and low pregnancy weight gain on children's psychomotor development. *Am. J. Obstet. Gynecol.* **1981**, *139*, 189–193. [CrossRef]
4. Stehbens, J.A.; Baker, G.L.; Kitchell, M. Outcome at ages 1, 3, and 5 years of children born to diabetic women. *Am. J. Obstet. Gynecol.* **1977**, *127*, 408–413. [CrossRef]
5. Gomez-Arango, L.F.; Barrett, H.L.; McIntyre, H.D.; Callaway, L.K.; Morrison, M.; Dekker Nitert, M.; Group, S.T. Connections Between the Gut Microbiome and Metabolic Hormones in Early Pregnancy in Overweight and Obese Women. *Diabetes* **2016**, *65*, 2214–2223. [CrossRef] [PubMed]
6. Koren, O.; Goodrich, J.K.; Cullender, T.C.; Spor, A.; Laitinen, K.; Backhed, H.K.; Gonzalez, A.; Werner, J.J.; Angenent, L.T.; Knight, R.; et al. Host remodeling of the gut microbiome and metabolic changes during pregnancy. *Cell* **2012**, *150*, 470–480. [CrossRef] [PubMed]
7. Louis, P.; Young, P.; Holtrop, G.; Flint, H.J. Diversity of human colonic butyrate-producing bacteria revealed by analysis of the butyryl-CoA:acetate CoA-transferase gene. *Environ. Microbiol.* **2010**, *12*, 304–314. [CrossRef] [PubMed]
8. Roediger, W.E. Role of anaerobic bacteria in the metabolic welfare of the colonic mucosa in man. *Gut* **1980**, *21*, 793–798. [CrossRef] [PubMed]
9. Roediger, W.E. Utilization of nutrients by isolated epithelial cells of the rat colon. *Gastroenterology* **1982**, *83*, 424–429.
10. Kasahara, K.; Krautkramer, K.A.; Org, E.; Romano, K.A.; Kerby, R.L.; Vivas, E.I.; Mehrabian, M.; Denu, J.M.; Backhed, F.; Lusis, A.J.; et al. Interactions between Roseburia intestinalis and diet modulate atherogenesis in a murine model. *Nat. Microbiol.* **2018**, *3*, 1461–1471. [CrossRef]
11. Yu, Z.; Morrison, M. Improved extraction of PCR-quality community DNA from digesta and fecal samples. *Biotechniques* **2004**, *36*, 808–812. [CrossRef] [PubMed]
12. Zakrzewski, M.; Proietti, C.; Ellis, J.J.; Hasan, S.; Brion, M.J.; Berger, B.; Krause, L. Calypso: A user-friendly web-server for mining and visualizing microbiome–environment interactions. *Bioinformatics* **2017**, *33*, 782–783. [CrossRef] [PubMed]
13. Karlsson, F.H.; Tremaroli, V.; Nookaew, I.; Bergstrom, G.; Behre, C.J.; Fagerberg, B.; Nielsen, J.; Backhed, F. Gut metagenome in European women with normal, impaired and diabetic glucose control. *Nature* **2013**, *498*, 99–103. [CrossRef] [PubMed]
14. Qin, J.; Li, Y.; Cai, Z.; Li, S.; Zhu, J.; Zhang, F.; Liang, S.; Zhang, W.; Guan, Y.; Shen, D.; et al. A metagenome-wide association study of gut microbiota in type 2 diabetes. *Nature* **2012**, *490*, 55–60. [CrossRef] [PubMed]
15. Remely, M.; Aumueller, E.; Merold, C.; Dworzak, S.; Hippe, B.; Zanner, J.; Pointner, A.; Brath, H.; Haslberger, A.G. Effects of short chain fatty acid producing bacteria on epigenetic regulation of FFAR3 in type 2 diabetes and obesity. *Gene* **2014**, *537*, 85–92. [CrossRef] [PubMed]
16. Tims, S.; Derom, C.; Jonkers, D.M.; Vlietinck, R.; Saris, W.H.; Kleerebezem, M.; de Vos, W.M.; Zoetendal, E.G. Microbiota conservation and BMI signatures in adult monozygotic twins. *ISME J.* **2012**, *7*, 707. [CrossRef] [PubMed]
17. Duncan, S.H.; Belenguer, A.; Holtrop, G.; Johnstone, A.M.; Flint, H.J.; Lobley, G.E. Reduced dietary intake of carbohydrates by obese subjects results in decreased concentrations of butyrate and butyrate-producing bacteria in feces. *Appl. Environ. Microbiol.* **2007**, *73*, 1073–1078. [CrossRef] [PubMed]
18. Li, H.; Gao, Z.; Zhang, J.; Ye, X.; Xu, A.; Ye, J.; Jia, W. Sodium butyrate stimulates expression of fibroblast growth factor 21 in liver by inhibition of histone deacetylase 3. *Diabetes* **2012**, *61*, 797–806. [CrossRef] [PubMed]

19. Fisher, F.M.; Maratos-Flier, E. Understanding the Physiology of FGF21. *Annu. Rev. Physiol.* **2016**, *78*, 223–241. [CrossRef]
20. Bajer, L.; Kverka, M.; Kostovcik, M.; Macinga, P.; Dvorak, J.; Stehlikova, Z.; Brezina, J.; Wohl, P.; Spicak, J.; Drastich, P. Distinct gut microbiota profiles in patients with primary sclerosing cholangitis and ulcerative colitis. *World J. Gastroenterol.* **2017**, *23*, 4548–4558. [CrossRef] [PubMed]
21. Shaw, K.A.; Bertha, M.; Hofmekler, T.; Chopra, P.; Vatanen, T.; Srivatsa, A.; Prince, J.; Kumar, A.; Sauer, C.; Zwick, M.E.; et al. Dysbiosis, inflammation, and response to treatment: A longitudinal study of pediatric subjects with newly diagnosed inflammatory bowel disease. *Genome Med.* **2016**, *8*, 75. [CrossRef] [PubMed]
22. Chen, J.; Chia, N.; Kalari, K.R.; Yao, J.Z.; Novotna, M.; Paz Soldan, M.M.; Luckey, D.H.; Marietta, E.V.; Jeraldo, P.R.; Chen, X.; et al. Multiple sclerosis patients have a distinct gut microbiota compared to healthy controls. *Sci. Rep.* **2016**, *6*, 28484. [CrossRef] [PubMed]
23. Moon, J.Y.; Zolnik, C.P.; Wang, Z.; Qiu, Y.; Usyk, M.; Wang, T.; Kizer, J.R.; Landay, A.L.; Kurland, I.J.; Anastos, K.; et al. Gut microbiota and plasma metabolites associated with diabetes in women with, or at high risk for, HIV infection. *EBioMedicine* **2018**, *37*, 392–400. [CrossRef] [PubMed]
24. Kuang, Y.S.; Lu, J.H.; Li, S.H.; Li, J.H.; Yuan, M.Y.; He, J.R.; Chen, N.N.; Xiao, W.Q.; Shen, S.Y.; Qiu, L.; et al. Connections between the human gut microbiome and gestational diabetes mellitus. *Gigascience* **2017**, *6*, 1–12. [CrossRef] [PubMed]
25. Metzger, B.E.; Ravnikar, V.; Vileisis, R.A.; Freinkel, N. "Accelerated starvation" and the skipped breakfast in late normal pregnancy. *Lancet* **1982**, *319*, 588–592. [CrossRef]
26. Herrera, E. Lipid metabolism in pregnancy and its consequences in the fetus and newborn. *Endocrine* **2002**, *19*, 43–55. [CrossRef]
27. Newbern, D.; Freemark, M. Placental hormones and the control of maternal metabolism and fetal growth. *Curr. Opin. Endocrinol. Diabetes Obes.* **2011**, *18*, 409–416. [CrossRef] [PubMed]
28. Cunnane, S.C.; Menard, C.R.; Likhodii, S.S.; Brenna, J.T.; Crawford, M.A. Carbon recycling into de novo lipogenesis is a major pathway in neonatal metabolism of linoleate and alpha-linolenate. *Prostaglandins Leukot. Essent. Fat. Acids* **1999**, *60*, 387–392. [CrossRef]

16

Dietary Patterns and Dietary Adaptations in Women with and without Gestational Diabetes: Evidence from the Growing Up in New Zealand Study

Robyn L. Lawrence [1], Clare R. Wall [2] and Frank H. Bloomfield [1,*]

1 The Liggins Institute, University of Auckland, Private Bag 92019, Auckland 1142, New Zealand; robyn.lawrence@auckland.ac.nz

2 Discipline of Nutrition and Dietetics, School of Medical Sciences, University of Auckland, Private Bag 92019, Auckland 1142, New Zealand; c.wall@auckland.ac.nz

* Correspondence: f.bloomfield@auckland.ac.nz

Abstract: Diet is a cornerstone of the management of gestational diabetes (GDM). We investigated differences in dietary patterns and dietary adaptations among pregnant women with and without GDM participating in the Growing Up in New Zealand study. Presence of GDM was determined using coded clinical data and plasma glucose results meeting the New Zealand Society for the Study of Diabetes diagnostic criteria. Women answered a food frequency questionnaire and questions regarding dietary changes and information received during pregnancy. Women with GDM had lower adherence scores than those without GDM for 'Junk' (mean (SD) score −0.28 (0.95) versus 0.02 (1.01) $p < 0.0005$) and 'Traditional/White bread' dietary patterns (−0.18 (0.93) versus 0.01 (1.01) $p = 0.002$). More women with GDM reported avoiding foods high in fat or sugar (25.3% versus 5.7%, $p < 0.05$) compared to women without GDM. A greater proportion of women with GDM compared with those without GDM received information from dietitians or nutritionists (27.0% versus 1.7%, $p < 0.05$) or obstetricians (12.6% versus 7.5%, $p < 0.05$). More women diagnosed before the antenatal interview received advice from dietitians or nutritionists compared with those diagnosed after (46.9% versus 6.0%, $p < 0.05$). Women with GDM appear to make positive changes to their diet in response to advice received from health care professionals.

Keywords: gestational diabetes; dietary patterns; pregnancy; maternal nutrition; dietary adaptations

1. Introduction

Pregnancy is a time when women frequently pay extra attention to their diet in order to promote the health and well-being of themselves and their baby [1–4]. Women receive information from a range of sources [2,3] and make a number of dietary adaptations during pregnancy [5]. Diet is thought to play a critical role in the development of gestational diabetes mellitus (GDM), a form of carbohydrate intolerance first diagnosed in pregnancy [6], and a number of dietary components have been associated with an increased or decreased risk of GDM [7–11]. GDM poses significant health risks to both mother and infant [12–14] extending beyond the pregnancy and neonatal period [15,16]. Rates of GDM-affected pregnancies are increasing, thought to be at least in part due to concomitant increasing prevalence of overweight and obesity [17–19]. Globally, reported prevalence of GDM ranges between 1% and 45% of pregnancies [20–22]. In New Zealand, GDM has been estimated to affect approximately 6% of pregnancies [23].

Dietary pattern analysis has become a popular tool for exploring dietary associations with GDM, as it is thought to better reflect real eating behaviours by considering the eating pattern as a whole [24]. A number of studies have found dietary patterns characterised by high intakes of red and processed meats, fried foods and added sugars to be associated with an increased risk of GDM, while dietary patterns characterised by high consumption of fruit, vegetables, wholegrains and nuts or 'Mediterranean'-style dietary patterns to be associated with a lower risk of developing GDM [25–35]. Nonetheless, research of dietary patterns and risk of GDM has primarily been conducted in largely Caucasian populations [11,25,30,34,36], with many using data from the same cohort of women from the Nurses' Health Study II [25,28,36]. Ethnicity is a widely accepted risk factor for GDM [37], with women of non-European descent disproportionately affected [38]. Different ethnic populations tend to have different diets [39], which may further influence the risk of developing GDM. Dietary patterns and adherence to nutrition recommendations have been reported to differ amongst pregnant women of different ethnicities within New Zealand [40,41]; however, associations between diet and the development of GDM have not been explored in the New Zealand population. Whether women who develop GDM make similar dietary adaptations during pregnancy to those who do not develop GDM is also unknown. The aim of this study was therefore to explore differences in dietary patterns and dietary adaptations among women with and without a diagnosis of GDM during pregnancy in New Zealand.

2. Materials and Methods

2.1. Study Population

Data used for the analyses in this study were derived from 6822 women enrolled in the Growing Up in New Zealand study (www.growingup.co.nz), a pre-birth, longitudinal cohort study exploring multidisciplinary determinants of health and development for children born in New Zealand [42]. Pregnant women with an estimated due date between 25th April 2009 and 25th March 2010 residing in an area defined by the geographical boundaries of three regional health boards in the upper-mid North Island of New Zealand were eligible to participate in the study. The geographical area of recruitment was chosen for its ethnic, socioeconomic and urban and rural residency diversity with the aim of having a study cohort that was broadly generalizable to the rest of New Zealand [42]. Ethical approval was provided by the Ministry of Health Northern Y Regional Ethics Committee (reference NTY/08/06/055) and written informed consent was obtained from all participating women.

2.2. Data Collection

Data collection during the antenatal period comprised a face-to-face interview, collecting information on maternal demographics, health and pregnancy history, smoking status, dietary intake and physical activity. A total of 6822 women consented and completed the antenatal interview (most often during the third trimester of pregnancy) and 6657 consented to access to their routine health records through use of their unique National Hospital Identifier (NHI).

2.3. Measurements

2.3.1. Diabetes Status during Pregnancy

The methods used to identify women with GDM in the cohort have been described previously [23]. Briefly, participant NHIs were used to obtain data on diabetes status during pregnancy from the Ministry of Health's National Minimum Dataset, the three regional health boards, and laboratories servicing the recruitment catchment area. Coded clinical data were collected from the Ministry of Health and the three regional health boards. Laboratories provided fasting plasma glucose concentration, glucose challenge test results and glucose tolerance test results. Women were classified as having GDM if they had a clinical code for GDM or if they had a blood glucose result (between 12 weeks' gestation to the end of pregnancy) meeting the diagnostic criteria for GDM in use by their regional health board at the time. All three regional health boards used the New Zealand Society for the Study of Diabetes criteria [43,44] to diagnose GDM: fasting plasma glucose of ≥ 5.5 mmol/L or a 2 h plasma glucose ≥ 9.0 mmol/L post 75 g oral glucose tolerance test (OGTT) [45–48]. One regional health board also considered a 60 min plasma glucose result on the 50 g glucose challenge test (GCT) of ≥ 11.1 mmol/L to be indicative of GDM [45]. Women identified as having pre-existing diabetes or impaired glucose tolerance were excluded from analyses.

2.3.2. Dietary Patterns and Dietary Habits

A semi-quantitative 44 item food frequency questionnaire (FFQ) administered as part of the antenatal interview was used to collect information on dietary intake and has been described in detail elsewhere [40,41]. The purpose of the antenatal FFQ was to describe the frequency of consumption over the previous four weeks of the four core food groups as recommended by the New Zealand Ministry of Health's guidelines for pregnant women [49]: fruits and vegetables; breads and cereals; milk, milk products, lean meat, meat alternatives and eggs, and foods likely to be high in fats, sugars and/or salt. Four dietary patterns have previously been identified in the cohort using principal component analysis as described by Wall et al. [41]. The dietary patterns identified were labelled as 'Junk', 'Health conscious', 'Traditional/White bread' and 'Fusion/Protein'. Food items with factor loadings of 0.3 or greater in the principal component analysis were considered to be strongly associated with the identified pattern. The 'Junk' dietary pattern had high loadings of confectionary, snacks, takeaways, hot chips, processed meats, soft and energy drinks, battered fried fish or seafood, ice-cream and cakes or biscuits. The 'Health conscious' dietary pattern had high loadings of vegetables, cheese, brown wholemeal bread, non-citrus fruits, yoghurt, dried fruits, high fibre cereal, and Vegemite™ or Marmite™. The 'Traditional/White bread' had high factor loadings for whole or standard milk, white bread, margarine, jam honey marmalade, peanut butter, Nutella™ and low fibre and/or high sugar cereals. The 'Fusion/Protein' had high factor loadings for noodles, rice, pasta, seafood, chicken, green leafy vegetables, eggs and red meat. Summary scores for each dietary pattern were available for 5664 women who had antenatal dietary data. A higher score indicates a stronger adherence to that dietary pattern.

The antenatal questionnaire also included open questions regarding foods or drinks deliberately avoided or added to the diet due to pregnancy [50] and were categorised as 'breads and cereals', 'lean meat, chicken, seafood, eggs, cooked dried beans, peas', 'milk and milk products', 'fruit and vegetables', 'supplement', 'chocolate', 'foods high in fat or sugar', 'alcohol', 'soft drinks' and 'other'. Women were asked whether they had received any information or been told anything that led them to make dietary changes while pregnant. If they answered 'yes' to this question they were asked to select from a list of information sources including 'family/whānau', 'friends', 'GP (Family doctor)', 'midwife', 'obstetrician', 'dietitian/nutritionist', alternative health practitioner', 'antenatal class', 'the internet', 'radio', 'TV', 'books, magazines, newspaper', or 'other'.

2.3.3. Covariates

Questions relating to maternal socio-demographic, health and lifestyle characteristics were also included in the antenatal interview. Self-reported ethnicity was allocated to one of six Level 1 categories (i) European; (ii) Māori; (iii) Pacific Peoples; (iv) Asian; (v) Middle Eastern/Latin American/African (MELAA), and (vi) Other ethnicity according to the coding criteria used by Statistics New Zealand [51]. If women identified with multiple ethnicities but did not self-prioritise a primary ethnicity, the prioritisation methodology employed by Statistics New Zealand between 1991 to 2004 [52] was used, as mutually exclusive ethnic groups were required for statistical analyses. The 'MELAA' and 'Other' ethnic groups were combined into the 'Other' ethnic group due to small numbers in these groups. The New Zealand Deprivation Index (NZDep06) [53] was used as a measure of social deprivation. The index is divided into deciles from 1 (least deprived) to 10 (most deprived). Pre-pregnancy weight and height were self-reported and used to calculate pre-pregnancy body mass index (BMI). Weight gain during pregnancy up to the point of the antenatal interview was assessed in a question asking about weight change during pregnancy in 5 kg increments. Women were also asked whether they were actively dieting or trying to lose weight during the 6 months prior to pregnancy and whether or not they lost any weight during that time. Physical activity was assessed using questions from the International Physical Activity Questionnaire (IPAQ). Participants were asked about intensity (moderate or vigorous), duration (<30, 30 to 60, or >60 min) and frequency (days per week) of activity [54]. To be classified as participating in moderate or vigorous activity women had to have engaged in moderate activity for at least 30 min for at least five days per week or vigorous activity for at least 30 min on at least two days per week. Women were asked whether they received any treatment to assist them in becoming pregnant and, if women answered 'yes', this question was followed by a multiple response question relating the type of treatment given, which included 'fertility awareness and weight loss'.

2.4. Statistical Analyses

Maternal socio-demographic, health and lifestyle characteristics and dietary patterns are reported as the frequency (%) for categorical variables and the mean ± standard deviation (SD) for continuous variables. In accordance with Growing Up in New Zealand data policy, cells where $n < 10$ are reported as <10 rather than the actual number. Differences in maternal characteristics and dietary patterns were tested using Chi squared or Fisher's exact test and unadjusted and adjusted logistic regression for categorical variables and independent samples t-test for continuous variables. Results are reported as the mean (SD), frequency (%) or odds ratios (OR) or adjusted odds ratios (aOR) and 95% confidence intervals (CI). Maternal age (<35 and ≥35 years), ethnicity (European, Māori, Pacific, Asian, Other) NZDep06 score (1–3, 4–7 and 8–10), pre-pregnancy BMI (<25, 25–29.9 and ≥30 kg/m^2), pre-pregnancy and first trimester physical activity (at least 150 min per week of moderate to vigorous physical activity), smoking pattern (continued smoking during pregnancy, stopped smoking during pregnancy, non-smoker), alcohol consumption (continued drinking during pregnancy, stopped drinking during pregnancy, non-drinker) and dietary pattern score were included in adjusted models. These variables were selected as they either were associated with GDM in univariate or multivariate analyses or are commonly considered to be associated with the risk of developing GDM in the literature. Analyses were conducted using SPSS version 21. A two-sided p value of <0.05 was considered statistically significant.

3. Results

The characteristics of women participating in the Growing Up in New Zealand study have been described previously [42]. The selection of participants included in this study is shown in Figure 1. Socio-demographic, health and lifestyle characteristics of the 5384 women included in the analyses of this study are shown in Table 1. GDM was identified in 280 (5.2%) of women. There were significant differences in maternal age, ethnicity, socioeconomic deprivation, pre-pregnancy BMI, physical activity pre-pregnancy and during the first trimester, pre-pregnancy dieting status, smoking patterns and alcohol consumption between women with and without GDM (Table 1).

Dietary pattern scores differed between women diagnosed with GDM and those without GDM (Table 2). Women with GDM had significantly lower mean scores for 'Junk' and 'Traditional/White bread' dietary patterns and a significantly higher mean score for the 'Fusion Protein' dietary pattern. Logistic regression analysis showed higher scores on the 'Junk' OR (per 1 SD change) 0.61 (95% CI; 0.51, 0.74) $p \leq 0.0005$ and the 'Traditional/White bread' dietary patterns OR 0.89 (0.71, 0.93) $p = 0.002$ were associated with a decreased odds of having GDM and higher scores on the 'Fusion/Protein' dietary pattern OR 1.25 (1.13, 1.38) $p \leq 0.0005$ were associated with an increased odds of having GDM. Although not statistically significant, there was a strong trend of a higher score on the 'Health conscious' dietary pattern to be associated with a reduced likelihood of having GDM OR 0.89 (0.78, 1.00) $p = 0.055$ in unadjusted analyses. After adjusting for maternal age, ethnicity, socioeconomic deprivation, pre-pregnancy BMI, pre-pregnancy and first trimester physical activity, smoking patterns, alcohol consumption and dietary pattern score on alternative dietary patterns, higher scores on 'Junk' aOR 0.64 (0.52, 0.80) $p = 0.001$ and 'Traditional/White bread' aOR 0.66 (0.55, 0.78) $p \leq 0.0005$ dietary patterns remained significantly associated with a reduced likelihood of having GDM, while the relationship between scores on the 'Fusion/Protein' and 'Health conscious' dietary patterns were attenuated and not significantly associated with GDM status aOR 1.04 (0.90, 1.2) $p = 0.269$ and aOR 1.11 (0.96, 1.29) $p = 0.378$ respectively.

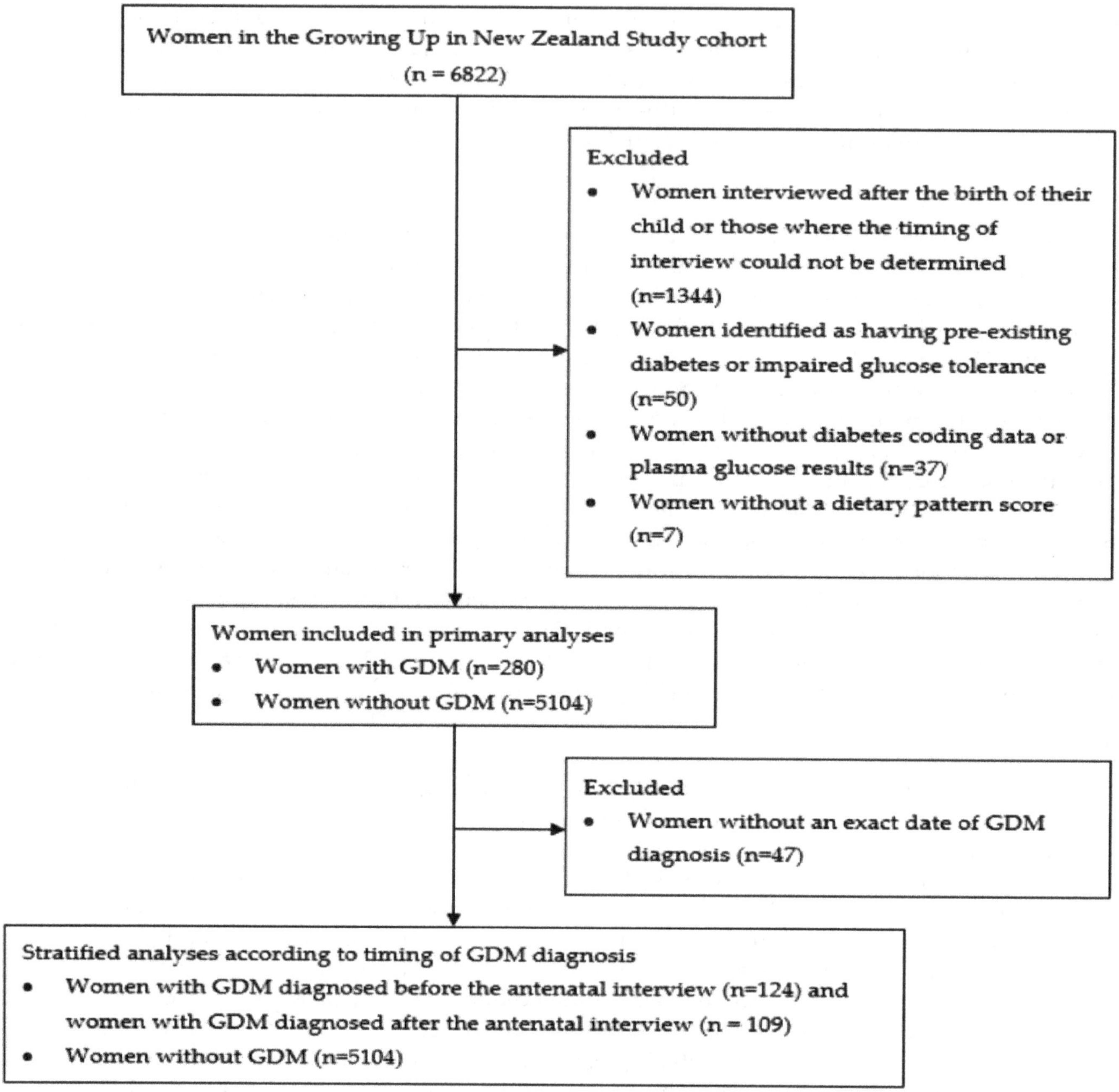

Figure 1. Flowchart showing selection of participants included in primary and secondary analyses of dietary patterns and dietary adaptations in women with and without GDM from the Growing Up in New Zealand study.

Table 1. Characteristics of women in the Growing Up in New Zealand cohort according to gestational diabetes mellitus (GDM) diagnosis [1].

	Women Without GDM	Women With GDM	*p*-Value
n (%)	5104 (94.8)	280 (5.2)	
Age group (years)			<0.0005
<20	259 (5.1)	<10 (1.8)	
20–24	747 (14.6)	28 (10.0)	
25–29	1267 (24.8)	51 (18.2)	
30–34	1616 (31.7)	95 (33.9)	
35–39	1039 (20.4)	81 (28.9)	
40 and over	176 (3.4)	20 (7.1)	
Self-prioritised ethnicity			<0.0005
European	2913 (57.2)	103 (36.8)	
Māori	686 (13.5)	22 (7.9)	
Pacific	630 (12.4)	55 (19.6)	
Asian	681 (13.4)	84 (30.0)	
Other	186 (3.6)	16 (5.7)	
Parity			0.628
First child	2167 (42.5)	123 (43.9)	
Subsequent child	2937 (57.5)	157 (56.1)	
Pregnancy planning			0.857
Planned	3144 (61.8)	171 (61.3)	
Unplanned	1941 (38.2)	108 (38.7)	
Fertility treatment			0.090
Yes	299 (9.5)	23 (13.5)	
No	2844 (90.5)	148 (86.5)	
Fertility treatment: fertility awareness and weight loss			0.169
Yes	26 (8.7)	<10 (17.4)	
No	272 (91.3)	19 (82.6)	
Socioeconomic deprivation			0.021
1 to 2 (least deprived)	864 (16.9)	30 (10.7)	
3 to 4	978 (19.2)	45 (16.1)	
5 to 6	909 (17.8)	61 (21.8)	
7 to 8	1050 (20.6)	63 (22.5)	
9 to 10 (most deprived)	1301 (25.5)	81 (28.9)	
Highest education			0.266
No secondary school	319 (6.3)	14 (5.0)	
Secondary school/NCEA* 1–4	1187 (23.3)	77 (27.6)	
Diploma/Trade certificate/NCEA* 5–6	1550 (30.4)	76 (27.2)	
Bachelor's degree	1178 (23.1)	58 (20.8)	
Higher degree	861 (16.9)	54 (19.4)	
Pre-pregnancy BMI (kg/m^2)			<0.0005
<18.5	192 (4.2)	<10 (2.8)	
18.5–24.9	2558 (56.2)	103 (41.4)	
25–29.9	1034 (22.7)	60 (24.1)	
30 and over	767 (16.9)	79 (31.7)	
Gestational weight gain			0.005
Gained ≥5 kg	4455 (88.9)	229 (83.0)	
Gained <5 kg	376 (7.5)	32 (11.6)	
No change	43 (0.9)	<10 (1.1)	
Lost <5 kg	74 (1.5)	10 (3.6)	
Lost ≥5 kg	62 (1.2)	<10 (0.7)	
Actively dieting pre-pregnancy	1272 (24.9)	104 (37.1)	<0.0005
Pre-pregnancy dieting weight loss			0.300
Yes	1032 (82.7)	81 (78.6)	
No	216 (17.3)	22 (21.4)	

Table 1. *Cont.*

	Women Without GDM	Women With GDM	*p*-Value
Physical activity†			
Physically active pre-pregnancy	2578 (50.5)	119 (42.5)	0.009
Physically active during first trimester	1459 (28.6)	62 (22.1)	0.020
Physically active during second and third trimesters	1147 (22.5)	59 (21.1)	0.584
Smoking patterns			0.012
Continued smoking during pregnancy	508 (10.0)	13 (4.6)	
Stopped smoking during pregnancy	494 (9.7)	31 (11.1)	
Non-smoker	4088 (80.3)	236 (84.3)	
Alcohol consumption			<0.0005
Any drinking during pregnancy	1536 (30.1)	42 (15.0)	
Stopped drinking during pregnancy	2276 (44.6)	100 (35.7)	
Non-drinker	1287 (25.2)	138 (49.3)	

[1] Includes only women interviewed before the birth of their child and excludes women with other forms of diabetes or for whom diabetes status could not be determined or those without dietary pattern scores; data presented as number of participants (percentages), missing values have not been included in the column%; *NCEA is the primary national qualification for secondary school students in New Zealand; †Engaged in moderate or vigorous physical activity for at least 150 min per week; BMI, Body Mass Index; NCEA, National Certificate of Educational Achievement.

Table 2. Dietary pattern scores among women with and without GDM.

Dietary Pattern	Women Without GDM n = 5104	Women With GDM n = 280	*p*-Value
Junk	0.02 (1.01)	−0.28 (0.95)	<0.0005
Health conscious	0.01 (1.00)	−0.11 (0.95)	0.055
Traditional/White bread	0.01 (1.01)	−0.18 (0.93)	0.002
Fusion Protein	−0.02 (0.99)	0.26 (1.09)	<0.0005

Data presented as the mean (SD).

Comparing scores in the highest versus the lowest tertile for each dietary pattern showed similar results (Table 3). Women with dietary pattern scores in the highest tertiles of 'Junk' were 62% less likely, and 'Traditional/White bread' 40% less likely to have GDM compared to women in the lowest tertiles. Having a score in the highest tertile of the 'Fusion Protein' dietary pattern almost doubled the likelihood of having a GDM diagnosis in unadjusted analyses. After adjusting for potential confounders (maternal age, ethnicity, socioeconomic deprivation, pre-pregnancy BMI, pre-pregnancy and first trimester physical activity, smoking pattern, alcohol consumption and dietary pattern score on alternative dietary patterns), women with scores in the highest tertiles of the 'Junk' and 'Traditional/White bread' dietary patterns were half as likely to have a diagnosis of GDM compared to women with scores in the lowest tertiles. The higher likelihood of GDM for those with scores in the highest tertile of the 'Fusion Protein' dietary pattern compared to the lowest tertile was attenuated and no longer statistically significant in the adjusted model. The 'Health conscious' dietary pattern was not significantly associated with GDM in both the unadjusted and adjusted models when comparing women with scores in the highest versus the lowest tertiles; however, the relationship of a reduced likelihood of GDM in the unadjusted model was reversed to an increased likelihood of GDM in the adjusted model.

Table 3. Unadjusted and adjusted odds of having GDM for women with intakes in the highest tertile compared to those with intakes in the lowest tertile of each dietary pattern.

Dietary Pattern	*n*	OR (95% CI)	*p*-Value	*n*	aOR (CI)	*p*-Value
Junk	3581	0.38 (0.28, 0.52)	<0.0005	3154	0.49 (0.34, 0.70)	<0.0005
Health conscious	3580	0.80 (0.60, 1.08)	0.141	3134	1.24 (0.87, 1.77)	0.244
Traditional/White bread	3597	0.60 (0.44, 0.81)	0.001	3157	0.47 (0.32, 0.68)	<0.0005
Fusion Protein	3589	1.93 (1.42, 2.62)	<0.0005	3160	1.25 (0.87, 1.81)	0.231

OR (95% CI) from unadjusted logistic regression; aOR (95% CI) from adjusted logistic regression (maternal age group, ethnicity, socioeconomic deprivation, pre-pregnancy BMI, pre-pregnancy and first trimester physical activity, smoking, alcohol consumption and dietary patterns included in the model).

In analyses stratified according to the timing of GDM diagnosis, the relationship between higher scores on 'Junk' and 'Traditional/White bread' dietary patterns with a reduced likelihood of GDM strengthened when comparing women without GDM to women with GDM diagnosed before the antenatal interview (Table 4). In analyses comparing women diagnosed with GDM after the antenatal interview to women without GDM, only the association of a higher score on the 'Junk' dietary pattern with a reduced likelihood of GDM diagnosis remained significant, although this was attenuated.

Table 4. Adjusted odds of having GDM for women with intakes in the highest tertile compared to those with intakes in the lowest tertile of each dietary pattern stratified according to timing of diagnosis.

	GDM Diagnosed Before Interview			GDM Diagnosed After Interview		
Dietary Pattern	*n*	aOR (CI)	*p*-Value	*n*	aOR (CI)	*p*-Value
Junk	3050	0.27 (0.15, 0.50)	<0.0005	3037	0.54 (0.30, 0.96)	0.036
Health conscious	3043	0.95 (0.54, 1.68)	0.860	3035	1.44 (0.81, 2.58)	0.214
Traditional/White bread	3072	0.21 (0.12, 0.38)	<0.0005	3045	0.64 (0.35, 1.18)	0.153
Fusion Protein	3062	1.13 (0.64, 1.99)	0.676	3055	0.67 (0.38, 1.18)	0.169

aOR (95% CI) from adjusted logistic regression (maternal age group, ethnicity, socioeconomic deprivation, pre-pregnancy BMI, pre-pregnancy and 1st trimester physical activity, smoking, alcohol consumption and dietary patterns included in the model).

Differences in the types of foods or drinks avoided or added due to pregnancy between women with and without GDM and between women diagnosed before or after the antenatal interview are shown in Table 5. Significantly more women with GDM avoided chocolate, foods high in fat or sugar and soft drinks and added milk or milk products to their diets during pregnancy compared to women without GDM. Significantly more women with GDM diagnosed before the antenatal interview avoided high fat or sugar foods and added milk or milk products compared to women with GDM diagnosed after the antenatal interview.

Almost three-quarters (71.6%) of women reported receiving information that resulted in making changes to their diet. Sources of information leading to dietary change in women with and without GDM are presented in Table 6. Significantly more women with GDM reported receiving information from a dietitian or nutritionist or an obstetrician and significantly fewer from friends, antenatal class, or books, magazines and newspapers compared to women without GDM. Compared to women without GDM, the magnitude of these differences was greater in women with GDM diagnosed before the antenatal interview than those with GDM diagnosed after the antenatal interview. Almost eight times more women with GDM diagnosed before the antenatal interview reported receiving information from a dietitian or nutritionist compared to women with GDM diagnosed after the antenatal interview.

Table 5. Foods and drinks avoided or added during pregnancy.

	Women Without GDM	Women With GDM	GDM Diagnosed before Interview	GDM Diagnosed after Interview
Foods/drinks avoided	$n = 4456$	$n = 241$	$n = 104$	$n = 96$
Chocolate	29 (0.7)	<10 (3.7) [a]	<10 (4.8) [a]	<10 (3.1) [a]
High fat or sugar foods	252 (5.7)	61 (25.3) [a]	37 (35.6) [a,b]	11 (11.5) [a,b]
Alcohol	2876 (64.5)	109 (45.2) [a]	52 (50.0) [a]	42 (43.8) [a]
Soft drinks	742 (16.7)	78 (32.4) [a]	30 (28.8) [a]	33 (34.4) [a]
Foods/drinks added	$n = 2129$	$n = 116$	$n = 50$	$n = 48$
Vegetables and fruit	108 (5.1)	<10 (1.7)	<10 (0.0)	<10 (2.1)
Breads and cereals	126 (5.9)	<10 (7.8)	<10 (10.0)	<10 (6.3)
Milk or milk products	779 (36.6)	62 (53.4) [a]	32 (64.0) [a,b]	21 (43.8) [b]
Lean meat, chicken, seafood, eggs, cooked dried beans or peas	766 (36.0)	45 (38.8)	18 (36.0)	23 (47.9)
Fluids	831 (39.0)	28 (24.1) [a]	10 (20.0) [a]	13 (27.1)
Supplements	446 (20.9)	24 (20.7)	<10 (12.0)	12 (25.0)
Other	337 (15.8)	13 (11.2)	<10 (12.0)	<10 (8.3)

Data presented as number of participants (percentages), missing have not been included in the column%; [a] Significantly different in women with GDM compared to women without GDM ($p < 0.05$); [b] Significantly different between women with GDM diagnosed before vs. after the antenatal interview ($p < 0.05$).

Table 6. Information leading to dietary changes.

	Women Without GDM	Women With GDM	Women With GDM Diagnosed before Interview	Women With GDM Diagnosed after Interview
n	5100	280	124	109
Received information leading to dietary changes	3652 (71.6)	215 (76.8)	98 (79.0)	83 (76.1)
Sources of information				
Family/whānau	873 (23.9)	36 (16.7)	14 (14.3) [a]	16 (19.3)
Friends	853 (23.4)	30 (14.0) [a]	15 (15.3)	11 (13.3) [a]
GP	1274 (34.9)	71 (33.0)	31 (31.6)	29 (34.9)
Midwife	2703 (74.1)	151 (70.2)	62 (63.3) [a]	63 (75.9)
Obstetrician	273 (7.5)	27 (12.6) [a]	16 (16.3) [a]	<10 (10.8)
Dietitian or nutritionist	61 (1.7)	58 (27.0) [a]	46 (46.9) [a,b]	<10 (6.0) [a,b]
Alternative health practitioner	58 (1.6)	<10 (1.9)	<10 (1.0)	<10 (3.6)
Antenatal class	247 (6.8)	<10 (2.8) [a]	<10 (1.0) [a]	<10 (4.8)
The internet	681 (18.7)	33 (15.3)	13 (13.3)	17 (20.5)
Radio	26 (0.7)	<10 (0.5)	<10 (0.0)	<10 (1.2)
TV	123 (3.4)	<10 (1.4)	<10 (2.0)	<10 (1.2)
Books, magazines, newspaper	1117 (30.6)	48 (22.3) [a]	18 (18.4) [a]	25 (30.1)
Other	127 (3.5)	10 (4.7)	<10 (7.1) [b]	<10 (0.0) [b]

Data presented as number of participants (percentages), missing have not been included in the column%; [a] Significantly different between women with GDM compared to women without GDM ($p < 0.05$); [b] Significantly different between women with GDM diagnosed before versus after the antenatal interview ($p < 0.05$).

4. Discussion

In this cohort of New Zealand women, we found women with a diagnosis of GDM had significantly lower adherence to 'Junk' and 'Traditional/White bread' dietary patterns compared to women without a diagnosis of GDM. These findings are in contrast to a number of studies exploring dietary patterns associated with GDM [26,28–30] in which dietary patterns characterized by higher intakes of processed meats, fried foods, cakes and biscuits, confectionary, jams, full-fat dairy and salty snacks, similar to the 'Junk' and 'Traditional/White bread' dietary patterns identified in the Growing Up in New Zealand cohort, have been associated with an increased risk of GDM. Together with our finding that a significantly greater proportion of women with GDM than of those without GDM reported receiving information from a dietitian or nutritionist or obstetrician and avoiding foods or drinks high in fat or sugar, these results are strongly suggestive of a treatment effect. This is particularly evident when looking at stratified analyses according to timing of diagnosis in which these relationships were strongest in women diagnosed with GDM before the antenatal interview compared to those diagnosed after, suggesting that these women with GDM are likely to have received advice on the management of GDM and made dietary adaptations prior to the completion of the food frequency questionnaire.

Diet is considered pivotal in the management of GDM [55–57] and New Zealand guidelines recommend women with a diagnosis of GDM are referred to a specialist diabetes in pregnancy service where they receive specialist care from a multidisciplinary team, including input from a dietitian and obstetrician [58]. Dietary guidelines for the management of GDM frequently recommend a low glycaemic index diet or the avoidance of simple sugars [59–63] and some encourage a reduction in saturated fats [58,59,63]. In our previous work exploring dietetic practice in the management of GDM, dietitians frequently reported discussing healthy eating, core food group requirements, carbohydrate quantity and distribution, simple sugars and fat with women with GDM [64]. These recommendations are consistent with the changes that women reported making to their diets and the differences seen in dietary patterns. For example, advice to limit intake of simple carbohydrates and saturated fats could result in lower scores on the 'Junk' and 'Traditional/White bread' dietary patterns as foods with these characteristics had high factor loadings in these patterns. Similarly, associations of higher intakes on the 'Fusion/Protein' dietary patterns in women with GDM diagnosed before the antenatal interview could be due to the foods with high factor loadings in this pattern being noodles, rice, or pasta (potentially low glycaemic index foods), seafood, chicken, red meat, eggs and green leafy vegetables, which women may have been encouraged to consume when receiving dietary advice for GDM. The 'Health Conscious' dietary pattern included high factor loadings for dried fruits and non-citrus fruits, which some women may limit after learning of their diagnosis of GDM due to the sugar content of these foods. This may partly explain non-significant and inconsistent findings for this dietary pattern. The smaller proportion of women avoiding soft drink in those with GDM diagnosed before the antenatal interview compared to those diagnosed after the antenatal interview could be explained by the finding that dietitians in New Zealand frequently provide advice on artificial sweeteners [64]. It is possible that women receiving this type of advice choose artificially sweetened soft drinks rather than avoiding them. Dietitians in our survey of dietetic practice also commonly reported discussing calcium and core food group requirements with women with GDM [64], consistent with a greater proportion of women with GDM reporting adding milk and milk products to their diets.

The relationship between higher adherence to the 'Junk' and 'Traditional/White bread' dietary patterns and a reduced likelihood of having a diagnosis of GDM, even in analyses including only women with GDM diagnosed after the interview and, therefore, presumably unaware of their diagnosis, may be explained by the finding that there was still a greater proportion of women diagnosed with GDM after the interview who reported receiving information from a dietitian or nutritionist compared to women without GDM. In our survey of dietetic practice in the management of GDM, 76% of dietitians reported that women had already received nutrition information prior to their first encounter with a dietitian [64]. Furthermore, a greater proportion of women with GDM reported a pre-pregnancy BMI in the overweight and obese category, receiving fertility treatment, including weight loss advice, and to be actively dieting pre-pregnancy compared to women without GDM. It is possible that women with GDM may have been identified or self-identified as having risk factors for GDM or other pregnancy complications and were therefore already actively making changes to their diets prior to receiving a diagnosis of GDM.

The diagnosis of GDM has been described as a 'teachable moment', in which a diagnosis of GDM may motivate women to make health-related behavioural changes [65]. These findings and ours are supported by studies in which nutrition counselling in pregnant women with or at risk of GDM have resulted in favourable dietary changes [66–68]. In a cluster-randomized controlled trial, Kinnunen et al. (2014) investigated the impact of intensified dietary counselling on food habits of 399 women at risk of GDM. The intervention consisted of five individual counselling sessions on gestational weight gain, physical activity and diet by public health nurses during routine visits to maternity clinics in Finland and resulted in improvements in consumption of fruit and vegetables, high fibre bread and low fat cheese and in the quality of dietary fat intake when compared to women in the usual care group. In a group of Canadian women, 17 with GDM and 27 with normal glucose tolerance, Morisset et al. (2014) demonstrated that a multidisciplinary medical and nutrition intervention, including counselling from a registered dietitian, was effective in the achieving prescribed macronutrient distributions and controlling gestational weight gain in women with GDM. Other studies have demonstrated further benefits of dietetic input in women with GDM, including reduced insulin use and improvements in glycated haemoglobin [69] and reduced likelihood of infant admission to neonatal intensive care or special care units [70].

Strengths of this study include the large, ethnically diverse sample size and the availability of information on factors likely to impact on dietary intake such as sources of information leading to dietary change during pregnancy. In the comparisons of women with GDM diagnosed before and those diagnosed after the antenatal interview, only women with a GDM diagnosis according to laboratory results were included in analyses, as clinical coding data did not include the exact date of diagnosis. A limitation to our findings is that data were not collected on actual input received during pregnancy to confirm our hypotheses. We also had insufficient data on history of GDM in a previous pregnancy to determine whether this may have contributed to dietary changes during the pregnancy reported on during this study.

5. Conclusions

Our study found women with GDM had significantly lower adherence scores on 'Junk' and 'Traditional/White bread' dietary patterns compared to women without GDM. A greater proportion of women with GDM avoided foods and drinks high in fat or sugar and reported receiving dietary information from a dietitian or nutritionist or an obstetrician compared to women without GDM. Women with GDM appear to make significant changes to their diet during pregnancy, most likely as a result of advice from dietitians or nutritionists and obstetricians.

Author Contributions: Conceptualization, R.L.L., C.R.W. and F.H.B.; methodology, R.L.L., C.R.W. and F.H.B.; formal analysis, R.L.L., C.R.W. and F.H.B.; writing—original draft preparation, R.L.L.; writing—review and editing, C.R.W. and F.H.B. All authors have read and agreed to the published version of the manuscript.

Acknowledgments: The Growing Up in New Zealand study was designed and conducted by the Growing Up in New Zealand Study Team, led by the University of Auckland. The authors thank the women, children and families participating in the Growing Up in New Zealand study. They also thank all members of the Growing Up in New Zealand team, including the research and operations teams, as well as the Kaitaki and Scientific Advisory Groups. The authors acknowledge the contributions of the original study investigators: Susan M.B. Morton, Polly E. Atatoa Carr, Cameron C. Grant, Arier C. Lee, Dinusha K. Bandara, Jatender Mohal, Jennifer M. Kinlock, Johanna M. Schmidt, Mary R. Hedges, Vivienne C. Ivory, Te Kani R. Kingi, Renee Liang, Lana M. Perese, Elizabeth Peterson, Jan E. Pryor, Elaine Reese, Elizabeth M. Robinson, Karen E. Waldie and Clare R. Wall. The views reported in this paper are those of the authors and do not necessarily represent the views of the Growing Up in New Zealand investigators. The authors would also like to thank all those involved in the facilitation of data collection for this study, particularly Lynn C. Sadler, Jade Tamatea, Meisha Nicolson, Arlo Upton, John Woodford, Mehreen Naveed, Noureen Rahim, Rashida Member and Andrea O'Brien. The authors thank Khan Safayet Hossin for his assistance with data management and Blake Seers and Christopher Triggs for statistical support.

References

1. Szwajcer, E.M.; Hiddink, G.J.; Koelen, M.A.; Van Woerkum, C.M.J. Nutrition-related information-seeking behaviours before and throughout the course of pregnancy: Consequences for nutrition communication. *Eur. J. Clin. Nutr.* **2005**, *59*, S57–S65. [CrossRef]
2. Lewallen, L.P. Healthy behaviors and sources of health information among low-income pregnant women. *Public Health Nurs.* **2004**, *21*, 200–206. [CrossRef]
3. Szwajcer, E.M.; Hiddink, G.J.; Maas, L.; Koelen, M.A.; van Woerkum, C.M.J. Nutrition-related information-seeking behaviours of women trying to conceive and pregnant women: Evidence for the life course perspective. *Fam. Pract.* **2009**, *25*, i99–i104. [CrossRef] [PubMed]

4. Szwajcer, E.; Hiddink, G.J.; Maas, L.; Koelen, M.; Van Woerkum, C. Nutrition awareness before and throughout different trimesters in pregnancy: A quantitative study among Dutch women. *Fam. Pr.* **2012**, *29*, i82–i88. [CrossRef] [PubMed]
5. Hillier, S.E.; Olander, E.K. Women's dietary changes before and during pregnancy: A systematic review. *Midwifery* **2017**, *49*, 19–31. [CrossRef] [PubMed]
6. *World Health Organization Diagnostic Criteria and Classification of Hyperglycaemia First Detected in Pregnancy*; World Health Organization: Geneva, Switzerland, 2013.
7. Bowers, K.; Yeung, E.; Williams, M.A.; Qi, L.; Tobias, D.K.; Hu, F.B.; Zhang, C. A prospective study of prepregnancy dietary iron intake and risk for gestational diabetes mellitus. *Diabetes Care* **2011**, *34*, 1557–1563. [CrossRef]
8. Bowers, K.; Tobias, D.K.; Yeung, E.; Hu, F.B.; Zhang, C. A prospective study of prepregnancy dietary fat intake and risk of gestational diabetes. *Am. J. Clin. Nutr.* **2012**, *95*, 446–453. [CrossRef]
9. Chen, L.; Hu, F.B.; Yeung, E.; Willett, W.; Zhang, C. Prospective study of pre-gravid sugar-sweetened beverage consumption and the risk of gestational diabetes mellitus. *Diabetes Care* **2009**, *32*, 2236–2241. [CrossRef]
10. Zhang, C.; Williams, M.A.; Sorensen, T.K.; King, I.B.; Kestin, M.M.; Thompson, M.L.; Leisenring, W.M.; Dashow, E.E.; Luthy, D.A. Maternal plasma ascorbic Acid (vitamin C) and risk of gestational diabetes mellitus. *Epidemiology* **2004**, *15*, 597–604. [CrossRef]
11. Zhang, C.; Liu, S.; Solomon, C.G.; Hu, F.B. Dietary fibre intake, dietary glycemic load, and the risk for gestational diabetes mellitus. *Diabetes Care* **2006**, *29*, 2223–2230. [CrossRef]
12. González-Quintero, V.H.; Istwan, N.B.; Rhea, D.J.; Rodriguez, L.I.; Cotter, A.; Carter, J.; Mueller, A.; Stanziano, G.J. The impact of glycemic control on neonatal outcome in singleton pregnancies complicated by gestational diabetes. *Diabetes Care* **2007**, *30*, 467–470. [CrossRef] [PubMed]
13. The HAPO Study Cooperative Research Group. Hyperglycemia and adverse pregnancy outcomes. *N. Engl. J. Med.* **2008**, *358*, 1991–2002. [CrossRef] [PubMed]
14. Vambergue, A.; Nuttens, M.C.; Goeusse, P.; Biausque, S.; Lepeut, M.; Fontaine, P. Pregnancy induced hypertension in women with gestational carbohydrate intolerance: The diagest study. *Eur. J. Obstet. Gynecol. Reprod. Biol.* **2002**, *102*, 31–35. [CrossRef]
15. Boney, C.M. Metabolic syndrome in childhood: Association with birth weight, maternal obesity, and gestational diabetes mellitus. *Pediatrics* **2005**, *115*, 290–296. [CrossRef]
16. Cho, N.H.; Silverman, B.L.; Rizzo, T.A.; Metzger, B.E. Correlations between the intrauterine metabolic environment and blood pressure in adolescent offspring of diabetic mothers. *J. Pediatrics* **2000**, *136*, 587–592. [CrossRef]
17. Hunt, K.J.; Schuller, K.L. The increasing prevalence of diabetes in pregnancy. *Obstet. Gynecol. Clin. North Am.* **2007**, *34*, 173–199. [CrossRef]
18. Ignell, C.; Claesson, R.; Anderberg, E.; Berntorp, K. Trends in the prevalence of gestational diabetes mellitus in southern Sweden, 2003–2012. *Acta Obstet. Gynecol. Scand.* **2014**, *93*, 420–424. [CrossRef]
19. Lavery, J.A.; Friedman, A.M.; Keyes, K.M.; Wright, J.D.; Ananth, C.V. Gestational diabetes in the United States: Temporal changes in prevalence rates between 1979 and 2010. *BJOG* **2016**, *124*, 804–813. [CrossRef]
20. Zhu, Y.; Zhang, C. Prevalence of gestational diabetes and risk of progression to Type 2 Diabetes: A global perspective. *Curr. Diabetes Rep.* **2016**, *16*, 7. [CrossRef]
21. Agarwal, M.; Dhatt, G.; Othman, Y. Gestational diabetes: Differences between the current international diagnostic criteria and implications of switching to IADPSG. *J. Diabetes Complicat.* **2015**, *29*, 544–549. [CrossRef]
22. Buckley, B.S.; Harreiter, J.; Damm, P.; Corcoy, R.; Chico, A.; Simmons, D.; Vellinga, A.; Dunne, F. On behalf of the DALI Core Investigator group Gestational diabetes mellitus in Europe: Prevalence, current screening practice and barriers to screening. A review. *Diabet. Med.* **2012**, *29*, 844–854. [CrossRef] [PubMed]
23. Lawrence, R.L.; Wall, C.R.; Bloomfield, F.H. Prevalence of gestational diabetes according to commonly used data sources: An observational study. *BMC Pregnancy Childbirth* **2019**, *19*, 349–359. [CrossRef] [PubMed]
24. Hu, F.B. Dietary pattern analysis: A new direction in nutritional epidemiology. *Curr. Opin. Lipidol.* **2002**, *13*, 3–9. [CrossRef] [PubMed]
25. Tobias, D.K.; Zhang, C.; Chavarro, J.; Bowers, K.; Rich-Edwards, J.; Rosner, B.; Mozaffarian, D.; Hu, F.B. Prepregnancy adherence to dietary patterns and lower risk of gestational diabetes mellitus. *Am. J. Clin. Nutr.* **2012**, *96*, 289–295. [CrossRef]

26. Schoenaker, D.A.J.M.; Soedamah-Muthu, S.S.; Callaway, L.K.; Mishra, G.D. Pre-pregnancy dietary patterns and risk of gestational diabetes mellitus: Results from an Australian population-based prospective cohort study. *Diabetologia* **2015**, *58*, 2726–2735. [CrossRef]
27. Zareei, S.; Homayounfar, R.; NaghiZadeh, M.M.; Ehrampoush, E.; Rahimi, M. Dietary pattern in pregnancy and risk of gestational diabetes mellitus (GDM). *Diabetes Metab. Syndr. Clin. Res. Rev.* **2018**, *12*, 399–404. [CrossRef]
28. Zhang, C.; Schulze, M.B.; Solomon, C.G.; Hu, F.B. A prospective study of dietary patterns, meat intake and the risk of gestational diabetes mellitus. *Diabetologia* **2006**, *49*, 2604–2613. [CrossRef]
29. Sedaghat, F.; Akhoondan, M.; Ehteshami, M.; Aghamohammadi, V.; Ghanei, N.; Mirmiran, P.; Rashidkhani, B. Maternal dietary patterns and gestational diabetes risk: A case-control study. *J. Diabetes Res.* **2017**, *2017*, 1–8. [CrossRef]
30. Donazar-Ezcurra, M.; Burgo, C.L.-D.; Martinez-Gonzalez, M.A.; Basterra-Gortari, F.J.; De Irala, J.; Bes-Rastrollo, M. Pre-pregnancy adherences to empirically derived dietary patterns and gestational diabetes risk in a Mediterranean cohort: The Seguimiento Universidad de Navarra (SUN) project. *Br. J. Nutr.* **2017**, *118*, 715–721. [CrossRef]
31. Gicevic, S.; Gaskins, A.J.; Fung, T.T.; Rosner, B.; Tobias, D.K.; Isanaka, S.; Willett, W.C. Evaluating pre-pregnancy dietary diversity vs. dietary quality scores as predictors of gestational diabetes and hypertensive disorders of pregnancy. *PLoS ONE* **2018**, *13*, e0195103. [CrossRef]
32. Izadi, V.; Tehrani, H.; Haghighatdoost, F.; Dehghan, A.; Surkan, P.J.; Azadbakht, L.; Tehrani, H. Adherence to the DASH and Mediterranean diets is associated with decreased risk for gestational diabetes mellitus. *Nutrition* **2016**, *32*, 1092–1096. [CrossRef] [PubMed]
33. He, J.-R.; Yuan, M.-Y.; Chen, N.-N.; Lu, J.-H.; Hu, C.-Y.; Mai, W.-B.; Zhang, R.-F.; Pan, Y.-H.; Qiu, L.; Wu, Y.-F.; et al. Maternal dietary patterns and gestational diabetes mellitus: A large prospective cohort study in China. *Br. J. Nutr.* **2015**, *113*, 1292–1300. [CrossRef] [PubMed]
34. Tryggvadottir, E.A.; Medek, H.; Birgisdottir, B.E.; Geirsson, R.T.; Gunnarsdottir, I. Association between healthy maternal dietary pattern and risk for gestational diabetes mellitus. *Eur. J. Clin. Nutr.* **2016**, *70*, 237–242. [CrossRef] [PubMed]
35. Shin, D.; Lee, K.W.; Song, W.O. Dietary patterns during pregnancy are associated with risk of gestational diabetes mellitus. *Nutrition* **2015**, *7*, 9369–9382. [CrossRef]
36. Bao, W.; Bowers, K.; Tobias, D.K.; Olsen, S.F.; Chavarro, J.; Vaag, A.; Kiely, M.; Zhang, C. Prepregnancy low-carbohydrate dietary pattern and risk of gestational diabetes mellitus: A prospective cohort study. *Am. J. Clin. Nutr.* **2014**, *99*, 1378–1384. [CrossRef]
37. Hedderson, M.M.; Darbinian, J.A.; Ferrara, A. Disparities in the risk of gestational diabetes by race-ethnicity and country of birth. *Paediatr. Périnat. Epidemiol.* **2010**, *24*, 441–448. [CrossRef]
38. National Women's Health National Women's Health Annual Clinical Report 2018. Available online: https://nationalwomenshealth.adhb.govt.nz/assets/Womens-health/Documents/ACR/NWH-Annual-Clinical-Report-2018-final.pdf (accessed on 8 October 2019).
39. Blumfield, M.L.; Hure, A.J.; Smith, R.; Collins, C.E.; MacDonald-Wicks, L. Systematic review and meta-analysis of energy and macronutrient intakes during pregnancy in developed countries. *Nutr. Rev.* **2012**, *70*, 322–336. [CrossRef]
40. Morton, S.M.; Grant, C.C.; Wall, C.R.; Carr, P.E.A.; Bandara, D.K.; Schmidt, J.M.; Ivory, V.; Inskip, H.M.; Camargo, C.A. Adherence to nutritional guidelines in pregnancy: Evidence from the Growing Up in New Zealand birth cohort study. *Public Health Nutr.* **2014**, *17*, 1919–1929. [CrossRef]
41. Wall, C.R.; Gammon, C.S.; Bandara, D.K.; Grant, C.C.; Carr, P.E.A.; Morton, S.M.B. Dietary patterns in pregnancy in New Zealand—Influence of maternal socio-demographic, health and lifestyle factors. *Nutrition* **2016**, *8*, 300. [CrossRef]
42. Morton, S.M.; Atatoa Carr, P.E.; Grant, C.C.; Robinson, E.M.; Bandara, D.K.; Bird, A.; Ivory, V.C.; Kingi, T.K.; Liang, R.; Marks, E.J.; et al. Cohort profile: Growing Up in New Zealand. *Int. J. Epidemiol.* **2013**, *42*, 65–75. [CrossRef]
43. New Zealand Society for the Study of Diabetes Screening for diabetes in asymptomatic individuals. *N. Z. Med. J.* **1995**, *108*, 464–465.
44. Simmons, D.; Wolmarans, L.; Cutchie, W.; Johnson, E.; Haslam, A.; Roodt, C.; Rowan, J. Gestational diabetes mellitus: Time for consensus on screening and diagnosis. *N. Z. Med. J.* **2006**, *119*, 1228.

45. Winnard, A.P.; MacLennan, L.; Okesene-Gafa, K.D. Diabetes in Pregnancy in CMDHB: Trends over Time, A 2011 Snapshot and Service Implications. Available online: https://countiesmanukau.health.nz/assets/About-CMH/Reports-and-planning/Diabetes/2011-Diabetes-in-Pregnancy-Trends-2011-snapshot.pdf (accessed on 12 July 2017).
46. National Women's Health National Women's Annual Clinical Report 2009. Available online: http://nationalwomenshealth.adhb.govt.nz/Portals/0/AnnualReports/NWAnnualClinicalReport2009.pdf (accessed on 24 August 2018).
47. National Women's Health National Women's Annual Clinical Report 2010. Available online: http://nationalwomenshealth.adhb.govt.nz/Portals/0/AnnualReports/AnnualClinicalReport2011.pdf (accessed on 24 August 2018).
48. Tamatea, J. Personal Communication, 2017.
49. Ministry of Health. *Food and Nutrition Guidelines for Healthy Pregnant and Breastfeeding Women: A Background Paper*; Ministry of Health: Wellington, New Zealand, 2008; ISBN 9780478317794.
50. Morton, S.M.; Atatoa Carr, P.E.; Bandara, D.K.; Grant, C.C.; Ivory, V.C.; Kingi, T.R.; Liang, R.; Perese, L.M.; Peterson, E.; Pryor, J.E.; et al. *Growing Up in New Zealand: A Longitudinal Study of New Zealand Children and Their Families. Report 1: Before We are Born*; The University of Auckland: Auckland, New Zealand, 2010.
51. *Statistics New Zealand Statistical Standard for Ethnicity 2005*; Statistics New Zealand: Wellington, New Zealand, 2005.
52. *Statistics New Zealand Report of the Review of the Measurement of Ethnicity June 2004*; Statistics New Zealand: Wellington, New Zealand, 2004.
53. Salmond, C.E.; Crampton, P.; Atkinson, J. *NZDep2006 Index of Deprivation*; Department of Public Health, University of Otago: Wellington, New Zealand, 2007.
54. Craig, C.L.; Marshall, A.L.; Sjöström, M.; Bauman, A.E.; Booth, M.L.; Ainsworth, B.E.; Pratt, M.; Ekelund, U.; Yngve, A.; Sallis, J.F.; et al. International Physical Activity Questionnaire: 12-country reliability and validity. *Med. Sci. Sports Exerc.* **2003**, *35*, 1381–1395. [CrossRef] [PubMed]
55. American Diabetes Association 14. Management of diabetes in pregnancy: Standards of medical care in diabetes—2020. *Diabetes Care* **2019**, *43*, S183–S192.
56. Metzger, B.E.; Buchanan, T.A.; Coustan, D.R.; De Leiva, A.; Dunger, P.D.; Hadden, D.R.; Hod, M.; Kitzmiller, J.L.; Kjos, S.L.; Oats, J.N.; et al. Summary and recommendations of the Fifth International Workshop-Conference on Gestational Diabetes Mellitus. *Diabetes Care* **2007**, *30*, 251–260. [CrossRef]
57. Simmons, D.; Rowan, J.; Reid, R.; Campbell, N. On behalf of the National GDM Working Party Screening, diagnosis and services for women with gestational diabetes mellitus (GDM) in New Zealand: A technical report from the National GDM Technical Working Party. *N. Z. Med. J.* **2008**, *121*, 74–86.
58. Ministry of Health. *Screening Diagnosis and Management of GDM in NZ: A Clinical Practice Guideline*; Ministry of Health: Wellington, New Zealand, 2014.
59. *Dietitians New Zealand Guideline: Standard of Care for the Nutritional Management of Gestational Diabetes Mellitus*; Dietitians New Zealand: Wellington, New Zealand, 2016.
60. National Institute for Health and Care Excellence Diabetes in pregnancy: Management from Preconception to the Postnatal Period. Available online: https://www.nice.org.uk/guidance/NG3 (accessed on 17 October 2019).
61. International Diabetes Federation Global Guideline: Diabetes and Pregnancy. Available online: File:///C:/Users/rcoe006/Downloads/Pregnancy_EN_RTP.pdf (accessed on 17 October 2019).
62. American Diabetes Association. Management of diabetes in pregnancy. *Diabetes Care* **2015**, *38*, S779. [CrossRef]
63. *Dietitians New Zealand Nutritional Management of Gestational Diabetes in Adults*; Dietitians New Zealand: Wellington, New Zealand, 2010.
64. Lawrence, R.L.; Wall, C.R.; Bloomfield, F.H.; Crowther, C.A. Dietetic management of gestational diabetes in New Zealand: A cross-sectional survey. *Nutr. Diet.* **2016**, *74*, 95–104. [CrossRef]
65. Okely, J.; Mason, C.; Collier, A.; Dunnachie, N.; Swanson, V. Diagnosis of gestational diabetes: A 'teachable moment'. *Diabet. Med.* **2019**, *36*, 184–194. [CrossRef]
66. Kinnunen, T.I.; Puhkala, J.; Raitanen, J.; Ahonen, S.; Aittasalo, M.; Virtanen, S.M.; Luoto, R. Effects of dietary counselling on food habits and dietary intake of Finnish pregnant women at increased risk for gestational diabetes–a secondary analysis of a cluster-randomized controlled trial. *Matern. Child Nutr.* **2014**, *10*, 184–197. [CrossRef]

67. Morisset, A.-S.; Côté, J.A.; Michaud, A.; Robitaille, J.; Dubé, M.-C.; Veillette, J.; Weisnagel, S.J.; Tchernof, A. Dietary Intakes in the Nutritional Management Of Gestational Diabetes Mellitus. *Can. J. Diet. Pr. Res.* **2014**, *75*, 64–71. [CrossRef] [PubMed]
68. Korpi-Hyovalti, E.; Schwab, U.; Laaksonen, D.E.; Linjama, H.; Heinonen, S.; Niskanen, L. Effect of intensive counselling on the quality of dietary fats in pregnant women at high risk of gestational diabetes mellitus. *Br. J. Nutr.* **2012**, *108*, 910–917. [CrossRef] [PubMed]
69. Reader, D.; Splett, P.; Gunderson, E.P. For the Diabetes Care and Education Dietetic Practice Group Impact of gestational diabetes mellitus nutrition practice guidelines implemented by registered dietitians on pregnancy outcomes. *J. Am. Diet. Assoc.* **2006**, *106*, 1426–1433. [CrossRef] [PubMed]
70. Absalom, G.; Zinga, J.; Margerison, C.; Van Der Pligt, P. Associations of dietetic management with maternal and neonatal health outcomes in women diagnosed with gestational diabetes: A retrospective cohort study. *J. Hum. Nutr. Diet.* **2019**, *32*, 728–736. [CrossRef]

Permissions

All chapters in this book were first published by MDPI; hereby published with permission under the Creative Commons Attribution License or equivalent. Every chapter published in this book has been scrutinized by our experts. Their significance has been extensively debated. The topics covered herein carry significant findings which will fuel the growth of the discipline. They may even be implemented as practical applications or may be referred to as a beginning point for another development.

The contributors of this book come from diverse backgrounds, making this book a truly international effort. This book will bring forth new frontiers with its revolutionizing research information and detailed analysis of the nascent developments around the world.

We would like to thank all the contributing authors for lending their expertise to make the book truly unique. They have played a crucial role in the development of this book. Without their invaluable contributions this book wouldn't have been possible. They have made vital efforts to compile up to date information on the varied aspects of this subject to make this book a valuable addition to the collection of many professionals and students.

This book was conceptualized with the vision of imparting up-to-date information and advanced data in this field. To ensure the same, a matchless editorial board was set up. Every individual on the board went through rigorous rounds of assessment to prove their worth. After which they invested a large part of their time researching and compiling the most relevant data for our readers.

The editorial board has been involved in producing this book since its inception. They have spent rigorous hours researching and exploring the diverse topics which have resulted in the successful publishing of this book. They have passed on their knowledge of decades through this book. To expedite this challenging task, the publisher supported the team at every step. A small team of assistant editors was also appointed to further simplify the editing procedure and attain best results for the readers.

Apart from the editorial board, the designing team has also invested a significant amount of their time in understanding the subject and creating the most relevant covers. They scrutinized every image to scout for the most suitable representation of the subject and create an appropriate cover for the book.

The publishing team has been an ardent support to the editorial, designing and production team. Their endless efforts to recruit the best for this project, has resulted in the accomplishment of this book. They are a veteran in the field of academics and their pool of knowledge is as vast as their experience in printing. Their expertise and guidance has proved useful at every step. Their uncompromising quality standards have made this book an exceptional effort. Their encouragement from time to time has been an inspiration for everyone.

The publisher and the editorial board hope that this book will prove to be a valuable piece of knowledge for researchers, students, practitioners and scholars across the globe.

List of Contributors

Simone Garzon
Department of Obstetrics and Gynecology, "Filippo del Ponte" Hospital, University of Insubria, 21100 Varese, Italy

Michele Fichera and Marco Marzio Panella
Department of General Surgery and Medical Surgical Specialties, University of Catania, 95124 Catania, Italy

Ursula Catena
Division of Gynecologic Oncology, Fondazione Policlinico Universitario Agostino Gemelli, IRCCS, 00168 Rome, Italy

Antonio Schiattarella and Pasquale de Franciscis
Department of Woman, Child and General and Specialized Surgery, University of Campania "Luigi Vanvitelli", 81100 Naples, Italy

George Vilos
Department of Obstetrics and Gynecology, Division of Reproductive Endocrinology and Infertility, Western University, London, ON N6H5W9, Canada

Jan Tesarik
MARGen Clinic, 18006 Granada, Spain

Péter Török
Faculty of Medicine, Institute of Obstetrics and Gynaecology, University of Debrecen, H-4032 Debrecen, Hungary

Giuseppe Grosso
Department of Biomedical and Biotechnological Sciences, University of Catania, 95123 Catania, Italy

Carla Gianfrancesco
Nutritional Epidemiology Group, School of Food Science and Nutrition, University of Leeds, Leeds LS2 9JT, UK
Sheffield Diabetes and Endocrine Centre, Sheffield Teaching Hospitals NHSF Trust, Sheffield S5 7AU, UK

Zoe Darwin and Linda McGowan
School of Healthcare, University of Leeds, Leeds LS2 9JT, UK

Debbie M. Smith
School of Social and Health Sciences, Leeds Trinity University, Leeds LS18 5HD, UK

Roz Haddrill
Department of Nursing, Midwifery & Health, Northumbria University, Newcastle upon Tyne NE7 7XA, UK

Michelle Carter and Janet E. Cade
Nutritional Epidemiology Group, School of Food Science and Nutrition, University of Leeds, Leeds LS2 9JT, UK

Eleanor M. Scott
Leeds Institute of Cardiovascular and Metabolic Medicine, University of Leeds, Leeds LS2 9JT, UK

Nisreen A. Alwan
Academic Unit of Primary Care and Population Sciences, Faculty of Medicine, University of Southampton, Southampton General Hospital, Southampton SO16 6YD, UK
NIHR Southampton Biomedical Research Centre, University of Southampton and University Hospital Southampton NHS Foundation Trust, Southampton SO16 6YD, UK

Michelle A. Morris
Leeds Institute for Data Analytics, School of Medicine, University of Leeds, Leeds LS2 9JT, UK

Salwa A. Albar
Department of Food Science and Nutrition, King Abdul-Aziz University, Jeddah 21551, Saudi Arabia

Stephanie M. Krige, Sharmilah Booley and Janetta Harbron
Division of Human Nutrition, Department of Human Biology, Faculty of Health Sciences, University of Cape Town, Cape Town 7925, South Africa

Naomi S. Levitt
Division of Diabetes and Endocrinology, Department of Medicine, Faculty of Health Sciences, University of Cape Town, Cape Town 7925, South Africa
Chronic Disease Initiative for Africa, Department of Medicine, Faculty of Health Sciences, University of Cape Town, Cape Town 7925, South Africa

Katherine Murphy
Chronic Disease Initiative for Africa, Department of Medicine, Faculty of Health Sciences, University of Cape Town, Cape Town 7925, South Africa

Tawanda Chivese
Chronic Disease Initiative for Africa, Department of Medicine, Faculty of Health Sciences, University of Cape Town, Cape Town 7925, South Africa
MRC/Wits Developmental Pathways for Health Research Unit, Department of Paediatrics, Faculty of Medicine and Health Sciences, University of the Witwatersrand, Johannesburg 2000, South Africa
Biostats Unit, Division of Epidemiology and Biostatistics, Faculty of Medicine and Health Sciences, Stellenbosch University, Cape Town 7599, South Africa

Tiziana Filardi, Francesca Panimolle, Andrea Lenzi and Susanna Morano
Department of Experimental Medicine, "Sapienza" University, Viale del Policlinico 155, 00161 Rome, Italy

Clara Crescioli
Department of Movement, Human and Health Sciences, Section of Health Sciences, Unit of Endocrinology, Università degli Studi di Roma "Foro Italico", 00135 Rome, Italy

Vikkie A. Mustad
R&D Department, Abbott Nutrition, Columbus, OH 43219, USA

Dieu T.T. Huynh
R&D Department, Abbott Nutrition, Singapore 138668, Singapore

José M. López-Pedrosa and Ricardo Rueda
R&D Department, Abbott Nutrition, 18004 Granada, Spain

Cristina Campoy
Department of Paediatrics, University of Granada, 18071 Granada, Spain; EURISTIKOS Excellence Centre for Paediatric Research, University of Granada, 18071 Granada, Spain

Jia-Yi Dong, Satoyo Ikehara and Meishan Cui
Public Health, Department of Social Medicine, Osaka University Graduate School of Medicine, Osaka 5650871, Japan

Takashi Kimura
Department of Public Health, Hokkaido University Graduate School of Medicine, Sapporo 0608638, Japan

Yoko Kawanishi and Tadashi Kimura
Department of Obstetrics and Gynecology, Osaka University Graduate School of Medicine, Osaka 5650871, Japan

Kimiko Ueda
Maternal & Child Health Information Center, Osaka Women's and Children's Hospital, Osaka 5941101, Japan

Hiroyasu Iso
Public Health, Department of Social Medicine, Osaka University Graduate School of Medicine, Osaka 5650871, Japan
Department of Public Health Medicine, Faculty of Medicine, University of Tsukuba, Tsukuba 3058575, Japan

Delphine Mitanchez
Department of Neonatology, Bretonneau Hospital, François Rabelais University, F-37000 Tours, France
INSERM UMR_S 938 Centre de Recherche Saint Antoine, F-75012 Paris, France

Cécile Ciangura and Sophie Jacqueminet
Department of Diabetology, Institute of Cardiometabolism and Nutrition (ICAN), APHP, University Hospital Pitié-Salpêtrière, F-75013 Paris, France

Clive J. Petry, Ieuan A. Hughes and Carlo L. Acerini
Department of Paediatrics, University of Cambridge, Cambridge Biomedical Campus, Cambridge CB2 0QQ, UK

Ken K. Ong
Department of Paediatrics, University of Cambridge, Cambridge Biomedical Campus, Cambridge CB2 0QQ, UK
MRC Epidemiology Unit, University of Cambridge, Cambridge Biomedical Campus, Cambridge CB2 0QQ, UK
Institute of Metabolic Science, University of Cambridge, Cambridge Biomedical Campus, Cambridge CB2 0QQ, UK

David B. Dunger
Department of Paediatrics, University of Cambridge, Cambridge Biomedical Campus, Cambridge CB2 0QQ, UK
Institute of Metabolic Science, University of Cambridge, Cambridge Biomedical Campus, Cambridge CB2 0QQ, UK

Louise Rasmussen, Maria Lund Christensen and Jens Rikardt Andersen
Department of Nutrition, Exercise and Sports, University of Copenhagen, Rolighedsvej 26, 1958 Frederiksberg C, Copenhagen, Denmark

Charlotte Wolff Poulsen and Per Glud Ovesen
Department of Obstetrics and Gynecology, Aarhus University Hospital, Palle Juul-Jensens Boulevard 99, 8200 Aarhus N, Denmark

Charlotte Rud
Department of Hepatology and Gastroenterology, Aarhus University Hospital, Palle Juul-Jensens Boulevard 99, 8200 Aarhus N, Denmark

Alexander Sidelmann
Steno Diabetes Center Copenhagen, Niels Steensens Vej 2-4, 2820 Gentofte, Denmark
Clinic for Clinical Metabolic Research, Herlev and Gentofte Hospital, University of Copenhagen, Gentofte Hospitalsvej 7, 3. Sal, 2800 Hellerup, Denmark

Ulla Kampmann
Steno Diabetes Center Aarhus, Aarhus University Hospital, Hedeager 3, 8200 Aarhus N, Denmark

La'Shay Atakora
London School of Hygiene and Tropical Medicine, London WC1E 7HT, UK

Lucilla Poston and Angela C. Flynn
Department of Women and Children's Health, King's College London, London SE1 7EH, UK

Louise Hayes
Population Health Sciences Institute, Newcastle University, Newcastle upon Tyne NE2 4AX, UK

Sara L. White
Department of Women and Children's Health, King's College London, London SE1 7EH, UK
Guy's and St Thomas' NHS Foundation Trust, London SE1 7EH, UK

Gabriele Piuri and Mattia Cappelletti
Inflammation Society, 18 Woodlands Park, Bexley DA52EL, UK

Katia Basello, Andrea Costanzi and Emiliana Tognon
GEK lab–Cryolab, University of Rome Tor Vergata, Via Montpellier, 1—00133 Rome, Italy

Gabriele Rossi, Chiara Maria Soldavini, Silvia Duiella, Giulia Privitera and Angela Spadafranca
Obstetrical Unit, Woman-Child-Newborn Department, Fondazione IRCCS Ca' Granda, Ospedale Maggiore Policlinico, 20122 Milan, Italy

Paola Antonia Corsetto and Angela Maria Rizzo
Department of Pharmacological and Biomolecular Sciences, Università degli Studi di Milano, 20133 Milano, Italy

Attilio Francesco Speciani
Inflammation Society, 18 Woodlands Park, Bexley DA52EL, UK
GEK lab–Cryolab, University of Rome Tor Vergata, Via Montpellier, 1—00133 Rome, Italy

Enrico Ferrazzi
Inflammation Society, 18 Woodlands Park, Bexley DA52EL, UK
Obstetrical Unit, Woman-Child-Newborn Department, Fondazione IRCCS Ca' Granda, Ospedale Maggiore Policlinico, 20122 Milan, Italy
Fondazione IRCCS Cà Granda, Ospedale Maggiore Policlinico, Department of Clinical Sciences and Community Health, Università degli Studi di Milano, 20122 Milan, Italy

Antonio Pérez-Pérez, Teresa Vilariño-García and Víctor Sánchez-Margalet
Department of Medical Biochemistry and Molecular Biology, and Immnology, School of Medicine, Virgen Macarena University Hospital, 41009 Seville, Spain

Pilar Guadix and José L. Dueñas
Obstetrics and Gynecology Service, Virgen Macarena University Hospital, 41009 Seville, Spain

Chiara Peila, Enrico Bertino, Francesco Cresi and Alessandra Coscia
Complex Structure Neonatology Unit, Department of Public Health and Paediatric, University of Turin, 10100 Turin, Italy

Diego Gazzolo
Department of Maternal, Fetal and Neonatal Health, C. Arrigo Children's Hospital, 15121 Alessandria, Italy

Helen Robinson
Department of Obstetric Medicine, Royal Brisbane and Women's Hospital, Butterfield St, Herston, QLD 4029, Australia

Helen Barrett and H. David McIntyre
Mater Research Institute, The University of Queensland, Brisbane, QLD 4101, Australia

Luisa Gomez-Arango and Marloes Dekker Nitert
School of Chemistry and Molecular Biosciences, The University of Queensland, St Lucia, QLD 4072, Australia

Leonie Callaway
Women's and Newborn Services, Royal Brisbane and Women's Hospital, Butterfield St, Herston, QLD 4029, Australia

Robyn L. Lawrence and Frank H. Bloomfield
The Liggins Institute, University of Auckland, Auckland 1142, New Zealand

Clare R. Wall
Discipline of Nutrition and Dietetics, School of Medical Sciences, University of Auckland, Auckland 1142, New Zealand

Index

A

Adipose Tissue Inflammation, 168, 172-173, 182

Adiposity, 31, 53, 58, 64, 85, 88, 97-98, 101, 116, 133-136, 143, 145, 152, 178, 201

Alcohol Consumption, 48, 115, 213-214, 216-217

Antenatal Care, 1, 144-145, 147

Antioxidant Activity, 172, 174

B

Bioactive Compounds, 57, 141, 167, 175-177

Bioactive Food Compounds, 170, 172, 176

Blood Glucose Control, 44, 69-70, 152

Body Mass Index, 9, 14-15, 20, 48, 50, 52, 77-78, 80-81, 85, 99, 105, 129, 139, 143, 145, 156, 191, 197, 201, 203, 213, 216

Breastfeeding, 61, 71, 116, 185-186, 191, 196-198, 223

Butyricimonas, 200, 206-207

C

Caesarean Section, 6, 44, 52, 61, 129

Carbohydrate Distribution, 117-120, 126

Carbohydrate Intolerance, 75, 85, 186, 210, 221

Cohort Study, 29, 47, 50, 70-71, 74, 76-78, 81-83, 98, 101, 115, 133-135, 137, 141-143, 154, 177, 211, 222, 224

Colostrum, 190-192, 196-199

Continuous Glucose Monitoring, 60-61, 70, 75-76, 117, 127-128

D

Diabetes In Pregnancy, 9, 16, 27, 47-48, 57, 66, 74, 85, 99, 104, 115, 127, 140, 142, 153, 164, 186, 201, 219, 221, 223

Diabetes-specific Formula, 60, 68

Dietary Adaptations, 210-211, 214, 219

Dietary Assessment, 14-15, 24-25, 27-29, 34, 48, 78, 154

Dietary Carbohydrates, 57, 60-61, 64

Dietary Factors, 77, 79-81, 102-103, 111, 114

Dietary Fibre, 31, 44, 46, 221

Dietary Intake, 4, 16, 22-23, 25, 28, 30-31, 33-36, 41, 43, 46, 48-49, 83-84, 119, 144-145, 150-153, 206-208, 211-212, 220, 223

Dietary Intervention, 44, 47, 51, 53, 55, 58-59, 64, 73-74, 89, 97, 100, 138, 158, 162, 168

Dietary Patterns, 48, 74, 111, 115-116, 154, 210-214, 216-222

Drink Intake Frequency Ranks, 107-108, 110, 113

Drinking During Pregnancy, 213, 216

E

Eating Speed, 77-83

Eggerthella, 200, 206-207

Endocrine Disruptors, 129-130, 133, 137-140

Endocrine-disrupting Chemicals, 129-130, 140, 142-143

Energy Intake, 30, 34, 36, 43, 49-50, 52, 55, 78-79, 82-83, 93-94, 103, 126, 146, 150-151, 158, 169, 178

Excess Energy Intake, 78, 82

F

Flavonoids, 171-172, 179-180, 182

Food Frequency Questionnaire, 30, 34, 78, 102, 104, 107, 110, 112-113, 146, 201, 210, 212, 219

Food Intake Frequency Ranks, 111

Frequency Of Consumption, 103, 112, 212

G

Gestational Age, 5-8, 31-33, 35-36, 42-43, 53, 55, 61, 67, 78, 80, 86, 88, 106, 118, 121-122, 135, 142, 148, 158-159, 162, 197

Gestational Diabetes, 1-2, 5-6, 8-12, 14-15, 27, 29-31, 33, 36, 46-51, 56-61, 64, 68, 70-78, 81, 83-86, 90, 92, 99-102, 10 , 108, 114-118, 125, 127-129, 133, 159-160, 162, 164-167, 170, 176-177, 179-181, 185-186, 197-199, 201, 203, 209-210, 215, 221-224

Gestational Diabetes Mellitus, 1-2, 5, 8-12, 15, 30, 36, 46-51, 56-60, 71-78, 81, 83-85, 99-101, 114-118, 127-129, 133, 137, 140-141, 143, 148, 153-155, 159-160, 162, 164-167, 177, 179-181, 185-186, 197-199, 203, 209-210, 215, 221

Gestational Weight Gain, 43, 48, 52, 54, 61, 67-68, 74-75, 79-81, 85-86, 90, 92, 99-101, 122, 133, 144-145, 148, 151-154, 167, 176, 184, 215, 219-220

Glucose Metabolism, 2, 6, 12, 45, 62, 98, 101, 132, 158, 200, 206

Glycated Albumin, 155, 157-158, 160-162, 165-166

Glycemic Load, 47, 57-58, 221

Glycemic Variability, 70, 117-120, 122, 124-128

H

Human Milk, 138, 185-186, 196-199

Hyperglycaemia, 10, 30-32, 44-46, 71, 73, 99, 115, 127-128, 130, 134, 136, 144, 153, 221

I

Impaired Glucose Tolerance, 31-32, 98, 133, 141, 212

Insulin Concentrations, 57, 104-105, 191

Insulin Disposition Index, 102, 105, 108, 112

Insulin Levels, 55, 172, 191, 198

Insulin Secretion, 2-3, 10, 51, 62, 102-103, 105, 108, 112, 114-115, 133, 136, 156, 172, 174, 176

Insulin-dependent Diabetes Mellitus, 185-186, 197-199

K
Ketonuria, 200-208

L
Leptin Resistance, 167-171, 174-179, 183
Leptin Sensitivity, 168, 170-172, 174, 176, 178
Lipid Peroxidation, 172-173
Low Glycaemic Index, 15, 31, 44, 51-53, 58-59, 73-74, 145, 219

M
Macronutrient Distribution, 30-31, 34, 38, 44, 46, 52
Macrosomia, 15, 44, 53, 55-56, 58, 61, 63, 68, 71, 73-74, 78-81, 83, 85-86, 88, 90-91, 93-94, 96, 98, 168-170
Maternal Lifestyle Interventions, 85, 97
Mediation Analysis, 77, 79-82
Metabolic Dysfunction, 97-98, 133, 143, 172
Methanobrevibacter, 200, 205, 207
Microbiome, 63, 72, 183, 200-201, 203, 207-209
Milk Biochemical Markers, 185-186, 197

N
Neonatal Adiposity, 58, 97, 101
Nutrients Transport, 167, 170
Nutritional Epidemiology, 7, 14, 23-24, 27-28, 221

O
Obesity, 2-3, 10, 31, 51-52, 61-62, 68, 71-72, 75, 77-78, 82-87, 93, 96-103, 114-115, 129-130, 134, 136, 138-140, 143-146, 151-154, 156, 164-165, 167-183, 185, 196-200, 208, 210, 221
Oleuropein, 172, 181
Organic Food, 107-108, 110, 112, 131
Oxidative Stress, 12, 134, 142, 155-156, 163, 165, 172-173, 176, 181-182

P
Phascolarctobacterium, 200, 206-207
Plasma Glucose Concentrations, 104-105
Platelet-activating Factor, 155-156, 161, 165
Polyphenolic Compounds, 167, 171, 176
Pregnancy Nutrition, 30
Pregnancy Outcomes, 11, 47-48, 52, 54, 56-58, 69-70, 74-76, 78, 86, 93, 99-100, 114, 125, 127, 129, 133-137, 152-153, 168, 170, 175, 177, 184, 221, 224
Pregnancy Questionnaire, 104, 112
Preterm Delivery, 52, 129, 152, 186, 196-197
Preterm Newborn, 185

R
Roseburia, 200-201, 204-208

S
Self-reported Eating Speed, 77-78, 80-81
Smoking Patterns, 213, 216
Sugar Intake, 30, 38-39, 43, 45

www.ingramcontent.com/pod-product-compliance
Lightning Source LLC
LaVergne TN
LVHW060547210926
848485LV00005B/1274
* 9 7 8 1 6 3 9 2 7 6 7 6 9 *